Research Progress of Plant Compounds for Diabetes and Its Complications

Research Progress of Plant Compounds for Diabetes and Its Complications

Editors

Cosmin Mihai Vesa
Dana Zaha

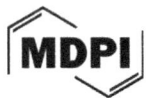

Basel • Beijing • Wuhan • Barcelona • Belgrade • Novi Sad • Cluj • Manchester

Editors
Cosmin Mihai Vesa
Preclinical Department
University of Oradea
Oradea
Romania

Dana Zaha
Preclinical Departmen
University of Oradea
Oradea
Romania

Editorial Office
MDPI
St. Alban-Anlage 66
4052 Basel, Switzerland

This is a reprint of articles from the Special Issue published online in the open access journal *Metabolites* (ISSN 2218-1989) (available at: www.mdpi.com/journal/metabolites/special_issues/ Plant_Compounds_Diabetes).

For citation purposes, cite each article independently as indicated on the article page online and as indicated below:

Lastname, A.A.; Lastname, B.B. Article Title. *Journal Name* **Year**, *Volume Number*, Page Range.

ISBN 978-3-7258-0500-6 (Hbk)
ISBN 978-3-7258-0499-3 (PDF)
doi.org/10.3390/books978-3-7258-0499-3

© 2024 by the authors. Articles in this book are Open Access and distributed under the Creative Commons Attribution (CC BY) license. The book as a whole is distributed by MDPI under the terms and conditions of the Creative Commons Attribution-NonCommercial-NoDerivs (CC BY-NC-ND) license.

Contents

About the Editors vii

Preface ix

Ni Kadek Santi Maha Dewi, Yan Ramona, Made Ratna Saraswati, Desak Made Wihandani and I Made Agus Gelgel Wirasuta
The Potential of the Flavonoid Content of *Ipomoea batatas* L. as an Alternative Analog GLP-1 for Diabetes Type 2 Treatment—Systematic Review
Reprinted from: *Metabolites* 2023, 14, 29, doi:10.3390/metabo14010029 1

Mădălina Moldovan, Ana-Maria Păpurică, Mara Muntean, Raluca Maria Bungărdean, Dan Gheban and Bianca Moldovan et al.
Effects of Gold Nanoparticles Phytoreduced with Rutin in an Early Rat Model of Diabetic Retinopathy and Cataracts
Reprinted from: *Metabolites* 2023, 13, 955, doi:10.3390/metabo13080955 24

Muhammad Khan, Muhammad Ajmal Shah, Mustafa Kamal, Mohammad Shamsul Ola, Mehboob Ali and Pharkphoom Panichayupakaranant
Comparative Antihyperglycemic and Antihyperlipidemic Effects of Lawsone Methyl Ether and Lawsone in Nicotinamide-Streptozotocin-Induced Diabetic Rats
Reprinted from: *Metabolites* 2023, 13, 863, doi:10.3390/metabo13070863 48

Irina-Camelia Chis, Carmen-Maria Micu, Alina Toader, Remus Moldovan, Laura Lele and Simona Clichici et al.
The Beneficial Effect of Swimming Training Associated with Quercetin Administration on the Endothelial Nitric Oxide-Dependent Relaxation in the Aorta of Rats with Experimentally Induced Type 1 Diabetes Mellitus
Reprinted from: *Metabolites* 2023, 13, 586, doi:10.3390/metabo13050586 65

Samuel Nzekwe, Adetoun Morakinyo, Monde Ntwasa, Oluwafemi Oguntibeju, Oluboade Oyedapo and Ademola Ayeleso
Influence of Flavonoid-Rich Fraction of *Monodora tenuifolia* Seed Extract on Blood Biochemical Parameters in Streptozotocin-Induced Diabetes Mellitus in Male Wistar Rats
Reprinted from: *Metabolites* 2023, 13, 292, doi:10.3390/metabo13020292 81

Arshad Husain Rahmani, Mohammed A. Alsahli, Amjad Ali Khan and Saleh A. Almatroodi
Quercetin, a Plant Flavonol Attenuates Diabetic Complications, Renal Tissue Damage, Renal Oxidative Stress and Inflammation in Streptozotocin-Induced Diabetic Rats
Reprinted from: *Metabolites* 2023, 13, 130, doi:10.3390/metabo13010130 92

Nandakumar Muruganathan, Anand Raj Dhanapal, Venkidasamy Baskar, Pandiyan Muthuramalingam, Dhivya Selvaraj and Husne Aara et al.
Recent Updates on Source, Biosynthesis, and Therapeutic Potential of Natural Flavonoid Luteolin: A Review
Reprinted from: *Metabolites* 2022, 12, 1145, doi:10.3390/metabo12111145 108

Min-Seong Ha, Jae-Hoon Lee, Woo-Min Jeong, Hyun Ryun Kim and Woo Hyeon Son
The Combined Intervention of Aqua Exercise and Burdock Extract Synergistically Improved Arterial Stiffness: A Randomized, Double-Blind, Controlled Trial
Reprinted from: *Metabolites* 2022, 12, 970, doi:10.3390/metabo12100970 126

Fatai Oladunni Balogun, Kaylene Naidoo, Jamiu Olaseni Aribisala, Charlene Pillay and Saheed Sabiu
Cheminformatics Identification and Validation of Dipeptidyl Peptidase-IV Modulators from Shikimate Pathway-Derived Phenolic Acids towards Interventive Type-2 Diabetes Therapy
Reprinted from: *Metabolites* **2022**, *12*, 937, doi:10.3390/metabo12100937 . . . . **141**

Muddaser Shah, Saif Khalfan Al-Housni, Faizullah Khan, Saeed Ullah, Jamal Nasser Al-Sabahi and Ajmal Khan et al.
First Report on Comparative Essential Oil Profile of Stem and Leaves of *Blepharispermum hirtum* Oliver and Their Antidiabetic and Anticancer Effects
Reprinted from: *Metabolites* **2022**, *12*, 907, doi:10.3390/metabo12100907 . . . . **158**

About the Editors

Cosmin Mihai Vesa

Cosmin Mihai Vesa is associate professor at the University of Oradea, Faculty of Medicine and Pharmacy. He teaches physiology of the renal, respiratory, and cardiovascular system. He is a medical doctor specialized in diabetes, nutrition and metabolic diseases, and he obtained his PhD diploma in 2019. His research interest include the pathophysiology of diabetes mellitus complications, insulin resistance, metabolic syndrome, obesity, and novel drugs in the treatment of diabetes mellitus. He serves as a guest editor in six MDPI Special Issues and is a reviewer of numerous journals.

Dana Zaha

Dana Carmen Zaha is a Professor (full) of Physiology at the Faculty of Medicine and Pharmacy, University of Oradea. She teaches blood, renal, respiratory and cardiac physiology. She is specialized in Laboratory medicine working in the Clinical County Emergency Hospital of Oradea. Currently, she is a PhD supervisor at the Doctoral School of Biomedical Sciences, University of Oradea. Her main research interests include antibiotic resistance, breast cancer, imunohistochemistry, and laboratory analysis in cardio-metabolic diseases.

Preface

Diabetes mellitus is one of the most prevalent chronic diseases in the modern world. Plant compounds have proven beneficial in in vitro and in vivo studies, reducing the systemic impact of the disease and acting via multiple mechanisms: the antioxidant effect, the anti-inflammatory effect, the hypoglycaemic effect, the lowering of blood lipids, and protection of the function of beta cells. Plant compounds are important adjuvants in diabetes mellitus treatment, helping to reduce the impact of hyperglycaemia and insulin resistance by acting at the molecular level on certain pathogenic mechanisms. It is important to remember that plant compounds research does not replace the classic medical treatment but is an adjuvant. Research in our Special Issue focusing mostly on diabetes rat models demonstrates that key plant compounds have beneficial effects in diabetic retinopathy, diabetic kidney disease, the vascular system as well as numerous biochemical parameters.

With 10 papers published, we consider this reprint as a valuable achievement for all of us, authors and editors.

Cosmin Mihai Vesa and Dana Zaha
Editors

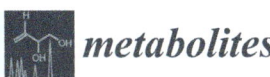

Systematic Review

The Potential of the Flavonoid Content of *Ipomoea batatas* L. as an Alternative Analog GLP-1 for Diabetes Type 2 Treatment—Systematic Review

Ni Kadek Santi Maha Dewi [1,2], Yan Ramona [3], Made Ratna Saraswati [4], Desak Made Wihandani [5] and I Made Agus Gelgel Wirasuta [2,6,*]

1. Doctoral Study Program, Faculty of Medicine, Udayana University, Denpasar 80232, Indonesia; santimahadewi@unud.ac.id
2. Pharmacy Department, Faculty of Mathematic and Natural Science, Udayana University, Kampus Bukit Jimbaran, Denpasar 80361, Indonesia
3. Biology Department, Faculty of Mathematic and Natural Science, Udayana University, Kampus Bukit Jimbaran, Denpasar 80361, Indonesia; yan_ramona@unud.ac.id
4. Department of Internal Medicine, Faculty of Medicine, Udayana University, Denpasar 80232, Indonesia; ratnasaraswati@unud.ac.id
5. Department of Biochemistry, Faculty of Medicine, Udayana University, Denpasar 80232, Indonesia; dmwihandani@unud.ac.id
6. Forensic Sciences Laboratory, Institute of Forensic Sciences and Criminology, Udayana University, Kampus Bukit Jimbaran, Denpasar 80361, Indonesia
* Correspondence: gelgel.wirasuta@unud.ac.id

Abstract: *Ipomoea batatas* L. (IBL) has gained significant popularity as a complementary therapy or herbal medicine in the treatment of anti-diabetes. This review seeks to explore the mechanism by which flavonoid compounds derived from IBL exert their anti-diabetic effects through the activation of GLP-1. The review article refers to the PRISMA guidelines. In order to carry out the literature search, electronic databases such as Science Direct, Crossref, Scopus, and Pubmed were utilized. The search query was based on specific keywords, including Ipomoea batatas OR sweet potato AND anti-diabetic OR hypoglycemic. After searching the databases, we found 1055 articles, but only 32 met the criteria for further review. IBL contains various compounds, including phenolic acid, flavonols, flavanols, flavones, and anthocyanins, which exhibit activity against anti-diabetes. Flavonols, flavanols, and flavones belong to a group of flavonoids that possess the ability to form complexes with $AlCl_3$ and Ca^{2+}. The intracellular L cells effectively retain Ca^{2+}, leading to the subsequent release of GLP-1. Flavonols, flavones, and flavone groups have been found to strongly interact with DPP-IV, which inhibits the degradation of GLP-1. The anti-diabetic activity of IBL is attributed to the mechanism that effectively increases the duration of GLP-1 in the systemic system, thereby prolonging its half-life.

Keywords: anti-diabetic; GLP-1; *Ipomoea batatas* L. flavonoid; pharmacology

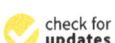

1. Introduction

The rise in diabetes cases worldwide can be attributed to several factors, including aging populations, population growth, and the increasing prevalence of the disease among different age groups [1]. According to projections made by the World Health Organization, DM is anticipated to rank as the seventh highest cause of mortality on a global scale by the year 2030. This forecast is based on the significant increase in the prevalence of this disease in recent times. In 2015, the International Diabetes Federation reported a staggering 415 million cases of diabetes worldwide. Alarming as it may be, this number is projected to climb even higher, reaching an estimated 642 million cases by the year 2040, according to their latest forecasts [2].

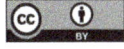

A total of 1055 publications have been identified to examine/report the potential of *Ipomoea batatas* L. (IBL) as an alternative method for diabetes treatment (Figure 1). These publications were categorized into 12 distinct research clusters, which were distinguished by the size of their nodes. The majority of the extensive cluster focused on *Ipomoea batatas* L. as an anti-diabetic and antioxidant, while a smaller portion delved into only one group, reporting on the mechanism of Glucagon-like peptide-1 (GLP-1) on IBL.

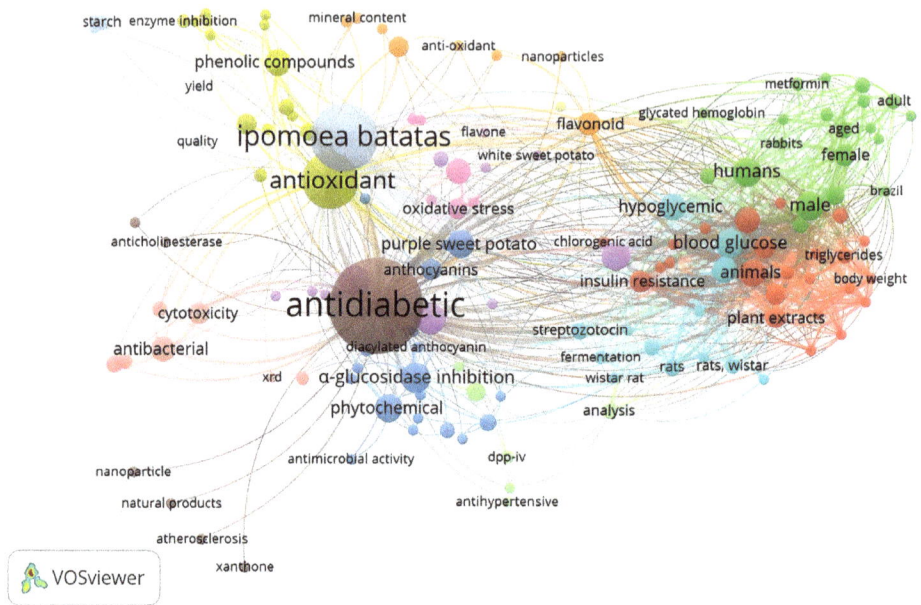

Figure 1. Keyword co-occurrence network.

All the published articles searched for our review mentioned that IBL contains various active compounds, including flavonoids, anthocyanins, phenolic acids, caffeoyl derivatives, triterpenoids, and alkaloids. Each compound is still discussable regarding its pharmacological mechanism. Recent reports indicated that flavonoid compounds have been demonstrated to have efficacy against diabetes mellitus (DM). The occurrence effect of flavonoid consumption to reduce DM is signaled by several signaling pathways, namely glucose transporters, liver enzymatic, tyrosine kinase inhibition, AMPK, PPARγ, and NF-κB [3–5]. At present, researchers have identified 27 IBL cultivars that possess anti-diabetic properties. These compounds exhibit pharmacological effects and target multiple sites of action, namely the pancreas, liver, skeletal muscle, and adipose tissue [6]. IBL's therapeutic effect on diabetes is achieved through a multifaceted pharmacological mechanism that acts on various chemical and pharmacological sites.

The compounds that have been identified were predicted to work in the gastrointestinal (GI) tract by α-glucosidase inhibition through the degradation of polysaccharides into monosaccharides and the secretion of GLP-1. It can lead to a reduction in gastric emptying, a decrease in gastrointestinal motility, and an increase in insulin secretion [7,8]. These findings also illustrated the effect on lowering blood pressure and cholesterol, both of which were identified as risk factors for DM based on the resulting outcome. A study IBL extract could induce the release of GLP-1, thereby making it an effective anti-diabetic agent [9]. This review article explores the potential and action mechanism of flavonoid compounds in IBL that can trigger GLP-1 activation.

2. Materials and Methods

2.1. Search Strategy

Consistent with the PRISMA criteria, we implemented a search strategy to conduct our study [10]. Searching for relevant articles, we conducted a systematic review of IBL's therapeutic potential in anti-diabetic treatment. We used several selected databases, such as Science Direct, Scopus, Crossref, and Pubmed, to search extensively for the literature. The keywords encompassed in the search query were (1) Ipomoea batatas OR sweet potato AND (2) anti-diabetic OR hypoglycemic.

2.2. Inclusion Criteria

We selected research articles that focused on the effects, anti-diabetic potentials, phytochemical compounds, and signaling mechanisms of *Ipomoea batatas*. English-written articles that relied on in vitro and in vivo studies formed the core of these research papers. The selected studies evaluated at least three essential measures: (1) *Ipomoea batatas*, (2) phytochemical compounds, and (3) the signaling mechanisms involved.

2.3. Exclusion Criteria

In order to proceed with our review, we excluded conference papers, thesis dissertations, review articles, papers published for conferences, and manuscripts without abstracts or that did not meet the inclusion requirements. Studies that looked into the relationship between *Ipomoea batatas* and other diseases were not part of this analysis.

2.4. Data Extraction and Management

To compile the articles for this study, a reference manager called Zotero was utilized. By examining the publications that met the inclusion criteria, we proceeded with our analysis. The information gathered included the (1) type/cultivar, (2) part of the plant, (3) identified compound, (4) bioactive compound, (5) site of action, and (6) anti-diabetic mechanism pharmacology activity of IBL.

2.5. Data Extraction Strategy

In this literature review, the outcomes of various in vitro and in vivo studies examining the influence of IBL on type 2 DM were presented. Sections 3 and 4 describe the results of the reports regarding the phytochemicals involved. In Section 5, we analyze the findings, considering the sites of action and pharmacological mechanisms of diabetes treatment.

3. Results

The Literature Search

The literature search identified 1055 articles relevant to the topic (Figure 1). Duplications were detected and removed, totaling 44 articles. Based on screening the titles and abstracts, 865 articles were removed. Then, 125 articles were further excluded based on the results of the screening of the inclusion criteria mentioned above. A total of 31 appropriate articles were reviewed in more depth in Table 1. The successful data extraction is shown in the flow diagram displayed in Figure 2.

Table 1. Type/cultivar of Ipomoea batatas, the predictive bioactive compounds, sites of action activity, and pharmacology mechanisms.

No	Type/Cultivar	Part of Plant	Identified Compound	Predictive Bioactive Compound	Analytical Method	Site of Action	Mechanism Pharmacology	Reference
1	IBL from cultivar Simon (Beijing, China)	Leaves	1-Caffeoylquinic acid; Neochlorogenic acid; Esculin; Protocatechualdehyde; Chlorogenic acid; Cryptochlorogenic acid; Caffeic acid hydroxycoumarin; Isochlorogenic acid A, B, and C; 3,4,5-Tricaffeoylquinic acid; Rutin; Hyperoside; Isoquercitrin; Astragalin; Quercetin; KAE; Diosmetin; Jaceosidin; Chrysin; and Pectolinarigenin	-	UHPLC-hybrid quadrupole-orbitrap/MS	Pancreas	• Inhibiting beta cell apoptosis and recovering the islet structure	[11]
				-		Liver	• Enhancing the AKT/PI3K/CSK-3β signaling pathway leads to a decline in dyslipidemia, an enhancement in insulin sensitivity, and an enhancement in glucose metabolism	
				-		Muscle	• The improvement of insulin sensitivity and the facilitation of glucose transport through upregulating the AKT/PI3K/GLUT-4 signaling pathway	
		Leaves		3,4,5-Tricaffeoylquinic acid; Cryptochlorogenic acid; Chlorogenic acid; Isochlorogenic acid A, B and C; Neochlorogenic acid; Esculin; Protocatechualdehyde; Caffeic acid; 7-hydroxycoumarin; Ethyl Caffeate; Rutin; Hyperoside; Isoquercitrin; Astragalin; Quercetin; Kampferol; Diosmetin; Jaceosidin; Chrysin; Pectolinarigenin; Hysperidin; Luteolin; and Catechin	UHPLC-hybrid quadrupole-orbitrap/MS	Gastrointestinal	• α-amylase inhibition • α-glucosidase inhibition	[12]
						Pancreas	• Protection of cell beta by antioxidant capacity using ABTS, DPPH, FRAP	
2	Purple IBL from in Luzhu District, Taoyuan City, Taiwan	Leaves	Methyl decanoate: Quercetin 3-O-β-D sophoroside; 4-Hydroxy-3-methoxy benzaldehyde; Quercetin; and Benzyl β-d-glucoside		GC-MS	Adipose	• GLUT-4 activation • PI3K/AKT pathway regulation in 3T3-L1 adipocytes	[13]

Table 1. Cont.

No	Type/Cultivar	Part of Plant	Identified Compound	Predictive Bioactive Compound	Analytical Method	Site of Action	Mechanism Pharmacology	Reference
3	IBL from the local market, India	Leaves		Acidic glycoprotein	-	Gastrointestinal	α-Glucosidase inhibition	[14]
4	IBL from Aan Village, Klungkung Regency, Bali Province, Indonesia	Leaves	-	Peonidin-caffeoyl-p-hydroxybenzoylsophorside-5-glucoside; Cyanidin 3-O-rutinoside (C3OR); Peonidin dirhamnoside; Cyanidin-3-glucoside isomer (C3G); Pelargonidin glucoside or cyanidin 3-O-rutinoside; and Peonidin dirhamnosaloyl-glucoside isomer	ESI-MS	Pancreas	Protection of pancreatic beta cell islet through the inhibition of intracellular nitric oxide (NO) and the reactive oxygen species (ROS) scavenging mechanism	[15]
5	Fresh orange-fleshed SPL (Jishu No. 16) collected from a farm in Yichun	Leaves	Trans-N-(p-coumaroyl) tyramine; 7,3′-Dimethylquercetin; 7-Hydroxy-5-methoxycoumarin; Caffeic acid ethyl ester; Trans-N-feruloyltyramine; Cis-N-feruloyltyramine; 3,4,5-Tricaffeoylquinic acid; 3,4-Dicaffeoylquinic acid; 4,5-Dicaffeoylquinic acid; 4,5-Feruloylcourmaoylquinic acid; Caffeic acid; Quercetin-3-O-α-D-glucopyranoside; and Indole-3-carboxaldehyde	3,4,5-Tricaffeoylquinic acid; 4,5-Dicaffeoylquinic acid; 3,4-Dicaffeoylquinic acid; Caffeic acid Quercetin-3-O-α-D-glucopyranoside; and 7,3′-dimethylquercetin

Trans-N-(p-coumaroyl) tyramine; Trans-N-feruloyltyramine; 7-Hydroxy-5-methoxycoumarin; Cis-N-feruloyltyramine; Caffeic acid ethyl ester; 3,4,5-Tricaffeoylquinic acid; and Indole-3-carboxaldehyde | HPLC, 1D NMR, 2D NMR, ESI-MS | Pancreas

Gastrointestinal | Protection of beta cell pancreas by decreasing ROS through radical scavenging DPPH

α-Glucosidase inhibition | [16] |
| 6 | IBL leaves from (Hebei province) in Autumn | Leaves | Flavone | | - | Pancreas | The beta cell acts as a safeguard by efficiently eliminating excessive free radicals, consequently decreasing the occurrence of lipid peroxidation | [17] |
| 7 | IBL from Slatina (central Croatia) | Leaves | Flavonoid; Phenol | | - | Pancreas | Protecting beta cell scavenging | [18] |

Table 1. Cont.

No	Type/Cultivar	Part of Plant	Identified Compound	Predictive Bioactive Compound	Analytical Method	Site of Action	Mechanism Pharmacology	Reference
8	IBL from Anguillara Veneta (Northern Italy)	Leaves	Catechin; Naringin; Epicatechin; Chlorogenic acid; p-OH benzoic acid; Vanillic acid; t-Ferulic acid; and o-Coumaric acid	Chlorogenic acid and Epicatechin	HPLC-PDA	Gastrointestinal	• α-glucosidase inhibition • Tyrosinase inhibition • α-amylase inhibition	[19]
						Pancreas	• Anti-apoptosis beta cells through suppressing the increasethe activation of caspase-3 and caspase-8	
9	Fresh leaves of IBL (family of clones B 00593) from Bandungan, Central Java Indonesia.	Leaves		Anthocyanins; Catechins; Quercetin; Proanthocyanidins; and Caffeic acid	-	Pancreas	• The preservation of beta cells involves the suppression of reactive oxygen species (ROS) production, the removal of ROS through scavenging processes, and the augmentation of antioxidant defense mechanisms. • In order to enhance insulin secretion and improve insulin sensitivity, it is crucial to inhibit the activation of NF-κB, thereby suppressing the production of TNF-α and inhibiting iNOS (inducible nitric oxide synthase).	[20]
10	'Suioh,' a IBL cultivar from Kumamoto prefecture, Japan	Leaves	Chlorogenic acid; 3,4,5-Tricaffeoylquinic acid; 3,4-Dicaffeoylquinic acid; 4,5-Dicaffeoylquinic acid; and 3,5-Dicaffeoylquinic acid	3,4,5-Tricaffeoylquinic acid	-	Gastrointestinal	• α-glucosidase inhibition • GLP-1 receptor activation, EGFRs are transactivated, thereby activating PI3K. This PI3K activation is essential for the cAMP/PKA-dependent pathway, which ultimately leads to the exocytosis of insulin. The exocytosis of insulin activates KATP channels, causing depolarization and an increase in Ca2+ levels, resulting in the secretion of insulin.	[9]
11	Purple IBL	-	Peonidin-3-glucoside (P3G); Cyanidin-3-rutinoside C3R); Cyanidin-3-glucoside (C3G); and Cyanidin-3,5-glucoside (C35G)	P3G; C3R; C3G; and C35G	-	Gastrointestinal	• Inhibition porcine pancreatic α-amylase	[21]

Table 1. Cont.

No	Type/Cultivar	Part of Plant	Identified Compound	Predictive Bioactive Compound	Analytical Method	Site of Action	Mechanism Pharmacology	Reference
12	'Bophelo' orange-fleshed IBL cultivar	Tubers and leaves	Isovanillic acid; Protocatechuic acid; Quercetin; Caffeic acid; Catechin; Hyperoside; Kaempferol; Rutin; and Vanillic acid	Isovanillic acid; Kaempferol; Protocatechuic acid; Caffeic acid; Catechin; Hyperoside; Rutin; Quercetin; and Vanillic acid	HPLC-MS	Pancreas	• Protecting beta cell melalui peningkatan antioxidant enzyme (catalase, CAT, glutathione peroxidase) dan uji antioxidant capacity using FRAP and TEAC	[22]
						Muscle	• Activation of GLUT-4 and improvement in glucose uptake • Expression of the genes NRF1, MEF2A, CPT1, and ACC2, and ultimately glucose uptake metabolism and the management of insulin resistance	
13	White potato Tainung No.10	Tubers and leaves	Arabinogalactan; and Epigallocatechin gallate	Arabinogalactan; and Epigallocatechin gallate	-	Muscle	• Activation of PI3K/Akt/GLUT-4 to increase insulin sensitivity and glucose uptake	[23]
14	Purple IBL (Cultivar Eshu No.12) from the Institute of Food Crops, Hubei Academy of Agricultural Sciences	Tubers	Peonidin-3-sophoroside-5-glucoside (P3SG); Cyanidin-3-sophoroside-5-glucoside (C3SG); Anthocyanins (containing one or two p-hydroxybenzoic, caffeic and/or ferulic acid); and 17 proteins (consisted of group: Acetylesterase, Proteinase inhibitor, Sporamin A, Superoxide dismutase [Cu-Zn], Beta-amylase, Sporamin B, preprosporamin, Polyphenol oxidase I chloroplastic, Purple acid phosphatase, and NBS-LRR protein and pectin)	P3SG; C3SG; Anthocyanins (containing one or two p-hydroxybenzoic, caffeic and/or ferulic acid); and 17 proteins (consisted of the group: Acetylesterase, Proteinase inhibitor, Sporamin A, Superoxide dismutase [Cu-Zn], Beta-amylase, Sporamin B, preprosporamin, Polyphenol oxidase I chloroplastic, Purple acid phosphatase, and NBS-LRR protein and pectin)	HPLC-DAD/ESI-MS	Pancreas	• Protecting cell beta through reducing ROS and improving antioxidant enzyme activities	[24]
						Liver	• Activation of AMPK/GLUT-2/GK and insulin receptor alfa (INSR) to increase the level of insulin and glucose transporter • The synthesis of glucose is diminished through the downregulation of gluconeogenic genes, specifically glucose-6-phosphatase (G6Pase) and phospoenolpyruvate carboxykinase (PEPCK)	
15	Purple IBL powder (cultivar Eshu No. 8)	Tubers	Diacylated anthocyanins	Peonidin-3-caffeoylferuloyl sophoroside-5-glucoside	-	Liver	Enhancing the secretion and sensitivity of the insulin elucidates mechanism: (i) inhibitor of liver XO activity; (ii) activation of the expression of SGLT2, GLUT-5, and GLUT-2; (iii) the suppression of the NF-κB pathway leads to a decrease in the expression of IL-1β and iNOS	[25]

Table 1. Cont.

No	Type/Cultivar	Part of Plant	Identified Compound	Predictive Bioactive Compound	Analytical Method	Site of Action	Mechanism Pharmacology	Reference
16	IBL (Linn.) Lam from Western Research Farm, National Root Crop Research Institute, Umudike, Abia state	Tubers	Flavonoid; Terpenoid; Tannin; Phenol		-	Pancreas	• Induction of beta cell regeneration or repairing and increasing the size and number of cells in the islet of Langerhans	[26]
						Gastrointestinal	• α-glucosidase inhibition	
						Adipose	• Activation of PI3K (Phosphoinositol-3-kinase), P38 MAPK (Mitogen-activated protein kinase), and GLUT-4 translocation. They have been seen to increase glucose uptake. • Insulin secretagogues, directly activating the K+ ATP channel through influx of Na+ and an outflow of K+	
17	Purple IBL cv. Ayamurasaki from the Kyushu National Agricultural Experiment Station in Miyazaki prefecture (Japan)	Tubers		Peonidin 3-O-[2-O-(6-O-E-feruloyl-β-D-glucopyranosyl)-6-O-E-caffeoyl-β-D-glucopyranoside]-5-O-β-D-glucopyranoside	-	Gastrointestinal	• α-Glucosidase inhibition	[27]
18	Korean red skin IBL (Ib 1) and Korean pumpkin IBL (Ib 2) from the market in Goyang, Republic of Korea	Peel-off tuber		α-carotene; β-carotene; zeaxanthin; and lutein	-	Gastrointestinal	• α-Glucosidase inhibition	[28]

Table 1. *Cont.*

No	Type/Cultivar	Part of Plant	Identified Compound	Predictive Bioactive Compound	Analytical Method	Site of Action	Mechanism Pharmacology	Reference
19	White IBL (Caiapo)	Tubers		Acidic glycoprotein	-	Gastrointestinal	• α-Glucosidase inhibition	[29]
						Adipose	• The translocation of GLUT-4, along with the promotion of lipolysis and the subsequent release of free fatty acids from adipose tissue, contributes to an increased glucose uptake in isolated adipocytes. This mechanism ultimately results in a reduction in HbA1c levels.	[30]
20	White-skinned sweet potato (WSSP) purchased from Kagawa, Japan, Prefectural Cooperative	Tubers	WSPP fraction consists of >50 kDa, 10–50 kDa, and ≤10 kDa	Caffeic acid	-	Adipose	• Improvement in the secretion and sensitivity of insulin through significant increases in the adiponectin expression	[31]
				≤10 kDa fraction	-	Muscle	• Improving insulin sensitivity and glucose uptake. Considerably increases AKT phosphorylation//GLUT-4	[32]
				>50 kDa fraction		Liver	• The inhibition of gluconeogenesis is achieved by suppressing the process itself and simultaneously promoting glycogen synthesis. This dual action leads to an increased uptake of glucose.	
21	Korean purple IBL (Shinzami, Saeungbone9, Gyeyae2469, Gyebone108, Saeungyae33, and Gyeyae2258)	Tubers	3-Caffeoyl-phydroxybenzoylsophoroside-5-glucoside; Peonidin 3-caffeoyl sophoroside-5-glucoside; Peonidin 3-(6″-caffeoyl-6‴-feruloyl sophoroside)-5-glucoside; and Peonidin 3-caffeoyl-phydroxybenzoylsophoroside-5-glucoside	Cyanidin 3-caffeoyl-p-hydroxybenzolsophoroside-5-glucoside and Peonidin 3-(6″-caffeoyl-6‴-feruloyl sophoroside)-5-glucoside	LC-DAD-ESI/MS	Liver	• Inhibition of hepatic gluconeogenesis in HepG2 cells can lead to an enhancement in insulin sensitivity by reducing glucose secretion • Protective beta cell by reducing ROS through radical scavenging	[33]

Table 1. *Cont.*

No	Type/Cultivar	Part of Plant	Identified Compound	Predictive Bioactive Compound	Analytical Method	Site of Action	Mechanism Pharmacology	Reference
22	Color-fleshed potatoes (Sinjami and Sinhwangmi)	Tubers	Lutein; Peonidin 3-(6″-caffeoyl-6″-feruloyl sophoroside)5-glucoside; Zeaxanthin; Cryptoxanthin; 13Z-ß-carotene; Peonidin 3-sophoroside-5-glucoside; Peonidin 3-p-hydroxybenzoyl sophoroside-5-glucoside; Cyanidin 3-p-hydroxybenzoyl sophoroside-5-glucoside; Cyanidin3-(6″-feruloyl sophoroside)-5-glucoside; Peonidin 3-(6″-feruloyl sophoroside)-5-glucoside; Cyanidin 3-(6″,6″-dicaffeoyl sophoroside)-5-glucoside; Cyanidin 3-caffeoyl-p-hydroxybenzoyl sophoroside-5-glucoside; Cyanidin3-(6″-caffeoyl6″-feruloyl sophoroside)-5-glucoside; Peonidin 3-caffeoyl sophoroside-5-glucoside; Peonidin 3-(6″,6″-dicaffeoyl sophoroside)-5glucoside; Peonidin 3-caffeoyl-p-hydroxybenzoyl sophoroside-5-glucoside; all-trans-ß-carotene; and 9Z-ß-carotene	Peonidin 3-caffeoyl-p-hydroxybenzoyl sophoroside-5-glucoside	UPLC-MS/MS (Q-TOF-ESI)	Adipose	• Stimulating adipogenesis through the inhibition of fat accumulation in adipocytes via the PPARγ expression. Activation of the PPARγ receptor will maintain glucose homeostasis	[34]

Table 1. *Cont.*

No	Type/Cultivar	Part of Plant	Identified Compound	Predictive Bioactive Compound	Analytical Method	Site of Action	Mechanism Pharmacology	Reference
23	IBL from Kagawa Prefecture, Japan	Tubers		Chlorogenic acid; and Caffeic acid and its derivatives	-	Pancreas	• Protection of beta cell from oxidative stress-related gene expression and peroxidation of the plasma membrane • Increase in the secretion insulin by the inhibited activation of the nuclear transcription factor and P38 MAP kinase pathway to decrease TNF-α production	[35]
24	White-skinned sweet potato (WSSP)	Tubers		Arabinogalactan protein	-	Liver	• Improving insulin sensitivity by the inhibition inflammatory cytokines such as IL-6 and TNF-α	[36]
25	Purple IBL Antin-3 cultivar from the BALITKABI Malang	Tubers	Anthocyanin group		-	Pancreas	• Regeneration and protecting beta cells through reducing oxidative stress using the radical scavenging DPPH method	[37]
26	White-skinned sweet potatoes (WSSP) from the local market Faisalabad (Pakistan)	Tubers		Carotenoid	-	Pancreas	• Protecting beta cells by decreasing oxidative stress, and induced elevated cytosolic free Ca^{2+} concentrations in beta cells further contribute to supraphysiological insulin release	[38]
		Tubers		Glicoprotein; Flavonoid; and Carotenoid	-	Liver	• Hepatoprotective mechanism due to a decrease in the glycation level prevents the formation of ROS—amplified activities of liver enzymes such as SGOT and SGPT.	[39]
27	Purple IBL from Padang, West Sumatra, Indonesia	Tubers		Peonidin; and Cyanidin	-	Gastrointestinal	• α-amylase inhibition	[40]

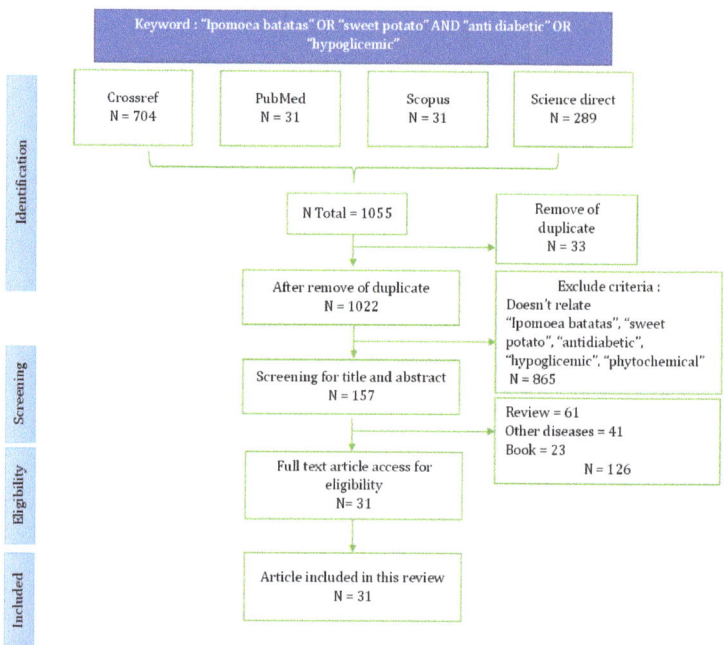

Figure 2. Flow chart identification and screening for the literature search.

4. Discussion

4.1. Type or Cultivar

IBL has several varieties. These varieties are differentiated based on tuber color, skin color, leaf color, texture, and size. The number of cultivars identified in this journal was 27, with several variations, such as orange [16,22,28,33], purple [12,14,19,21,24,25,27,33,34,40], and white IBL [8,9,14–16,18,21,24,27–30,34,36,37]. Differences in the cultivars will affect the phytochemical contents and their anti-diabetic activity.

4.2. Parts of Plant and Phytochemical Identified of IBL

Many reports mentioned that parts of IBL used for its anti-diabetic effects include the leaves, tubers, and tuber skin. Each part has different chemical compositions. In purple IBL tubers, the anthocyanin content commonly used as a marker is higher than in its leaves. The concentration of anthocyanins is also greater in purple IBL compared to white or orange IBL. The phenolic acid content, such as 3,4,5-Tricaffeoylquinic acid, chlorogenic acid, caffeic acid, Isochlorogenic acid C, Isochlorogenic acid A, and caffeoyl acid derivative [10,11,15,20], flavonoid groups such as C3R, C3G, C35G, cyanidin 3-caffeoyl-p-hydroxybenzolsophoroside-5-glucoside, P3G, peonidin 3-caffeoyl-p hydroxybenzoyl sophoroside-5-glucoside, peonidin 3-O-[2-O-(6-O-E-feruloyl-β-D-glucopyranosyl)-6-O-E-caffeoyl-β-D-glucopyranoside]-5-O-β-D-glucopyranoside [21,27], quercetin, epicatechin, protocatechualdehyde, rutin, kaemferol, isoquercitrin, and jaceosidin, have been identified in such type of potato. They directly serve as effective anti-diabetic agents [10,11,22,35]. Flavonol, a subclass of flavonoids, is extensively found in various natural sources. Flavonols, such as quercetin and epicacthecin, demonstrated their potential for increasing GLP-1 secretion in a tissue culture of GLUTag cells [41]. Ground triterpenoid, such as trans-N-feruloyltyramine, *trans-N-(p-coumaroyl)* tyramine, *cis-N-*feruloyltyramine, and 7-hydroxy-5-methoxycoumarin, and alkaloid groups such as Indole-3-carboxaldehyde also have potential as anti-diabetic agents [16].

4.2.1. Site of Action

GLP-1 is produced in the intestine through the posttranslational processing of proglucagon. The L cells, primarily found in the colon and ileum, are types of open-type epithelial cells that directly interact with nutrients in the intestinal lumen. The level of GLP-1 in circulation quickly rises due to nutrients such as carbohydrates, fats, proteins, and dietary fiber [42]. Glucose is taken up through GLUT-2, fructose through GLUT-5, and SCFAs are absorbed and metabolized intracellularly. The GLP-1 secretion is induced by the closure of KATP channels, which is a result of carbohydrate uptake through SGLT1, GLUT-2, and GLUT-5. Through intracellular metabolism, cell membrane depolarization is triggered, leading to the production of ATP and the closure of KATP channels. Additionally, this process facilitates the opening of voltage-gated Ca^{2+} channels. Furthermore, the uptake of free amino acids and peptides also induces depolarization and the subsequent activation of voltage-gated Ca^{2+} channels (VGCCs). The activation of VGCCs is brought about by the coupled transport of Na^+ for amino acids and PepT1 for peptides, leading to the stimulation of GLP-1 secretion. The release of GLP-1 is triggered by the influx of extracellular Ca^{2+} and the release of Ca^{2+} from intracellular reservoirs, resulting in additional depolarization and the subsequent activation of the exocytotic machinery [43,44]. The excessive production of GLP-1 within the cells results in its dispersion across the entire systemic system. It then attaches to the GLP-1R receptor found in different organ tissues, including the skeletal muscle, adipose tissue, liver, pancreas, and gastrointestinal tract. The binding of GLP-1 to the liver results in a decline in glucose production, while concurrently promoting an elevation in glucose uptake within adipose tissue and muscle [45,46].

Various flavonoid compounds, including hispidulin, epicatechin, quercetin, C3G, 5,7-dihydroxy-6-4-dimethoxyfavanone, and homoesperetin-7-rutinoside, have demonstrated their ability to enhance GLP-1 release both in vitro and in vivo. GLP-1 stimulation has been demonstrated in GLUTag cells when exposed to epicatechin, C3G, and hispidulin. Homoesperetin-7-rutinoside has also exhibited stimulation through molecular docking [47]. The chelation of Ca^{2+} by quercetin, similar to the chelation of $AlCl_3$, has been documented in various studies. Complexes between quercetin and metals are formed at the ortho positions O3/O4, O4/O5, and O3'/O4', as detailed by numerous reports in the literature (Figure 3) [48]. Compounds belonging to the flavonol, flavanol, and flavones groups exhibit activity against $AlCl_3$, resulting in a yellow color change. It is anticipated that these compounds will operate via a similar mechanism against Ca^{2+}. These compounds have the ability to prolong the half-life of GLP-1, leading to an elevation in insulin release and a modification in glucose absorption from systemic to cellular in the form of glycogen [49]. Furthermore, the A or B rings of flavonoids are capable of interacting with $AlCl_3$ through their ortho-dihydroxyl groups, resulting in the formation of complexes that are susceptible to acid [50].

Increased oxidative stress is largely responsible for the development and improvement of DM and its complications. Pancreatic islets have low expression levels of antioxidant enzymes, which make them more vulnerable to oxidative damage. Biomarkers such as MDA are used to assess oxidative stress, with increased levels indicating higher levels of lipid peroxidation. Oxidative stress in diabetes is reduced by GLP-1, which activates the cAMP, PI3K, and PKC pathways through receptors and Nrf-2. This also increases the antioxidant capacity. Conversely, oxidative stress can be reduced by suppressing ROS through radical scavenging and chelating mechanisms, thus protecting pancreatic beta cells [51].

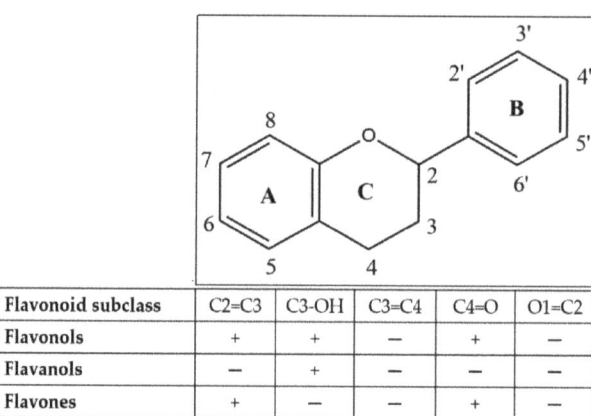

Flavonoid subclass	C2=C3	C3-OH	C3=C4	C4=O	O1=C2
Flavonols	+	+	−	+	−
Flavanols	−	+	−	−	−
Flavones	+	−	−	+	−

Figure 3. Flavonoid skeleton.

4.2.2. Gastrointestinal Tract

Regulation of Carbohydrate Metabolism

The inhibition of α-glucosidase influenced the capability of the small intestine to inhibit the absorption of carbohydrates. This particular enzyme inhibited the conversion of complex carbohydrates and was unable to be assimilated into simple carbohydrates [52]. The IC_{50} values of all the compounds were investigated to be in the range of 4.46 µM to 64.14 µM, which were observed in various studies on the efficacy of α-glucosidase inhibitors in comparison to acarbose. Ethyl caffeate could inhibit α-glucosidase more effectively (about 6.77 times more than acarbose). These flavonoid compounds had a potent inhibitory effect on α-glucosidase, such as rutine, isoquercitrin, quercetin, kaempferol, and hyperoside [12]. Compared to acarbose, Trans-N-(p-coumaroyl)tyramine, 3,4,5-Tricaffeoylquinic acid, trans-N-feruloyltyramine, and cis-N-feruloyltyramine inhibited α-glucosidase 37.9, 36.6, 18.7, and 11.8 times more effectively, respectively. Quercetin-3-O-glucosidase and 7-Hydroxy-5-methoxycoumarin, with respective IC_{50} values of 22.38 ± 1.73 µM and 64.14 ± 9.23 µM, also had good activity [16]. Chlorogenic acid was also predicted to have inhibition activities on α-glucosidase and tyrosinase. The docking results also supported that Chlorogenic acid binds to the active site of α-glucosidase and can act in a reversible competitive manner through hydrogen bonds [19]. Peonidin 3-O-[2-O-(6-O-E-feruloyl-β-D-glucopyranosyl)-6-O-E-caffeoyl-β-D-glucopyranoside]-5-O-β-D glucopyranoside showed that a potent maltase inhibition was preferred over sucrase inhibition [27]. The aqueous fraction contained an acidic glycoprotein (IC_{50} 53 µg/mL) that exhibited anti-diabetic properties and was predicted to have a mechanism of α-glicosidase inhibition, which is a significant breakthrough for the care of DM. This finding is particularly noteworthy when compared to acarbose [14].

Ethyl caffeic had an α-amylase activity that was 13.1 times stronger than acarbose. This was possibly due to the contribution of the OH group of the ethyl caffeic binding to the enzyme. The mixed-type inhibition of α-amylase by chlorogenic acid occurred as a result of the binding of chlorogenic acid to amino acid residues near the active site through hydrogen bonds. This binding process led to a modification in the secondary structure of the enzyme's protein, thereby inhibiting its activity [12]. C3G, C3R, C35G, and P3G had IC_{50} values of 0.024 ± 0.003 (mM), 0.040 ± 0.007 (mM), 0.031 ± 0.007 (mM), and 0.075 ± 0.007 (mM), respectively, for porcine pancreatic α-amylase inhibition These four anthocyanin compounds were proven in silico, and the active side of the compound was thought to be mediated by interacting with the carboxylate group of GLU233. C3G was the most potent inhibitor of the four compounds, with a low Ki of 0.0014 mM. The Ki values of the other compounds were much higher: 0.019 nM for C3R, 0.020 nM for C35G, and 0.045 nM for P3G. The inhibition activity was observed to be conferred by the shared key side chain GLU233 [21]. Each compound induced absorption that exclusively took place as fiber and was subsequently eliminated through the gastrointestinal tract.

Increased Insulin Secretion

GLP-1, a hormone known as incretin, is released by intestinal endocrine L cells, which exhibit an effect of eaten food. The enhancement of GLP secretion in the gastrointestinal tract can lead to an improvement in insulin secretion, a decrease in GI motility, and a delay in gastric emptying. Various studies have identified compounds belonging to the phenolic acid and flavonoid groups that exhibit potential for augmenting GLP-1 secretion [7,8].

The most potent chlogenic acid derivative was 3,4,5-Tricaffeoylquinic acid, which increased GLP-1 secretion around 10-fold compared to the sulfonylure control tested on GLUTag cells. The same effect was also produced during the in vivo test, where the treatment group produced more GLP-1 secretion compared to the sulfonylurea control group. Hence, GLP-1 has the ability to maintain glycemic balance without the potential of inducing hypoglycemia. The elevation of cAMP concentrations may lead to the stimulation of GLP-1 secretion in both in the vivo model and a cell line. The noticed elevations in GLP-1 production in L cells were caused by the activation of PKA and cAMP in the in vitro model using GLUTag cells [9]. Cyanidin 3-O-glucoside (C3OG) and epicatechin functioned through the activation of the cAMP/PKA and ERK $\frac{1}{2}$ pathways. Ca^{2+} chelation's mechanism of action led to an elevation in the intracellular Ca^{2+} concentration, consequently resulting in an augmentation of GLP-1 secretion. The activity of this compound seemed to be supported by the appearance of a $3'4'$ catechol group in the B ring, which was considered a crucial chemical structural component [41]. Hispidulin was also recognized as an effective anti-DM agent. Notably, the study demonstrated that hispidulin treatment led to an increase in the intracellular cAMP levels in L cells [47].

An alternative approach that has shown clinical benefits involves inhibiting DPP-4 to prolong the duration of GLP-1. Flavonoids, namely flavonol, flavanol, and flavone (Figure 3), displayed varying degrees of inhibitory activity, which were dependent on their concentration. Notably, narcissoside, myricetin, C3OG, hyperoside, and isoliquiritigenin demonstrated higher inhibitory activities. An analysis of the relationship between the structure and activity revealed that incorporating hydroxyl groups at positions $C3'$, $C4'$, and C6 in the flavonoid structure enhanced the effectiveness of DPP-4 inhibition. However, the addition of a hydroxyl group at position three of ring C in the flavonoid configuration was discovered to be disadvantageous for suppression. Additionally, the methylation of the hydroxyl groups at positions $C3'$, $C4'$, and C7 of the flavonoid conformation tended to reduce the inhibitory activity against the DPP-4 enzyme. Furthermore, it was determined that the presence of a 2,3-double bond and a 4-carbonyl group on ring C of the flavonoid configuration was crucial for achieving the inhibitory effect [53].

4.2.3. Pancreas

Inhibiting Apoptosis Beta Cell and Recovering the Islet Structure through Protective Cell Beta

Pancreatic beta cells have a crucial function in regulating glucose balance and serve as the primary producers of insulin. Their role encompasses the synthesis, storage, and secretion of insulin [54]. The research findings indicated that the IC_{50} value for total compound fell within the range of 9.69 ± 0.03 μM to IC_{50} 125 ± 0 μM for Vit C. This particular range demonstrated a significant efficacy for conferring natural antioxidant properties to the compound. An elevation in ROS was the sole factor responsible for harm to the beta cells. Antioxidants in abundance are believed to have the potential to diminish ROS, leading to the recovery of islet beta cells. This recovery process will enhance the insulin secretion process through protective cell beta.

Giving SPLP (sweet potato leave phenol) leaf extract from Beijing to T2DM mice for 4 weeks showed a recovery of pancreatic tissue with an increased area and complete islet structure, increased mass, and clear borders. Giving SPLP treatment inhibited beta cell apoptosis. Phenolic compounds, including 1-caffeoylquinic acid, chlorogenic acid, caffeac acid, and 3,4,5-tricaffeoylquinic acid, are believed to have the competence to govern the process of beta cell regeneration. The IC_{50} value of 3,4,5-Tricaffeoylquinic acid indicated a radical scavenging activity that was 10.8 times more potent than the control substance, cevitamic acid. Subsequently, the other compounds exhibiting greater strength than ascorbic acid included Isochlorogenic acid C, Isochlorogenic acid A, Isochlorogenic acid B, Caffeic acid ethyl ester, and Caffeic acid. Additional research has documented the presence of ABTS-induced antioxidant activity. Ethyl caffeate and 3,4,5-Tricaffeoylquinic acid have been identified as exhibiting commendable activity, with IC_{50} values comparable to that of ascorbic acid. The order of antioxidant potency, in terms of descending activity, can be arranged as follows: Isochlorogenic acid C exhibited the highest potency, followed by Chlorogenic acid, Neochlorogenic acid, caffeic acid, Cryptochlorogenic acid, Isochlorogenic acid A, 1-Caffeoylquinic acid, Isochlorogenic acid B, esculin, and finally 7-hydroxycoumarin.

Protocatechualdehyde exhibited the most potent antioxidant activity, surpassing that of ascorbic acid by a factor of 2.32. Quercetin exhibited the highest antioxidant activity among the flavonoid group, with a remarkable 4.14-fold increase compared to ascorbic acid. Following closely, kaemferol and jaceosidin demonstrated a commendable ABTS radical scavenging activity, which was nearly on par with cevitamic acid. In the DPPH radical scavenging test, protocatechualdehyde displayed the most potent DPPH activity, surpassing ascorbic acid by a significant factor of 2.69. Ethyl caffeate and 3,4,5-tricaffeoylquinic had a good DPPH activity. The descending order of DPPH antioxidant activity, ranging from high to low, is as follows: caffeic acid, isochlorogenic acid C, chlorogenic acid, 1-caffeoylquinic acid, neochlorogenic acid, isochlorogenic acid A, cryptochlorogenic acid, isochlorogenic acid B, 7-hydroxycoumarin, and esculin. Quercetin exhibited a significantly higher DPPH radical scavenging activity that was 1.8 times greater than that of cevitamic acid. Notably, isoquercitrin, hyperoside, kaempferol, and routine also demonstrated commendable scavenging capabilities. The remarkable DPPH radical scavenging capacity of caffeic acid could be attributed to its 1,2-phenolic diol group, as well as its conjugation involving the C=C and C=O bonds. Another mechanism using the FRAP method was that protocatechualdehyde had a 2.22 stronger activity than cevitamic acid. Ethyl caffeate, caffeac acid, 3,4,5-tricaffeoylquinic acid, and Isochlorogenic acid also had a good activity. For the flavonoid compounds, namely quercetin produced a stronger reducing power activity of 1.54 compared to vitamin C. Hyperoside, kaempferol, isoquercitrin, and rutine exhibited commendable FRAP capacities [11,16,55]. The IC_{50} values of SPLP were consistent with a prior study, indicating a more potent oxidative stress protection compared to polyphenols derived from tea and grape seed [56].

The significant increase in the enzymatic antioxidants SOD and GSH-Px were correlated with an antioxidant activity to reduce ROS. A decrease in ROS will cause the recovery of pancreatic beta cells. The compound suspected in this process was protein-bound anthocyanin from tuber. Anthocyanins that were identified from purple IBL and possibly bound to protein were peonidin-3-cyanidin-3-sophoroside-5-glucoside and sophoroside-5-glucoside [15,24,57]. Additional research indicated that Cyanidin 3-caffeoyl-p-hydroxybenzoyl-sophoriside-5-glucoside exhibited the most potent antioxidant properties among the various anthocyanin compounds. This finding was determined through the utilization of ascorbic acid and the ABTS and DPPH methods, as stated in the alternative investigations. Furthermore, peonidin 3-caffeoyl sophoroside-5-glucoside exhibited superior antioxidant activities compared to peonidin3-(6″-caffeoyl-6″-feruoyl sophoroside)-5-glucoside and peonidin3-caffeoyl-p-hydroxybenzoyl-sophoroside-5-glucoside [33].

Tuber extract and orange-fleshed IBL leaves as beta cell protectors can reduce lipid peroxidation through a radical scavenging mechanism and the results of measuring the antioxidant activity with FRAP and TEAC can significantly reduce ROS. The antioxidant capacity values using FRAP were, respectively, 299.8 ± 2.5 and 296.9 ± 7.4 (μM AAE/mg protein) and testing using the TEAC method were 127.9 ± 2.10 and 126.3 ± 2.51 (μM TE/mg Protein). The results of this test were greater than standard ascorbic acid, namely

271.0 ± 4.17 (μM AAE/mg protein) and 107.2 ± 1.68 (μM TE/mg protein). The compounds predicted to be contained in the extract that had radical scanning activity were caffeic acid, hyperoside, protocatechuic acid, quercetin, routine, and vanillic acid [22]. Caffeic acid was reported to be a compound with a potent antioxidant activity [58,59]. MAE (microwave assisted extraction) leaves of purple IBL cultivar antin-3, which were predicted to contain the anthocyanin group, produced an IC_{50} value of 61.91 ± 1.11 ppm [37].

This compound worked directly in increasing insulin secretion through the repair of islet beta cells. This compound was responsible for scavenging reactive oxygen species (ROS) and elevating the AMP/ATP ratio within beta cells. The alteration in the AMP/ATP ratio triggered the activation of mitochondrial targets, leading to the induction of mitogenesis and the stimulation of insulin secretion [60].

Suppression of the Anti-Inflammatory Pathway

The compounds identified from Bandungan, Java, Indonesia, were anthocyanin, catechin, quercetin, proanthocyanin, and caffeic acid. These compounds were predicted to work in the pancreas by inhibiting the anti-inflammatory mechanisms [20]. The administration of the leaf extract at a dose of 2.5 g/kgBW for a duration of 14 days demonstrated a noteworthy 50% augmentation in pancreatic islet cells in comparison to the control group. Conversely, the administration of caiapo at a dose of 5 g/KgBW over a period of 8 weeks substantially enhanced the beta cell mass by a two-fold increase when compared to the untreated diabetic control subjects ($p < 0.05$). The results indicated that increased dosages of the extract could potentially result in a more significant restoration of islet beta cells. It is important to highlight that the extract was thought to comprise quercetin, chlorogenic acid, caffeic acids, and their derivatives. The anti-inflammatory characteristics of these compounds are believed to play a crucial role in diminishing inflammation by inhibiting inflammatory mediators. Quercetin is known to inhibit tyrosine kinase activity, which has been shown to be anti-diabetic. The regulation of quercetin effects through the inhibition of the NF-κB activation of beta cells also helps to improve glucose-stimulated insulin secretion [14,61,62]. Apart from that, the content of chlorogenic acid, caffeic acids, and their derivatives is thought to be able to inhibit the JNK, P38 MAP, and NF-κB pathways and is also associated with various inflammatory mediators, including IL-6, CRP, and TNF-α. It has also been reported that inhibiting oxidative stress may also induce hypoglycemic effects [35].

4.2.4. Liver
Improving Insulin Secretion and Insulin Sensitivity by Reducing Glucose Synthesis

The primary structures of other acylated anthocyanins, namely C3S5G and P3S5G, are anticipated to play a vital role in improving glucose absorption and increasing insulin levels. According to the studies, this compound can lower glycolysis through p-AMPK activity impairment. The treatment group given 200 mg/kg of free anthocyanin compound of sweet potato (FAC-PSP) extract containing 40.74 ± 2.88 mg C3G/g for 4 weeks showed a substantial rise in the p-AMPK expression levels. In the liver, the insulin-responsive glucose transporter GLUT-2 is crucial for metabolism and glucose uptake. The manifestation of the GLUT-2 protein possesses the capability to amplify the re-uptake and usage of glucose in the liver [24]. Cyanidin 3-caffeoyl-p-hydroxybenzolsophoroside-5-glucoside and Peonidin 3-(6″-caffeoyl-6‴-feruloyl sophoroside)-5-glucoside have been found to restrain hepatic gluconeogenesis in HepG2 cells. However, the outcomes of an in vivo study investigating the effects of cyanidin revealed that oral administration significantly reduced fasting blood glucose levels from their initial high values at time zero (186–205 mg/dL, respectively [33].

According to earlier studies, it was found that blackcurrant extract, which consists of 45% anthocyanins and 82% total polyphenols, has potential to enhance plasma GLP-1 levels by approximately 30% and stimulate AMPK in the liver. Cyanidin 3-caffeoyl-p-hydroxybenzolsophoroside-5-glucoside and Peonidin 3-(6″-caffeoyl-6‴-feruloyl sophoroside)-5-glucoside have been reported to restrain hepatic gluconeogenesis in HepG2 cells. However, the outcomes of an in vivo study investigating the effects of cyanidin revealed that oral administration significantly reduced fasting blood glucose levels from their initial high values at time zero (186–205 mg/dL, respectively) [63,64]. The blocking of PEPCK and the G6Pase expression exhibited remarkable effectiveness in thwarting the escalation of blood glucose levels. This indicates that the process of gluconeogenesis will be suppressed, leading to a subsequent decrease in the production of glucose [65]. There is ongoing discussion regarding the mechanism by which GLP-1 affects hepatic gluconeogenesis and glycogen formation in the liver. Some argue that these effects are directly mediated by GLP-1R in hepatocytes, while others suggest that they may be indirectly mediated by the central nervous system (CNS) or insulin release. In vitro studies have shown that GLP-1 promotes glycogen synthesis and reduces gluconeogenesis by upregulating glycogen synthase, which is downstream of PI3K/PKB, PKC, and serine/threonine protein phosphatase 1. Additionally, GLP-1 decreased the expression of the gluconeogenetic enzyme phosphoenol pyruvate carboxykinase in rat hepatocytes [65].

The current research was primarily focused on the P13K/AKT pathway, which is considered to be one of the key insulin signaling pathways. [66]. Moreover, the PI3K/AKT/GSK-3ß signaling pathway activation not only improves insulin sensitivity and glucose metabolism, but also exerts a beneficial influence on dyslipidemia. A study conducted using high doses of sweet potato leaf polyphenols (SPLP) at 150 mg/kgBB demonstrated a more effective reduction in fasting blood glucose (FBG) over a period of 4 weeks compared to low-dose treatment. These findings suggested that the reduction in FBG by SPLP was both dose-dependent and time-dependent. The various components of SPLP, including 1-caffeoylquinic acid, 3,4,5-tricaffeoylquinic acid (3,4,5-triCQA), chlorogenic acid, caffeac acid derivative, quercetin, isoquercitrin, hyperoside, and rutin, play a crucial role in regulating hepatic glycogen synthesis in the liver. This regulation is mediated by insulin through the upregulation of PI3K/AKT and the downregulation of the GSK-3ß FOXO1 expression [11].

4.2.5. Muscle

Enhancing the Absorption of Glucose, Secretion, and Insulin Sensitivity

The regulation of glucose metabolism and the maintenance of energy homeostasis heavily relies on the insulin-stimulated uptake of glucose in skeletal muscle. The PI3K/Akt pathway is a critical target for the treatment of type 2 diabetes mellitus (T2DM) due to its involvement in modulating the signaling pathways associated with muscle function [66]. In this study, it was hypothesized that the presence of arabinogalactan and epigallocatechin in WSPP was expected to result in an elevation in the expression degrees of p-IR, p-Akt, and M-GLUT-4. Remarkably, the administration of high doses of DM + 30% WSP-Tuber and DM + 5% WSP-Leave resulted in a significant reduction in fasting blood glucose levels, thereby improving the fasting glucose tolerance [23]. Epigallocatechin has recently been demonstrated to enhance the secretion of GLP-1. By overexpressing GLP-1, it will be able to enter the systemic circulation and bind to the GLP-1R receptor in different tissues, including skeletal muscle. Consequently, this binding event can lead to an elevation in the level of cAMP signaling through the Gs protein, thereby promoting AMPK phosphorylation. By promoting the translocation of GLUT-4 from its intracellular depot to the sarcolemma, this process effectively stimulates glycogen synthesis and enables the uptake of glucose in skeletal muscle [45,67].

Insulin induced a notable rise in AKT phosphorylation in another fraction within the ≤ 10 kDA range from WSSp [32]. The expression of GLUT-4, the NRF1 gene, and MERF2a was observed to increase after subjecting C2C12 skeletal muscle cells to tissue culture testing. In this experiment, the cells were subjected to different concentrations of OSPT (orange sweet potato tubers) and OSPL (orange sweet potato leaves) for a period of 3 h. The doses used were 500 µg/mL of OSPT and 100 µg/mL of OSPL. The expression of GLUT-4, a key factor in glucose absorption, was regulated by the transcription factors MEF2a and NRF1. The metabolism of glucose absorption was significantly influenced by these transcription factors. The close relationship between the expression and activity of the GLUT-4 gene and the NRF1 and MEF2a genes, as well as their association with insulin sensitivity and glucose homeostasis in skeletal muscle, has been discovered. ACC2 and CPT1 play crucial roles as regulators of mitochondrial fatty acid oxidation, and therefore, any interventions that affect their expression can impact intracellular lipid levels and have therapeutic implications in managing insulin resistance. The enhanced expression of these genes in the treated cells indicated that a compound derived from aqueous methanol extracts of orange-fleshed IBL, containing caffeaic acid, catechin, hysperoside, kaemferol, rutin, isovanillic acid, quercetin, protocatechui acid, and vanillic acid, holds the potential for enhancing insulin sensitivity [22].

4.2.6. Adiposa

Increasing Glucose Uptake and Insulin Secretion

In vitro experiments have confirmed the effectiveness of a pure compound comprising quercetin 3-O-β-D sophoroside, quercetin, benzyl β-d-glucoside, 4-hydroxy-3-methoxybenzaldehyde, and methyl decanoate. This compound significantly increased the expression of PI3K, AKT, and GLUT-4 phosphorylation in 3T3-L1 adipocytes when tested at a dose of 0.01 mg/mL through a Western blot analysis. The activation of this gene increased GLUT-4 translocation so that glucose uptake also increased [13,68,69]. Caiapo containing aglycoprotein 4 g/day orally has been clinically tested on 30 patients and has been effective in reducing HbA1c progressively in diabetes patients for 1–2 months when compared to the placebo group [30]. Other studies also reported that caffeic acid could increase insulin secretion and sensitivity by increasing the adiponectin expression [31]. Adiponectin, a hormone that enhances insulin sensitivity and possesses anti-apoptotic and anti-inflammatory properties, is predominantly synthesized in adipose tissue. In individuals with obesity and type 2 diabetes, there has been a notable reduction in adiponectin levels. The administration of adiponectin has been shown to augment glucose uptake stimulated by insulin through the activation of AMPK in primary rat adipocytes. Moreover, adiponectin directly interacts with insulin receptor substrate-1 (IRS-1) and plays a pivotal role in facilitating insulin-mediated glucose uptake in adipocytes [70,71].

5. Conclusions and Future Perspective

IBL was reported to have variety and cultivars that contain chemicals with anti-diabetic properties. Such chemical compounds include flavonols, flavanol, flavones, antochyanin, phenolic acid, and triterpenoid groups. IBL can be considered as a multi-chemical and multi-pharmacological site since it functions in multiple organs through various ways. GLP-1 therapy for DM will prove to be quite advantageous in the future due to its efficacious nature. Flavonols, flavones, and flavone groups capable of forming complexes with $AlCl_3$ can also form complexes with Ca^{2+} through a chelation mechanism. Therefore, it is crucial to scientifically establish the correlation between chelated $AlCl_3$ + flavonoids, which have the potential to stimulate GLP-1 production. Additionally, it is important to determine whether the active $AlCl_3$–flavonoid compound can inhibit the DPP-IV enzyme, as GLP-1 has a short half-life due to the degradation by this enzyme. The group compounds play a crucial role in increasing GLP-1 activity and exerting its anti-diabetic effects, which would subsequently strengthen insulin production and the uptake of glucose into cells as glycogen from the systemic circulation.

Consequently, this research presents significant challenges that necessitate rigorous scientific validation. Once this hypothesis is confirmed, it will pave the way for the development of new drugs with well-defined pharmacological mechanisms. The results of the $AlCl_3$ + flavonoid complex require an isolation and structure elucidation process. It is hoped that the structure of the compound in IBL, a new drug candidate for treating DM, can be determined. Therefore, future research should involve in silico, in vitro, and in vivo testing of each isolated compound to strengthen the understanding of the pharmacological mechanisms involved. Subsequently, a chronic toxicity test should be conducted to ensure the safety and efficacy of the new drug candidate. The findings from this research are expected to be valuable for the pharmaceutical industry, which is interested in further developing it into drug formulations. Health professionals will gradually recognize that herbal medicines share similar pharmacological mechanisms with synthetic medicines, leading to an inclination towards prescribing herbal medicines for diabetes mellitus patients. Therefore, policymakers should consider legalizing the prescription of natural medicines among health professionals in order to provide patients with a sense of comfort when receiving DM medications made from herbal ingredients in the future.

Author Contributions: Conceptualization, N.K.S.M.D. and I.M.A.G.W.; methodology, N.K.S.M.D.; software, N.K.S.M.D.; validation, N.K.S.M.D., I.M.A.G.W. and D.M.W.; formal analysis, D.M.W.; investigation, M.R.S.; resources, N.K.S.M.D.; data curation, I.M.A.G.W.; writing—original draft preparation, N.K.S.M.D.; writing—review and editing, Y.R.; visualization, M.R.S.; supervision, D.M.W.; project administration, N.K.S.M.D. All authors have read and agreed to the published version of the manuscript.

Funding: This research received no external funding.

Data Availability Statement: The data to support the finding of this study can be made available by the corresponding authors upon request. The data are not publicly available due to privacy or ethical restrictions.

Acknowledgments: The authors express their gratitude to the rector of Universitas Udayana, Indonesia for providing access to their facilities during the course of this study.

Conflicts of Interest: The authors declare no conflict of interest.

References

1. Danaei, G.; Finucane, M.M.; Lu, Y.; Singh, G.M.; Cowan, M.J.; Paciorek, C.J.; Lin, J.K.; Farzadfar, F.; Khang, Y.H.; Stevens, G.A.; et al. National, regional, and global trends in fasting plasma glucose and diabetes prevalence since 1980: Systematic analysis of health examination surveys and epidemiological studies with 370 country-years and 2.7 million participants. *Lancet* **2011**, *378*, 31–40. [CrossRef]
2. Ogurtsova, K.; da Rocha Fernandes, J.D.; Huang, Y.; Linnenkamp, U.; Guariguata, L.; Cho, N.H.; Cavan, D.; Shaw, J.E.; Makaroff, L.E. IDF Diabetes Atlas: Global estimates for the prevalence of diabetes for 2015 and 2040. *Diabetes Res. Clin. Pract.* **2017**, *128*, 40–50. [CrossRef]
3. Al-Ishaq, R.K.; Abotaleb, M.; Kubatka, P.; Kajo, K.; Büsselberg, D. Flavonoids and their anti-diabetic effects: Cellular mechanisms and effects to improve blood sugar levels. *Biomolecules* **2019**, *9*, 430. [CrossRef]
4. Sen Tseng, P.; Ande, C.; Moremen, K.W.; Crich, D. Influence of Side Chain Conformation on the Activity of Glycosidase Inhibitors. *Angew. Chem.-Int. Ed.* **2023**, *62*, 2–6. [CrossRef]
5. Rajasekaran, P.; Ande, C.; Vankar, Y.D. Synthesis of (5,6 & 6,6)-oxa-oxa annulated sugars as glycosidase inhibitors from 2-formyl galactal using iodocyclization as a key step. *Arkivoc* **2022**, *2022*, 5–23.
6. Arisanti, C.I.S.; Wirasuta, I.M.A.G.; Musfiroh, I.; Ikram, E.H.K.; Muchtaridi, M. Mechanism of Anti-Diabetic Activity from Sweet Potato (Ipomoea batatas): A Systematic Review. *Foods* **2023**, *12*, 2810. [CrossRef]
7. Müller, T.D.; Finan, B.; Bloom, S.R.; D'Alessio, D.; Drucker, D.J.; Flatt, P.R.; Fritsche, A.; Gribble, F.; Grill, H.J.; Habener, J.F.; et al. Glucagon-like peptide 1 (GLP-1). *Mol. Metab.* **2019**, *30*, 72–130. [CrossRef]
8. Andersen, A.; Christensen, A.S.; Knop, F.K.; Vilsbøll, T. Glucagon-like peptide 1 receptor agonists for the treatment of Type 2 diabetes. *Ugeskr. Laeger* **2022**, *181*, 202–210. [CrossRef]
9. Nagamine, R.; Ueno, S.; Tsubata, M.; Yamaguchi, K.; Takagaki, K.; Hira, T.; Hara, H.; Tsuda, T. Dietary sweet potato (*Ipomoea batatas* L.) leaf extract attenuates hyperglycaemia by enhancing the secretion of glucagon-like peptide-1 (GLP-1). *Food Funct.* **2014**, *5*, 2309–2316. [CrossRef]
10. Hutton, B.; Salanti, G.; Caldwell, D.M.; Chaimani, A.; Schmid, C.H.; Cameron, C.; Ioannidis, J.P.A.; Straus, S.; Thorlund, K.; Jansen, J.P.; et al. The PRISMA extension statement for reporting of systematic reviews incorporating network meta-analyses of health care interventions: Checklist and explanations. *Ann. Intern. Med.* **2015**, *162*, 777–784. [CrossRef]
11. Luo, D.; Mu, T.; Sun, H. Sweet potato (*Ipomoea batatas* L.) leaf polyphenols ameliorate hyperglycemia in type 2 diabetes mellitus mice. *Food Funct.* **2021**, *12*, 4117–4131. [CrossRef]
12. Luo, D.; Mu, T.; Sun, H. Profiling of phenolic acids and flavonoids in sweet potato (*Ipomoea batatas* L.) leaves and evaluation of their anti-oxidant and hypoglycemic activities. *Food Biosci.* **2021**, *39*, 100801. [CrossRef]
13. Lee, C.L.; Lee, S.L.; Chen, C.J.; Chen, H.C.; Kao, M.C.; Liu, C.H.; Wu, Y.C. Characterization of secondary metabolites from purple Ipomoea batatas leaves and their effects on glucose uptake. *Molecules* **2016**, *21*, 745. [CrossRef]
14. Pal, S.; Gautam, S.; Mishra, A.; Maurya, R.; Srivastava, A.K. Antihyperglycemic and antidyslipidemic potential of ipomoea batatas leaves in validated diabetic animal models. *Int. J. Pharm. Pharm. Sci.* **2015**, *7*, 176–186.

15. Yustiantara, P.S.; Yustiantara, P.S.; Warditiani, N.K.; Armita Sari, P.M.N.; Anita Dewi, N.L.K.A.; Ramona, Y.; Jawi, I.M.; Wirasuta, I.M.A.G. Determination of TLC fingerprint biomarker of *Ipomoea batatas* (L.) Lam leaves extracted with ethanol and its potential as antihyperglycemic agent. *Pharmacia* 2021, *68*, 907–917. [CrossRef]
16. Zhang, L.; Tu, Z.-C.; Yuan, T.; Wang, H.; Xie, X.; Fu, Z.-F. Antioxidants and α-glucosidase inhibitors from Ipomoea batatas leaves identified by bioassay-guided approach and structure-activity relationships. *Food Chem.* 2016, *208*, 61–67. [CrossRef]
17. Zhao, R.; Li, Q.; Long, L.; Li, J.; Yang, R.; Gao, D. Antidiabetic activity of flavone from Ipomoea Batatas leaf in non-insulin dependent diabetic rats. *Int. J. Food Sci. Technol.* 2007, *42*, 80–85. [CrossRef]
18. Zovko, M.; Petlevski, R.; Kaloðera, Z.; Plantak, K. Antioxidant and antidiabetic activity of leaves of Ipomoea batatas grown in continental Croatia. *Planta Medica* 2008, *74*, PA135. [CrossRef]
19. Zengin, G.; Locatelli, M.; Stefanucci, A.; Macedonio, G.; Novellino, E.; Mirzaie, S.; Dvorácskó, S.; Carradori, S.; Brunetti, L.; Orlando, G.; et al. Chemical characterization, antioxidant properties, anti-inflammatory activity, and enzyme inhibition of *Ipomoea batatas* L. leaf extracts. *Int. J. Food Prop.* 2017, *20*, 1907–1919. [CrossRef]
20. Novrial, D.; Soebowo, S.; Widjojo, P. Protective Effect of Ipomoea batatas L Leaves Extract on Histology of Pancreatic Langerhans Islet and Beta Cell Insulin Expression of Rats Induced by Streptozotocin. *Molekul* 2020, *15*, 48. [CrossRef]
21. Sui, X.; Zhang, Y.; Zhou, W. In vitro and in silico studies of the inhibition activity of anthocyanins against porcine pancreatic α-amylase. *J. Funct. Foods* 2016, *21*, 50–57. [CrossRef]
22. Ayeleso, T.; Ramachela, K.; Mukwevho, E. Aqueous-Methanol Extracts of Orange-Fleshed Sweet Potato (Ipomoea batatas) Ameliorate Oxidative Stress and Modulate Type 2 Diabetes Associated Genes in Insulin Resistant C2C12 Cells. *Molecules* 2018, *23*, 2058. [CrossRef]
23. Shih, C.K.; Chen, C.M.; Varga, V.; Shih, L.C.; Chen, P.R.; Lo, S.F. White sweet potato ameliorates hyperglycemia and regenerates pancreatic islets in diabetic mice. *Food Nutr. Res.* 2020, *64*, 1–11. [CrossRef]
24. Jiang, T.; Shuai, X.; Li, J.; Yang, N.; Deng, L.; Li, S.; He, J. Protein-Bound Anthocyanin Compounds of Purple Sweet Potato Ameliorate Hyperglycemia by Regulating Hepatic Glucose Metabolism in High-Fat Diet/Streptozotocin-Induced Diabetic Mice. *J. Agric. Food Chem.* 2020, *68*, 1596–1608. [CrossRef]
25. Shen, L.; Yang, Y.; Zhang, J.; Feng, L.; Zhou, Q. Diacylated anthocyanins from purple sweet potato (*Ipomoea batatas* L.) attenuate hyperglycemia and hyperuricemia in mice induced by a high-fructose/high-fat diet. *J. Zhejiang Univ. Sci. B* 2023, *24*, 587–601. [CrossRef]
26. Okafor, C.S.; Ezekwesili, C.; Mbachu, N.; Onyewuchi, K.C.; Ogbodo, U.C. Anti-diabetic Effects of the Aqueous and Ethanol Extracts of Ipomoea batatas Tubers on Alloxan Induced Diabetes in Wistar Albino Rats. *Int. J. Biochem. Res. Rev.* 2021, *30*, 1–13. [CrossRef]
27. Matsui, T.; Ebuchi, S.; Kobayashi, M.; Fukui, K.; Sugita, K.; Terahara, N.; Matsumoto, K. Anti-hyperglycemic effect of diacylated anthocyanin derived from Ipomoea batatas cultivar Ayamurasaki can be achieved through the alpha-glucosidase inhibitory action. *J. Agric. Food Chem.* 2002, *50*, 7244–7248. [CrossRef]
28. Das, G.; Patra, J.K.; Basavegowda, N.; Vishnuprasad, C.N.; Shin, H.-S.H.-S.S. Comparative study on antidiabetic, cytotoxicity, antioxidant and antibacterial properties of biosynthesized silver nanoparticles using outer peels of two varieties of *Ipomoea batatas* (L.) Lam. *Int. J. Nanomed.* 2019, *14*, 4741–4754. [CrossRef] [PubMed]
29. Sakuramata, Y.; Oe, H.; Kusano, S.; Aki, O. Effects of combination of Caiapo® with other plant-derived substance on anti-diabetic efficacy in KK-Ay mice. *Biofactors* 2004, *22*, 149–152. [CrossRef] [PubMed]
30. Ludvik, B.; Neuffer, B.; Pacini, G. Efficacy of *Ipomoea batatas* (Caiapo) on Diabetes Control in Type 2 Diabetic. *Diabetes Care* 2004, *27*, 436–440. [CrossRef] [PubMed]
31. Kusano, S.; Tamasu, S.; Nakatsugawa, S. Effects of the White-Skinned Sweet Potato (*Ipomoea batatas* L.) on the Expression of Adipocytokine in Adipose Tissue of Genetic Type 2 Diabetic Mice. *Food Sci. Technol. Res.* 2005, *11*, 369–372. [CrossRef]
32. Kinoshita, A.; Nagata, T.; Furuya, F.; Nishizawa, M.; Mukai, E. White-skinned sweet potato (*Ipomoea batatas* L.) acutely suppresses postprandial blood glucose elevation by improving insulin sensitivity in normal rats. *Heliyon* 2023, *9*, e14719. [CrossRef] [PubMed]
33. Jang, H.; Kim, H.; Kim, S. In vitro and in vivo hypoglycemic effects of cyanidin 3-caffeoyl-p-hydroxybenzoylsophoroside-5-glucoside, an anthocyanin isolated from purple-fleshed sweet potato. *Food Chem.* 2019, *272*, 688–693. [CrossRef] [PubMed]
34. Kim, H.-J.; Koo, K.A.; Park, W.S.; Kang, D.-M.; Kim, H.S.; Lee, B.Y.; Goo, Y.-M.; Kim, J.-H.; Lee, M.K.; Woo, D.K.; et al. Anti-obesity activity of anthocyanin and carotenoid extracts from color-fleshed sweet potatoes. *J. Food Biochem.* 2020, *44*, e13438. [CrossRef] [PubMed]
35. Niwa, A.; Tajiri, T.; Higashino, H. Ipomoea batatas and Agarics blazei ameliorate diabetic disorders with therapeutic antioxidant potential in streptozotocin-induced diabetic rats. *J. Clin. Biochem. Nutr.* 2011, *48*, 194–202. [CrossRef]
36. Oki, N.; Nonaka, S.; Ozaki, S. The effects of an arabinogalactan-protein from the white-skinned sweet potato (*Ipomoea batatas* L.) on blood glucose in spontaneous diabetic mice. *Biosci. Biotechnol. Biochem.* 2011, *75*, 596–598. [CrossRef]
37. Wicaksono, L.A.; Yunianta, Y.; Widyaningsih, T.D. Anthocyanin extraction from purple sweet potato cultivar antin-3 (*Ipomoea batatas* L.) using maceration, microwave assisted extraction, ultrasonic assisted extraction and their application as anti-hyperglycemic agents in alloxan-induced wistar rats. *Int. J. PharmTech Res.* 2016, *9*, 181–192.
38. Kamal, S.; Akhter, N.; Khan, S.G.; Kiran, S.; Farooq, T.; Akram, M.; Zaheer, J. Anti-diabetic activity of aqueous extract of Ipomoea batatas L. in alloxan induced diabetic Wistar rats and its effects on biochemical parameters in diabetic rats. *Pak. J. Pharm. Sci.* 2018, *31*, 1539–1548.

39. Akhtar, N.; Akram, M.; Daniyal, M.; Ahmad, S. Evaluation of antidiabetic activity of Ipomoea batatas L. extract in alloxan-induced diabetic rats. *Int. J. Immunopathol. Pharmacol.* **2018**, *32*, 2058738418814678. [CrossRef]
40. Nurdjanah, S.; Astuti, S.; Yuliana, N. Inhibition Activity of α-amylase by Crude Acidic Water Extract from Fresh Purple Sweet Potato (Ipomoea batatas L.) and its Modified Flours. *Asian J. Sci. Res.* **2020**, *13*, 190–196. [CrossRef]
41. Cremonini, E.; Daveri, E.; Mastaloudis, A.; Oteiza, P.I. (−)-Epicatechin and Anthocyanins Modulate GLP-1 Metabolism: Evidence from C57BL/6J Mice and GLUTag Cells. *J. Nutr.* **2021**, *151*, 1497–1506. [CrossRef]
42. Hjørne, A.P.; Modvig, I.M.; Holst, J.J. The Sensory Mechanisms of Nutrient-Induced GLP-1 Secretion. *Metabolites* **2022**, *12*, 420. [CrossRef]
43. Kuhre, R.E.; Frost, C.R.; Svendsen, B.; Holst, J.J. Molecular mechanisms of glucose-stimulated GLP-1 secretion from perfused rat small intestine. *Diabetes* **2015**, *64*, 370–382. [CrossRef]
44. Jiang, Y.; Wang, Z.; Ma, B.; Fan, L.; Yi, N.; Lu, B.; Wang, Q.; Liu, R. GLP-1 improves adipocyte insulin sensitivity following induction of endoplasmic reticulum stress. *Front. Pharmacol.* **2018**, *9*, 1168. [CrossRef]
45. Wu, L.; Zhou, M.; Li, T.; Dong, N.; Yi, L.; Zhang, Q.; Mi, M. GLP-1 regulates exercise endurance and skeletal muscle remodeling via GLP-1R/AMPK pathway. *Biochim. Biophys. Acta-Mol. Cell Res.* **2022**, *1869*, 119300. [CrossRef]
46. Omotuyi, O.I.; Nash, O.; Inyang, O.K.; Ogidigo, J.; Enejoh, O.; Okpalefe, O.; Hamada, T. Flavonoid-rich extract of Chromolaena odorata modulate circulating GLP-1 in Wistar rats: Computational evaluation of TGR5 involvement. *3 Biotech* **2018**, *8*, 124. [CrossRef]
47. Wang, Y.; Wang, A.; Alkhalidy, H.; Luo, J.; Moomaw, E.; Neilson, A.P.; Liu, D. Flavone Hispidulin Stimulates Glucagon-Like peptide-1 secretion and Ameliorates Hyperglycemia in Streptozotocin-Induced Diabetic Mice. *Mol. Nutr. Food Res.* **2020**, *64*, e1900978. [CrossRef]
48. de Castilho, T.S.; Matias, T.B.; Nicolini, K.P.; Nicolini, J. Study of interaction between metal ions and quercetin. *Food Sci. Hum. Wellness* **2018**, *7*, 215–219. [CrossRef]
49. Horáková, L. Flavonoids in prevention of diseases with respect to modulation of Ca-pump function. *Interdiscip. Toxicol.* **2011**, *4*, 114–124. [CrossRef]
50. de Almeida, L.F.; Dos Santos, E.C.F.; Machado, J.C.B.; de Oliveira, A.M.; Napoleão, T.H.; Ferreira, M.R.A.; Soares, L.A.L. Phytochemical profile, in vitro activities, and toxicity of optimized Eugenia uniflora extracts. *Boletín Latinoam. Y Del Caribe De Plantas Med. Y Aromáticas* **2023**, *22*, 130–144. [CrossRef]
51. Oh, Y.S.; Jun, H.S. Effects of glucagon-like peptide-1 on oxidative stress and Nrf2 signaling. *Int. J. Mol. Sci.* **2017**, *19*, 26. [CrossRef]
52. Barber, E.; Houghton, M.J.; Williamson, G. Flavonoids as human intestinal α-glucosidase inhibitors. *Foods* **2021**, *10*, 1939. [CrossRef]
53. Pan, J.; Zhang, Q.; Zhang, C.; Yang, W.; Liu, H.; Lv, Z.; Liu, J.; Jiao, Z. Inhibition of Dipeptidyl Peptidase-4 by Flavonoids: Structure–Activity Relationship, Kinetics and Interaction Mechanism. *Front. Nutr.* **2022**, *9*, 892426. [CrossRef] [PubMed]
54. Ackermann, A.M.; Gannon, M. Molecular regulation of pancreatic β-cell mass development, maintenance, and expansion. *J. Mol. Endocrinol.* **2007**, *38*, 193–206. [CrossRef]
55. Wirasuta, I.M.A.G. Chemical profiling of ecstasy recovered from around Jakarta by High Performance Thin Layer Chromatography (HPTLC)-densitometry. *Egypt. J. Forensic Sci.* **2012**, *2*, 97–104. [CrossRef]
56. Xi, L.; Mu, T.; Sun, H. Preparative purification of polyphenols from sweet potato (Ipomoea batatas L.) leaves by AB-8 macroporous resins. *Food Chem.* **2015**, *172*, 166–174. [CrossRef]
57. Arisanti, C.; Sukawati, C.; Prasetia, I.G.N.J.A.; Wirasuta, I. Stability of Anthocyanins Encapsulated from Purple Sweet Potato Extract Affected by Maltodextrin Concentration. *Macromol. Symp.* **2020**, *391*, 1900127. [CrossRef]
58. Olivier, D.K.; van Wyk, B.E.; van Heerden, F.R. The chemotaxonomic and medicinal significance of phenolic acids in Arctopus and Alepidea (Apiaceae subfamily Saniculoideae). *Biochem. Syst. Ecol.* **2008**, *36*, 724–729. [CrossRef]
59. Masek, A.; Chrzescijanska, E.; Latos, M. Determination of antioxidant activity of caffeic acid and p-coumaric acid by using electrochemical and spectrophotometric assays. *Int. J. Electrochem. Sci.* **2016**, *11*, 10644–10658. [CrossRef]
60. Dhanya, R. Quercetin for managing type 2 diabetes and its complications, an insight into multitarget therapy. *Biomed. Pharmacother.* **2021**, *146*, 112560. [CrossRef] [PubMed]
61. Dai, X.; Ding, Y.; Zhang, Z.; Cai, X.; Li, Y. Quercetin and quercitrin protect against cytokine-induced injuries in RINm5F β-cells via the mitochondrial pathway and NF-κB signaling. *Int. J. Mol. Med.* **2012**, *31*, 265–271. [CrossRef]
62. Wirasuta, I.M.A.G.; Dewi, N.M.A.R.; Cahyadi, K.D.; Dewi, L.P.M.K.; Astuti, N.M.W.; Widjaja, I.N.K. Studying systematic errors on estimation decision, detection, and quantification limit on micro-TLC. *Chromatographia* **2013**, *76*, 1261–1269. [CrossRef]
63. Ben-Shlomo, S.; Zvibel, I.; Shnell, M.; Shlomai, A.; Chepurko, E.; Halpern, Z.; Barzilai, N.; Oren, R.; Fishman, S. Glucagon-like peptide-1 reduces hepatic lipogenesis via activation of AMP-activated protein kinase. *J. Hepatol.* **2011**, *54*, 1214–1223. [CrossRef]
64. Solverson, P. Anthocyanin Bioactivity in Obesity and Diabetes: And Periphery. *Cells* **2020**, *9*, 2515. [CrossRef]
65. Wang, T.; Jiang, H.; Cao, S.; Chen, Q.; Cui, M.; Wang, Z.; Li, D.; Zhou, J.; Wang, T.; Qiu, F.; et al. Baicalin and its metabolites suppresses gluconeogenesis through activation of AMPK or AKT in insulin resistant HepG-2 cells. *Eur. J. Med. Chem.* **2017**, *141*, 92–100. [CrossRef]
66. Chen, C.; Tan, S.; Ren, T.; Wang, H.; Dai, X.; Wang, H. Polyphenol from Rosaroxburghii Tratt Fruit Ameliorates the Symptoms of Diabetes by Activating the P13K/AKT Insulin Pathway in db/db Mice. *Foods* **2022**, *11*, 636. [CrossRef]

67. Warditiani, N.K.; Astuti, N.M.W.; Sari, P.M.N.A.; Swastini, D.A.; Wirasuta, I.M.A.G. Analysis of lipid profile and atherogenic index (Aip) in dyslipidemia rats given ipomea batatas tuber extract (ibte). *Res. J. Pharm. Technol.* **2021**, *14*, 4999–5002. [CrossRef]
68. Song, W.Y.; Aihara, Y.; Hashimoto, T.; Kanazawa, K.; Mizuno, M. (−)-Epigallocatechin-3-gallate induces secretion of anorexigenic gut hormones. *J. Clin. Biochem. Nutr.* **2015**, *57*, 164–169. [CrossRef]
69. Warditiani, N.K.T.; Astuti, K.W.; Sari, P.M.N.A.; Wirasuta, I.M.A.G. Antidyslipidemic Activity of Methanol, Ethanol and Ethyl Acetate Mangosteen rind (*Garcinia mangostana* L). *Res. J. Pharm. Technol.* **2020**, *13*, 261. [CrossRef]
70. Wang, Y.; Meng, R.W.; Kunutsor, S.K.; Chowdhury, R.; Yuan, J.M.; Koh, W.P.; Pan, A. Plasma adiponectin levels and type 2 diabetes risk: A nested case-control study in a Chinese population and an updated meta-analysis. *Sci. Rep.* **2018**, *8*, 406. [CrossRef]
71. Yanai, H.; Yoshida, H. Beneficial Effects of Adiponectin on Glucose and Lipid Metabolism and Atherosclerotic Progression: Mechanisms and Perspectives. *Int. J. Mol. Sci.* **2019**, *20*, 1190. [CrossRef]

Disclaimer/Publisher's Note: The statements, opinions and data contained in all publications are solely those of the individual author(s) and contributor(s) and not of MDPI and/or the editor(s). MDPI and/or the editor(s) disclaim responsibility for any injury to people or property resulting from any ideas, methods, instructions or products referred to in the content.

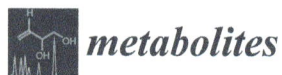

Article

Effects of Gold Nanoparticles Phytoreduced with Rutin in an Early Rat Model of Diabetic Retinopathy and Cataracts

Mădălina Moldovan [1,*], Ana-Maria Păpurică [1], Mara Muntean [2], Raluca Maria Bungărdean [3], Dan Gheban [3,4], Bianca Moldovan [5], Gabriel Katona [5], Luminița David [5] and Gabriela Adriana Filip [1]

[1] Department of Physiology, Iuliu Hatieganu University of Medicine and Pharmacy, Clinicilor Street, No. 1, 400006 Cluj-Napoca, Romania; papurica.ana.maria@elearn.umfcluj.ro (A.-M.P.); gabriela.filip@umfcluj.ro (G.A.F.)

[2] Department of Cell and Molecular Biology, Iuliu Hatieganu University of Medicine and Pharmacy, Pasteur Street, No. 6, 400349 Cluj-Napoca, Romania; muntean.mara@elearn.umfcluj.ro

[3] Department of Pathology, Iuliu Hatieganu University of Medicine and Pharmacy, Clinicilor Street, No. 3-5, 400340 Cluj-Napoca, Romania; maria.bungardean@elearn.umfcluj.ro (R.M.B.); dgheban@gmail.com (D.G.)

[4] Department of Pathology, Emergency Clinical Hospital for Children, Motilor Street, No. 41T-42T, 400370 Cluj-Napoca, Romania

[5] Faculty of Chemistry and Chemical Engineering, Babes-Bolyai University, Arany Janos Street, No. 11, 400028 Cluj-Napoca, Romania; bianca.moldovan@ubbcluj.ro (B.M.); gabik@chem.ubbcluj.ro (G.K.); luminita.david@ubbcluj.ro (L.D.)

* Correspondence: moldovan.madalina@elearn.umfcluj.ro

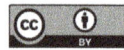

Citation: Moldovan, M.; Păpurică, A.-M.; Muntean, M.; Bungărdean, R.M.; Gheban, D.; Moldovan, B.; Katona, G.; David, L.; Filip, G.A. Effects of Gold Nanoparticles Phytoreduced with Rutin in an Early Rat Model of Diabetic Retinopathy and Cataracts. *Metabolites* **2023**, *13*, 955. https://doi.org/10.3390/metabo13080955

Academic Editors: Vesa Cosmin Mihai and Dana Carmen Zaha

Received: 31 July 2023
Revised: 12 August 2023
Accepted: 13 August 2023
Published: 18 August 2023

Copyright: © 2023 by the authors. Licensee MDPI, Basel, Switzerland. This article is an open access article distributed under the terms and conditions of the Creative Commons Attribution (CC BY) license (https://creativecommons.org/licenses/by/4.0/).

Abstract: Diabetic retinopathy (DR) and cataracts (CA) have an early onset in diabetes mellitus (DM) due to the redox imbalance and inflammation triggered by hyperglycaemia. Plant-based therapies are characterised by low tissue bioavailability. The study aimed to investigate the effect of gold nanoparticles phytoreduced with Rutin (AuNPsR), as a possible solution. Insulin, Rutin, and AuNPsR were administered to an early, six-week rat model of DR and CA. Oxidative stress (MDA, CAT, SOD) was assessed in serum and eye homogenates, and inflammatory cytokines (IL-1 beta, IL-6, TNF alpha) were quantified in ocular tissues. Eye fundus of retinal arterioles, transmission electron microscopy (TEM) of lenses, and histopathology of retinas were also performed. DM was linked to constricted retinal arterioles, reduced endogen antioxidants, and eye inflammation. Histologically, retinal wall thickness decreased. TEM showed increased lens opacity and fibre disorganisation. Rutin improved retinal arteriolar diameter, while reducing oxidative stress and inflammation. Retinas were moderately oedematous. Lens structure was preserved on TEM. Insulin restored retinal arteriolar diameter, while increasing MDA, and amplifying TEM lens opacity. The best outcomes were obtained for AuNPsR, as it improved fundus appearance of retinal arterioles, decreased MDA and increased antioxidant capacity. Retinal edema and disorganisation in lens fibres were still present.

Keywords: diabetic retinopathy; cataracts; gold nanoparticles; Rutin; antioxidant; early; incipient

1. Introduction

Research on ocular complications of diabetes mellitus (DM), including diabetic retinopathy (DR) and cataracts (CA), is currently shifting its focus towards early detection and therapy [1,2]. This is a shift from what is now regarded as the standard method, which primarily focuses on late-phase treatment. These strategies have a painful and limited curative ability for DR, and pose a significant economic burden for CA [3,4]. Moreover, CA surgery, despite being a customary practice, was found to be associated with an increased risk of DR development in diabetic patients [5]. The transition from advanced-stage management to early-stage prevention is being made possible, firstly by advancements in screening [6,7].

Numerous studies have emphasized the pressing issue of timely detection at subclinical stages, defined by the presence of morphophysiological alterations with limited characteristic symptoms. One study on diabetic patients [2] described peripheral spoke-like lesions on the eye lens through slit-lamp examination, typically associated with cortical CA (a type often linked to diabetes). These lesions only became symptomatic with accumulation in the centre of the lens, leading to impaired vision, correctable by surgery. Likewise, subclinical abnormalities in DR resulting from early microvascular and neuronal degeneration were measured using spectral domain optical coherence tomography and optical coherence tomography angiography [8].

Thus, the impact of subclinical diagnosis by various screening methods could be increased by subsequent treatment. At present, lifestyle changes are primarily recommended, specifically blood glucose management. A metanalysis study [9] found that, despite being guideline advocated, strict glycaemic control could not be correlated to significant benefits against microvascular complications. To address this research gap, recent studies have postulated the use of plant-derived antioxidants as effective remedies for diabetes-induced complications. This can be justified by the existing understanding of pathophysiology. According to Brownlee's hypothesis [10], there is a singular common mechanism that causes both diabetes and its complications—increased production of reactive oxygen species (ROS). This model states that the typical diabetes-linked reduced amount of insulin and/or its effects trigger a systematic chain of events. Firstly, the ensuing hyperglycaemia stimulates an increased flux through the major pathways responsible for diabetes damage—polyol, hexosamine, protein kinase C (PKC), advanced glycation end-product formation (AGEs) and activation of Poly(ADP-ribose) polymerase. Secondly, vulnerable glial cells, such as astrocytes, Müller cells and microglia, enter a state of oxidative stress, which is coupled with an increase in the secretion of proinflammatory cytokines, TNF-α, IL-1β, and IL-6 [11]. Furthermore, it has been proposed [12] that the retinal glia hosts a resident renin-angiotensin system (RAS), which produces local Angiotensin II (Ang II). Intraocular levels of Ang II have been shown to rise in diabetes and were associated with an increased inflammatory and oxidative stress response. Ang II has also been found to stimulate the retinal microglia through the Angiotensin type 1 receptor (AT1), leading to a decrease in retinal blood flow, independent of systemic changes [13]. Similarly, RAS modulators have demonstrated anticataract properties, possibly by inhibiting the AT1-mediated production of ROS [14].

A variety of antioxidant plant compounds have been suggested as potential treatments for diabetic ocular complications, each presenting individual strengths and weaknesses. Among these compounds, Rutin, a flavonol from the flavonoid subclass of dietary polyphenols, shows promising properties for managing DM. Rutin is known for its antioxidant and anti-inflammatory abilities [15]. Additionally, a recent study has demonstrated that Rutin can act as an inhibitor of AT1 receptors [16]. Moreover, it can lower glycaemia by inhibiting carbohydrate absorption and gluconeogenesis, and it can promote insulin secretion and the cellular uptake of glucose [15]. This compound has also been shown to decrease serum triglycerides, LDL, and VLDL, with high HDL levels in experimental models [15].

The main disadvantage of Rutin is its low bioavailability, attributed to its highly hydrophilic nature, which hinders diffusion through cell membranes. After ingestion, Rutin is hydroxylated to quercetin, a compound quickly metabolised in the body, resulting in limited bioavailability [17].

Delivering therapeutic agents to the eye poses an additional challenge. As such, barriers exist for both topical administrations, the tear layer and corneal epithelium with tight junctions [18], and systemic delivery, including the blood–aqueous barrier and blood–retina barrier [19].

Considering the systemic nature of diabetes, and Rutin's multiorgan action, oral administration, together with a nanotechnology-based formulation, were proposed to overcome delivery and bioavailability issues. Nanoparticles are accepted as efficient drug delivery systems for both lens and retinal pathologies. Gold nanoparticles (AuNPs) have been used in previous medical studies due to their ease of functionalisation with various active molecules [20]. A recent study [21] demonstrated significant uptake of AuNPs functionalised with resveratrol, a stilbene from the subclass of dietary polyphenols, in ocular lens epithelial cells, in both in vitro and in vivo models of CA, with no dose-dependent toxicity. Similarly, improvements were demonstrated in a Wistar rat model of diabetic retinopathy when treated with AuNPs phytoreduced with resveratrol [22]. Other authors [23] revealed increased in vitro glucose uptake by adipocytes using AuNPs prepared with vicenin-2, a compound from the same flavonoid subclass as Rutin.

In the present study, we hypothesized that the administration of gold nanoparticles conjugated with Rutin (AuNPsR) in an early rat model of DR and CA may present beneficial therapeutic effects. The effects were evaluated by oxidative stress investigation in serum and ocular tissues, and inflammatory cytokines levels in eye homogenates. Eye fundus assessment of retinal arterioles, transmission electron microscopy (TEM) of eye lenses, and histopathological examination of retinas were also performed.

2. Materials and Methods

2.1. Reagents

Tetrachloroauric acid trihydrate, 2-thiobarbituric acid, Bradford reagent, sodium hydroxide, and Folin–Ciocalteu reagent were obtained from Merck (Darmstadt, Germany). O-phthalaldehyde, osmium tetroxide and glutaraldehyde were purchased from Sigma-Aldrich (Taufkirchen, Germany). IL1β, TNFα, and IL6 were measured in eye homogenates by ELISA assays using the Elabscience ELISA kits (Houston, TX, USA), according to the producer instructions. Results were expressed as pg/mg protein.

2.2. Gold Nanoparticles Synthesis and Characterisation

The synthesis of AuNPsR was carried out as follows: to a mixture of 61 mg Rutin and 100 mL distilled water, 2 M aqueous solution of NaOH was added dropwise (approximately 4 mL), until Rutin was totally dissolved, and the colour of the obtained solution turned yellow-orange. An amount of 100 mL of 1 mM tetra chloroauric solution was added over the Rutin solution and the mixture was stirred at room temperature for one hour. The obtained AuNPsR were purified via centrifugation at 10,000 rpm followed by washing of the resulting pellet twice with distilled water. The pellet was resuspended and used for biological determination. The obtained AuNPsR were characterised using classical methods. UV-Vis spectroscopy was applied to follow the progress of the reaction; to this end, a Perkin Elmer Lambda 25 spectrometer was used. The absorbance of gold colloidal solution was scanned between 300 and 800 nm, in a 1 cm quartz cuvette, with distilled water being used as blank. Transmission electron microscopy (TEM), by using a Hitachi H-7650 transmission microscope, made possible the morphological characterisation of AuNPsR. The ImageJ 1.53 t [24] software was used to measure the mean size of the synthesized AuNPsR, from at least 100 AuNPsR. The zeta potential and hydrodynamic diameter of AuNPsR were assessed using a Malvern Zetasizer Nanoseries compact scattering spectrometer. The crystal structure and the crystalline grain size of the obtained gold nanoparticles were analysed via X-ray crystallography. X-ray diffraction (XRD) data were acquired with a Smart Lab Rigaku diffractometer with a graphite monochromator with Cu-Kα radiation (k 1/4 1:54 Å) X-ray source: Anode Cu, 9 kW at room temperature over the 2Theta range from 10 to 90 degrees, with a 0.01-degree step. For the Rietveld refinement, the Integrated X-ray Powder Diffraction (PDXL) software was used.

2.3. Experimental Design

The study adhered to the ethical standards regarding animal research and received approval from the University Ethical Board and the Veterinary and Food Safety Direction (project authorisation no. 294/09.03.2022). Sixty-eight Wistar albino female rats, three months old, weighing 300 $\pm$ 10 g, were provided by the Experimental Animal Facility of Iuliu Hatieganu University of Medicine and Pharmacy in Cluj-Napoca, Romania. Rats were housed in cages under standard environmental conditions, with a temperature of 21 $\pm$ 2 °C, a relative humidity of 55% $\pm$ 5%, and a 12 h light/12 h dark cycle. Conventional food and water were provided ad libitum.

The experiment consisted of three stages: induction of diabetes, development of incipient ocular complications, and administration of treatment. The experimental design is illustrated in Figure 1.

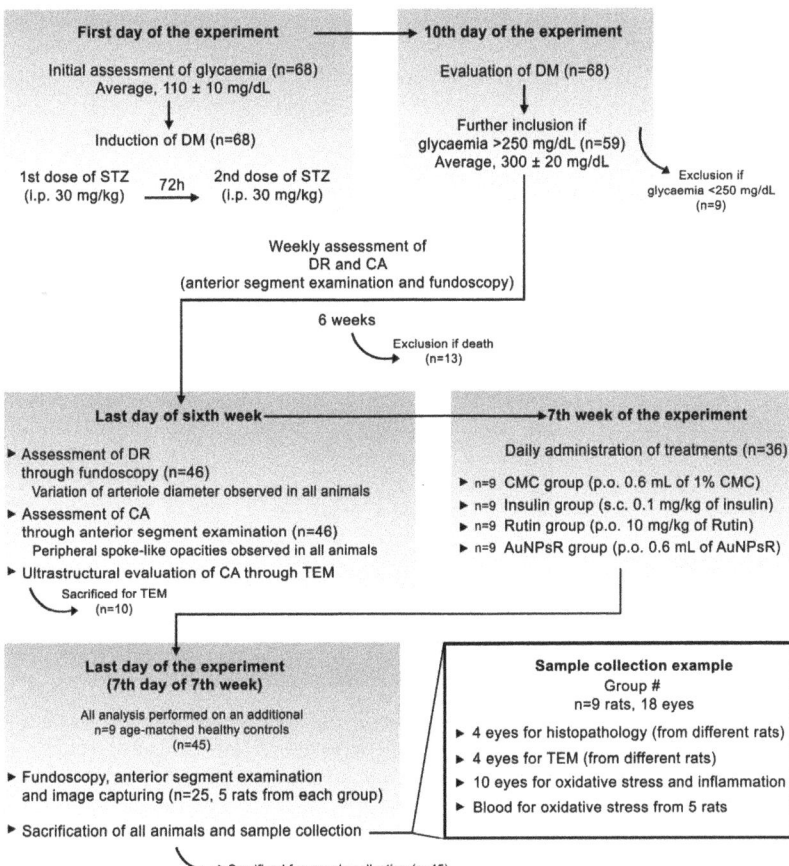

Figure 1. Illustrative representation of the experimental design; DM = diabetes mellitus; STZ = streptozotocin; i.p. = intraperitoneal; DR = diabetic retinopathy; CA = cataracts; TEM = transmission electron microscopy; CMC = carboxymethylcellulose; s.c. = subcutaneous; p.o. = per os.

Prior to the induction of DM, blood samples were drawn from 68 animals to assess glycaemic levels, which were found to be within the normal range (average of 110 ± 10 mg/dL). To induce DM, two doses of streptozotocin (STZ) were administered to all 68 rats by intraperitoneal injection: 30 mg/kg STZ on day zero and 30 mg/kg STZ after 72 h. Animals were included in the study if their blood glucose levels exceeded 250 mg/dL on the seventh days after the last dose of STZ. At this point, nine rats were excluded because their glycaemic level was below 250 mg/dL. The average glycaemic value obtained for the remaining 59 animals was 300 ± 20 mg/dL.

In the following six weeks after induction of DM, weekly anterior segment examination and fundoscopy were performed to assess the incipient development of CA and DR. In this timeframe, 13 animals were excluded due to death. On the last day of the sixth week, 46 rats survived and were further analysed. Early DR was defined through variations in retinal arteriole diameter and was detected in all surviving animals. Similarly, all animals exhibited the first signs of CA formation, including swollen fibres and subcapsular opacities, according to a previously described grading system of lens opacity [25]. Ten randomly selected diabetic animals were sacrificed and used for the ultrastructural evaluation of CA through TEM. Additionally, the same evaluation was performed for age-matched healthy rats, which were considered controls. A side-by-side view of the anterior segment photography and the corresponding TEM micrographs is presented in Figure 2.

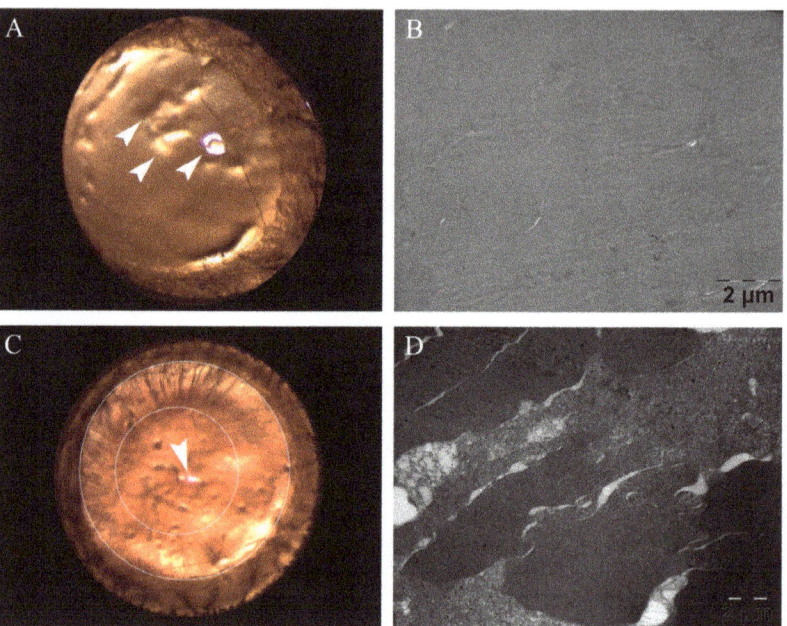

Figure 2. Side-by-side images obtained from a healthy rat and a six-week diabetic rat; (**A**) anterior segment photography of healthy eye lens. (**B**) Transmission electron microscopy (TEM) micrograph of healthy eye lens with lens fibres tightly packed together, separated by thin spaces. (**C**) Anterior segment photography depicting peripheral spoke-like opacities of incipient cataracts; the larger oval outlines the internal limit of the iris, while the smaller oval outlines the internal border of cataracts lesions, more visible in the upper left quadrant (from eleven to one clockwise). (**D**) TEM micrograph of eye lens with notable lens fibre disorganisation, characteristic of incipient cataracts. Arrowheads point towards microscope reflection, not to be confused with central opacity.

Subsequently, 36 animals with signs of incipient diabetic ocular complications were included in the study and were randomly divided in the following four treatment groups (nine animals/group): CMC group (0.6 mL/day of 1% carboxymethylcellulose vehicle solution), Insulin group (0.1 mg/kg of insulin), Rutin group (10 mg/kg/day), and AuNPsR group (0.6 mL/day of AuNPsR). A fifth group with nine healthy age-matched animals, without DM and treated only with CMC, was considered the Control group. Treatments were administered daily for seven days, via oral gavage, between 7 a.m. and 8 a.m., except for insulin, which was administered subcutaneously.

After seven days of treatment, five randomly selected animals/group were completely sedated in order to perform fundoscopy, anterior segment evaluation, and image collection. Then, all specimens (n = 45) were sacrificed by overdose as to not damage the eye from the increased pressure. For microscopic studies, a total of eight eyes, from four animals/group, were enucleated. These eight eyes/group were distributed evenly between histopathology and TEM processing. Specifically, each of the four animals contributed one eye to TEM processing and another eye to histopathology processing. This approach ensured that all eyes subjected to microscopic studies were sourced from distinct animals, randomly chosen from each group. From five animals/group, blood was used to assess oxidative stress levels, whilst their ten eyes were collected for biochemical analysis.

All eyes were collected using a technique specifically developed to maintain structural integrity. The soft tissues overlaying the skull were removed. Then, an incision was made along the frontonasal suture, and the dorsal part of the skull was gently lifted. This exposed the ocular globes and their respective optic nerves, which were easily enucleated and further processed.

2.4. Fundoscopy Examination

Fundus photographs were captured using a Leica Microsystems M320 T Surgical Training Microscope. Pupils were dilated with a drop of 1% tropicamide, and the vibrissae were trimmed to prevent them from obstructing the photographs. During the procedure, eyelids were completely retracted, and a mound of propylene glycol water-based viscous gel was applied to the external portion of the rodent's eye. A glass microscope slide was placed on top of the gel, and gentle pressure was exerted to flatten the cornea. The gel prevents the image from distorting and provides a practical alternative to liquid oil in this situation. The position of the specimen and the pressure applied to the glass slide were permanently adjusted to achieve the proper focus. The specimen's position and angle were altered accordingly to examine different areas of the fundus. All photographs were captured using the built-in camera of the surgical microscope.

2.5. Fundus Photography Processing and Analysis

Fundus photographs were analysed using ImageJ version 1.53 k [24]. Firstly, arterioles were differentiated from venules based on the anatomical model described by McLenachan et al. [26]. Thus, an alternating pattern was observed, with each arteriole being situated next to a venule. Following the approach outlined by Miri et al. [27], the darker red vessels were considered as venous in nature.

To facilitate the visualisation of red colour variance, all photographs were imported into ImageJ, converted to the RGB format, and then split into greyscale colour channels. For the red channel, brighter greys indicated higher red amounts, while darker greys meant lower red amounts or no red. As a result, arterioles, associated with a bright red colour due to oxygenated blood, appeared as washed-out brighter grey, while venules, associated with a dark red colour due to deoxygenated blood, appeared as clearly distinguishable dark grey. This facilitated successful arteriole isolation.

For measurements, the raw fundus photographs were used, as depicted in Figure 3. Fundus photographs were obtained from both eyes of five randomly selected animals of every group. For each eye, three arterioles were measured, resulting in 30 measurements for every group (three arterioles × two eyes per animal × five animals per group). The selected measurement area was within a disc diameter of 0.5 to 0.25 from the edge of the fundoscopy disc margin. This area was chosen to account for the curvature of the eye and to ensure measurement consistency across photographs. A central line was drawn following the long axis of the vessel. To assess diameter, five distinct measurement lines perpendicular to the central line were created. The width of each measurement line was calculated, and the five values were averaged.

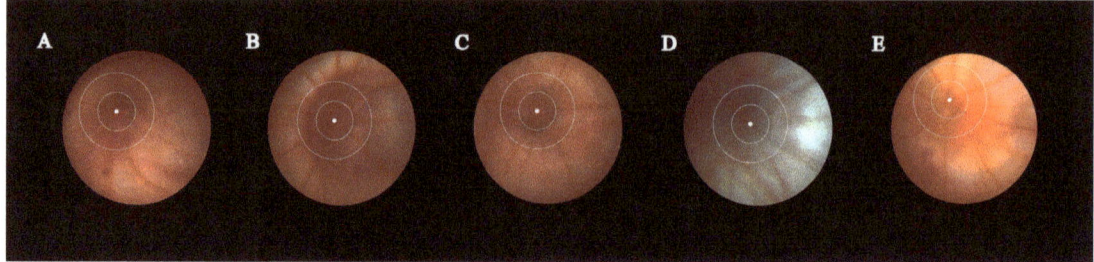

Figure 3. A representative fundus photography from each group, in controls (**A**) and in rats with six weeks of diabetes and one week of treatment as follows: CMC (carboxymethylcellulose) (**B**), insulin (**C**), Rutin (**D**), AuNPsR (gold nanoparticles phytoreduced with Rutin) (**E**). The selected region for measuring retinal arteriole diameter is defined as the area enclosed between the smaller circle and the larger circle.

2.6. Oxidative Stress Investigation and Inflammation Assessment

Oxidative stress was evaluated in serum and eye homogenates by quantification of malondialdehyde (MDA), as a marker of lipid peroxidation, using Conti's method [28]. Additionally, catalase (CAT) activity was measured through Pippenger's method [29]. Superoxide dismutase (SOD) activity was assessed through the method described by Beauchamp and Fridovich [30]. Inflammation from eye homogenates was evaluated via ELISA tests, and the results were expressed as pg/mg protein.

2.7. Retina Histopathological Examination

Extraocular tissues were excised immediately after enucleation, to ensure proper penetration of the fixative. Then, the eyes underwent a two-step fixation process. For this purpose, a 10% formaldehyde solution was utilized, at ten times the volume of the tissue being studied. For the first 24 h, the ocular globes were submerged in the fixation solution, as a whole. Subsequently, they were briefly removed from the fixative, and sectioned in half, along the anatomical sagittal plane (with the blade placed perpendicular to the superior and inferior rectus muscles). Then, the obtained halves were fixed for a second 24 h period, in the same solution. Through employing a preliminary fixation of the entire globe, collapse upon halving was avoided. Ultimately, samples were embedded in paraffin and sectioned at 5 µ, then stained with haematoxylin-eosin and examined using an Olympus BX43F light microscope (Olympus, Tokyo, Japan). Pictures of representative areas were captured using the microscope mounted camera (Olympus UC30 camera with the Olympus U-CMAD3 adapter).

2.8. Eye Lens Transmission Electron Microscopy

Following enucleation, eye lenses were removed as swiftly as possible. The ocular globe was held in place with toothed microsurgical forceps whilst the cornea was removed along the limbus, by gliding two surgical blades against each other and in opposing directions. After extraction, eye lenses were first fixed in a 2.7% glutaraldehyde solution in 0.1 M phosphate buffer, and then they were cut in halves. Afterward, samples were washed four times, in the same buffer. Subsequent to postfixation with 1.5% osmium tetroxide (OsO4) in 0.15 M phosphate buffer, eye lenses underwent dehydration in a series of acetone solutions of increasing concentrations (from 30%, up to 100%), infiltration and embedding in EMbed 812. Using a Diatome A382 diamond knife (Diatome, Hatfield, USA), 70–80 nm thick ultrathin sections were obtained on a Bromma 8800 ULTRATOME III (LKB, Stockholm, Sweden). These sections were then collected on 300 mesh copper grids, contrasted with uranyl acetate and lead citrate, and examined at 80 kV using a JEOL JEM-100CX II transmission electron microscope (JEOL, Tokyo, Japan). Images were captured with a MegaView G3 camera, equipped with a Radius 2.1 software (both from Emsis, Münster, Germany).

2.9. Eye Lens TEM Photography Processing and Analysis

To assess opacity modifications in eye lenses using TEM micrographs, an adapted protocol based on Wirahadikesuma et al. was implemented [31]. Micrographs were analysed using ImageJ version 1.53 k [24].

Twenty micrographs from each group were examined. For each micrograph, 20 regions of interest were measured by two blinded researchers, resulting in a total of 800 measurements for each group (20 photos per group × 20 measurements per micrograph × two independent researchers). Regions of interest were selected based on the homogeneity of lens tissue and were defined as a square area, with the calculated side length of 365 pixels, which would provide 95% coverage of each micrograph. As the measurement unit was not significant to our outcome, the standard pixel unit was utilised.

To measure pixel density, the .tif micrographs were converted to the commonly used 8-bit integer format, yielding a possible range of pixel densities from zero to 255. Following Ansel Adam's Zone System, zero represents pure black, and 255 represents pure white. Considering that the images are micrographs, where pure black corresponds to complete electron density, such as a perfect saturation of the employed TEM fixative and contrasting agent (OsO4), zero was considered the maximum opacity achievable by our tissue. Measurements from the control group were used as a reference. Hence, the maximum pixel density obtained in the control group was considered the transparency standard, with a value of 166.949 pixels/area. To facilitate visualisation of opacity measurements, the following formula was applied to convert pixel density to a percentage of opacity,

$$(255 - x)/255 \times 100. \tag{1}$$

Consequently, 100% opacity would correspond to zero pixels/area (maximum opacity), and 0% opacity would correspond to 166.949 pixels/area (minimum opacity or maximum transparency achievable). This conversion is depicted in Figure 4.

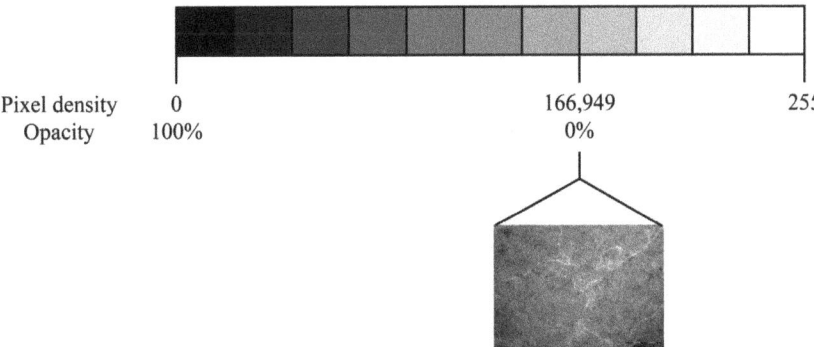

Figure 4. Depiction of Ansel Adam's Zone System according to a greyscale gradient, which ranges from zero pixels, or the equivalent of pure black, to 255 pixels, or the equivalent of pure white. For our experimental purpose of evaluating eye lens opacity using transmission electron microscopy micrographs, 100% opacity was attributed to zero pixels, and 0% opacity, or standard transparency, to 166.949 pixels. This value corresponds to the presented micrograph of a subject from the control group, which demonstrated the highest transparency.

Any heterogeneity caused by CA-induced morphological modifications would be indicated by higher electron density and consequently a tendency towards increased opacity.

2.10. Statistical Analysis

Data were analysed using GraphPad Prism version 9.0.0 for Windows, GraphPad Software, San Diego, CA USA, www.graphpad.com, accessed on 15 May 2021. All multi-group assessments were performed using the Kruskal–Wallis test for not normally distributed data. Outliers of TEM micrographs were identified using Robust regression and Outlier removal (ROUT) with Q set at the default 1%. To describe the quantitative data from arteriole diameter and eye lens opacity investigations, the minimum and maximum values, median, and interquartile range (Q1–Q3, the range between the 25th percentile and the 75th percentile) were graphed. Additionally, quantitative data from serum oxidative stress, eye tissue oxidative stress and inflammation examinations, was described through mean and standard deviation. A *p*-value equal to or lower than 0.05 was considered statistically significant. Photos were analysed using ImageJ 1.53 k [24].

3. Results

3.1. Characterisation of Gold Nanoparticles Functionalised with Rutin

In order to avoid the use of toxic solvents and the production of harmful waste, an environmentally friendly synthesis method was applied for the production of AuNPsR. Rutin was successfully used to reduce the gold ions at room temperature and also to prevent the aggregation of the synthesized nanoparticles by acting as a capping agent at their surface. The UV-Vis spectrophotometry was used to monitor the synthesis of AuNPsR and to confirm their obtaining after reduction of the gold ions from the $HAuCl_4$ solution, obtaining that was first visually confirmed by the colour change from yellow to purple-red. Figure 5 presents the recorded UV-Vis spectra of the Rutin solution and AuNPsR colloidal solution. It is easy to observe that the Vis typical absorption band of Rutin at 399 nm [32] disappeared during the progress of the synthesis, and the AuNPsR characteristic surface plasmon resonance SPR band at λ = 523 nm appeared [33].

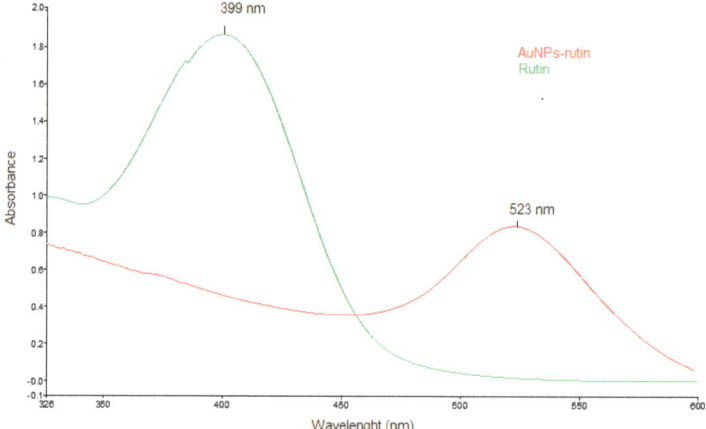

Figure 5. UV-Vis spectra of Rutin and gold nanoparticles phytoreduced with Rutin (AuNPsR).

The morphology, diameter, and size distribution of the AuNPsR were analysed using transmission electron microscopy (TEM). The TEM image, shown in Figure 6a, revealed that the obtained AuNPsR were mostly spherical in shape, presenting homogenous size distribution and an average diameter (Figure 6b) of 15 nm.

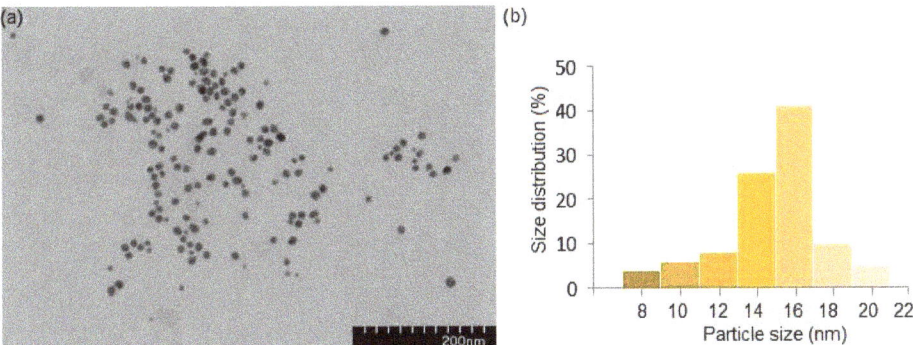

Figure 6. TEM image (**a**) and size distribution (**b**) of gold nanoparticles phytoreduced with Rutin (AuNPsR).

Dynamic light scattering (DLS) experiments allowed us to evaluate the stability of the AuNPsR solution and their surface charge and also to analyse their hydrodynamic diameter. The obtained negative zeta potential value, measured to be −19.0 eV (Figure 7), suggests that the resulting colloidal solution of AuNPsR presents a rather good stability. The negative surface charge of the AuNPsR is due to the Rutin molecules negatively charged that are present at the surface of the nanoparticles, which confer them a good stability [34].

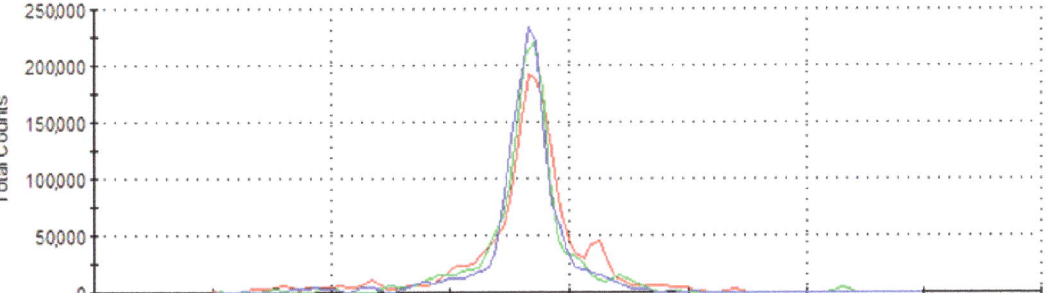

Figure 7. Zeta potential of gold nanoparticles phytoreduced with Rutin (AuNPsR). There are three distinct measurement sets, each consisting of thirty individual runs. Every coloured line corresponds to a singular measurement set.

The hydrodynamic diameter of the AuNPsR was found to be 78.48 nm.
X-ray diffraction analysis was used to determine the crystal structure of the obtained gold nanoparticles. Figure 8 presents the XRD diffractogram of AuNPsR.

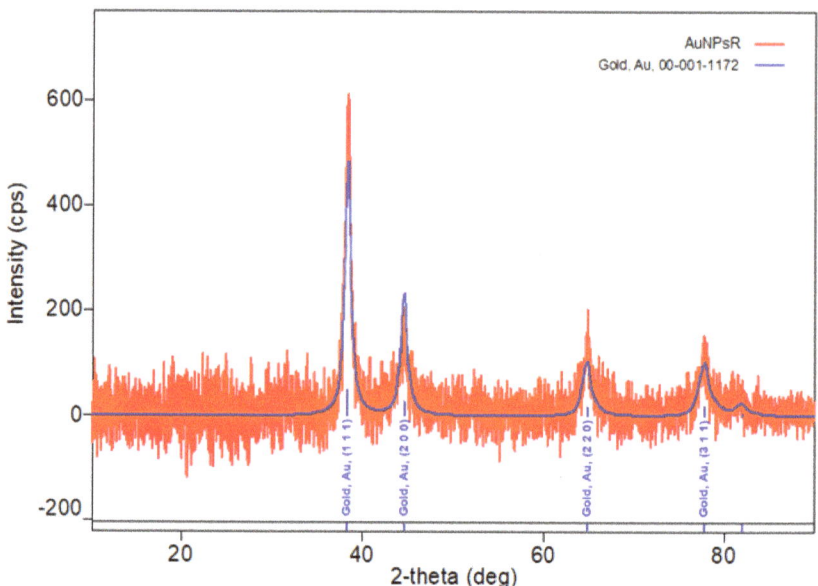

Figure 8. X-ray diffraction pattern of synthesized gold nanoparticles phytoreduced with Rutin (AuNPsR).

The presence of the four characteristic peaks at 2θ values of 38.28°, 44.52°, 64.74°, and 77.90°, corresponding to the reflection planes of (111), (200), (220), and (311) of faced centred cubic gold was observed (identification ICDD DB card 00-001-1172). The Williamson–Hall method was used to measure the crystallite size, which was found to be 58 Å, thus confirming the formation of gold nanoparticles.

3.2. Fundoscopy Examination

To evaluate arteriole diameter differences between groups, the Kruskal–Wallis test for not normally distributed data was used. The results are depicted in Figure 9.

In terms of arteriole diameter, diabetic specimens from CMC group demonstrated a significant vasoconstriction compared to controls ($p < 0.001$). The administration of insulin to diabetic rodents resulted in a statistically significant increase in arteriole diameter compared to CMC ($p < 0.001$). The same pattern was obtained after treatment of diabetic subjects with Rutin ($p < 0.01$). The administration of AuNPsR enhanced the diameter of arterioles for diabetics compared to CMC ($p < 0.001$). All treatments used proved a good effect on the retinal arteriole diameter. It is worth highlighting that administration of Rutin and AuNPsR displayed a significant spread of values in relation to their respective median lines.

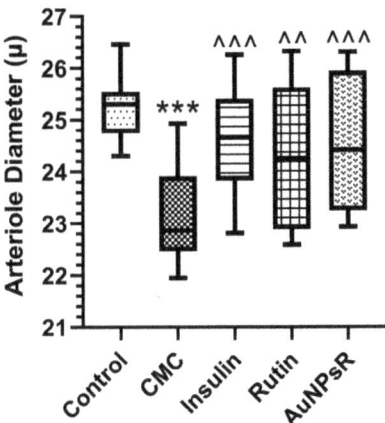

Figure 9. Retinal arterioles variation of diameter in Control group, and in rats with six-week diabetes, followed by one week of treatments: carboxymethylcellulose (CMC), insulin, Rutin, and gold nanoparticles phytoreduced with Rutin (AuNPsR). Parameters are expressed as minimum and maximum values, median, and interquartile range (Q1–Q3, the range between the 25th percentile and the 75th percentile), with *** $p < 0.001$ compared to Control group; ^^ $p < 0.01$, ^^^ $p < 0.001$ compared to CMC group.

3.3. Blood and Eye Tissue Oxidative Stress Investigation

Results from the oxidative stress investigation of blood samples are presented in Figure 10. Blood sample analysis revealed that animals with DM and treated with CMC had high levels of MDA compared to controls ($p < 0.001$). Similar results were obtained in the insulin treatment group. The administration of Rutin decreased blood MDA levels compared to CMC group ($p < 0.05$). Accordingly, the administration of AuNPsR in diabetic animals lowered MDA level in serum compared to CMC ($p < 0.01$). Notably, AuNPsR administration did not show statistical difference when compared to Rutin ($p > 0.05$). The activity of SOD in the CMC group decreased compared to controls ($p < 0.001$). Additionally, similar results were observed for the insulin-treated group. Only AuNPsR administration increased SOD activity compared to CMC group ($p < 0.05$). Catalase (CAT) activity diminished in CMC-treated rats when compared to controls, $p < 0.001$. Moreover, all treatments improved CAT activity when compared to the CMC group, as follows: insulin, $p < 0.05$; Rutin, $p < 0.05$; AuNPsR, $p < 0.05$.

The oxidative stress investigation outcomes of eye tissue homogenate are depicted in Figure 11. Malondialdehyde (MDA) levels in the eye homogenate increased significantly in the CMC group compared to controls ($p < 0.001$). Notably, similar results were observed in the insulin treatment group. Rutin administration decreased ocular MDA levels compared to CMC ($p < 0.05$). Similarly, AuNPsR-treated diabetics showed an important decrease in the ocular MDA level when compared to the CMC group ($p < 0.001$). Ocular superoxide dismutase (SOD) activity diminished in the CMC-treated diabetes group, when compared to controls ($p < 0.001$). The compounds administered had no favourable effects regarding ocular SOD activity. Eye homogenate catalase (CAT) activity decreased statistically in both CMC ($p < 0.001$) and insulin ($p < 0.001$) groups, when compared to controls.

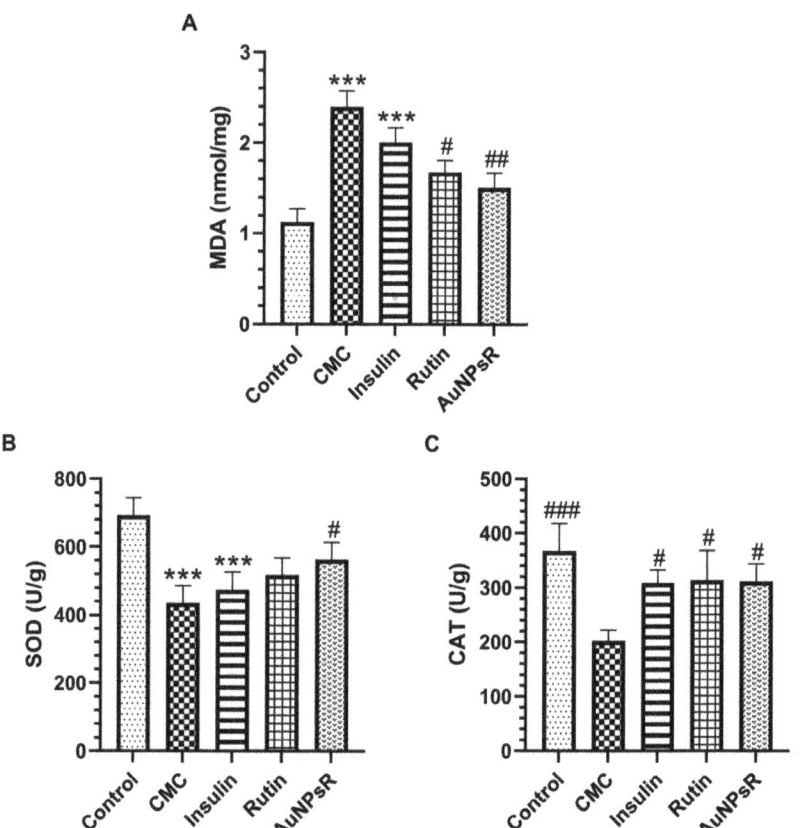

Figure 10. Blood oxidative stress assessment. (**A**) Malondialdehyde (MDA) levels, (**B**) superoxide dismutase (SOD) and (**C**) catalase (CAT) activities in controls, and in diabetic animals treated with CMC (carboxymethylcellulose), insulin, Rutin, and AuNPsR (gold nanoparticles phytoreduced with Rutin). Parameters are expressed as mean and standard deviation, with *** $p < 0.001$ compared to Control group; # $p < 0.05$, ## $p < 0.01$, and ### $p < 0.001$ compared to CMC group.

3.4. Eye Tissue Inflammation Investigation

Proinflammatory cytokines levels measured from eye homogenate are graphed in Figure 12. In the CMC group, TNF alpha secretion increased significantly when compared to controls ($p < 0.05$), while Rutin administration reduced TNF alpha levels, when compared to the CMC group ($p < 0.05$). Accordingly, IL-1 beta levels were significantly enhanced in CMC-treated diabetic animals, when compared to controls ($p < 0.05$), while insulin administration showed a notable decrease in IL-1 beta ($p < 0.001$). Remarkably, AuNPsR administration demonstrated a marked increase in IL-1 beta levels, when compared to insulin-treated diabetic animals ($p < 0.001$). Moreover, out of all treatments administered, AuNPsR showed the highest levels of IL-1 beta. In a similar manner to previous inflammatory cytokines, CMC-treated diabetics showed a statistical increase in IL-6 levels, when compared to controls ($p < 0.001$). Both insulin and AuNPsR yielded similar results, with a decrease in IL-6, compared to the CMC group, but without statistical significance. A favourable outcome was noted only in the Rutin group, which showed a statistically significant decrease in IL-6 when compared to CMC administered diabetics ($p < 0.05$).

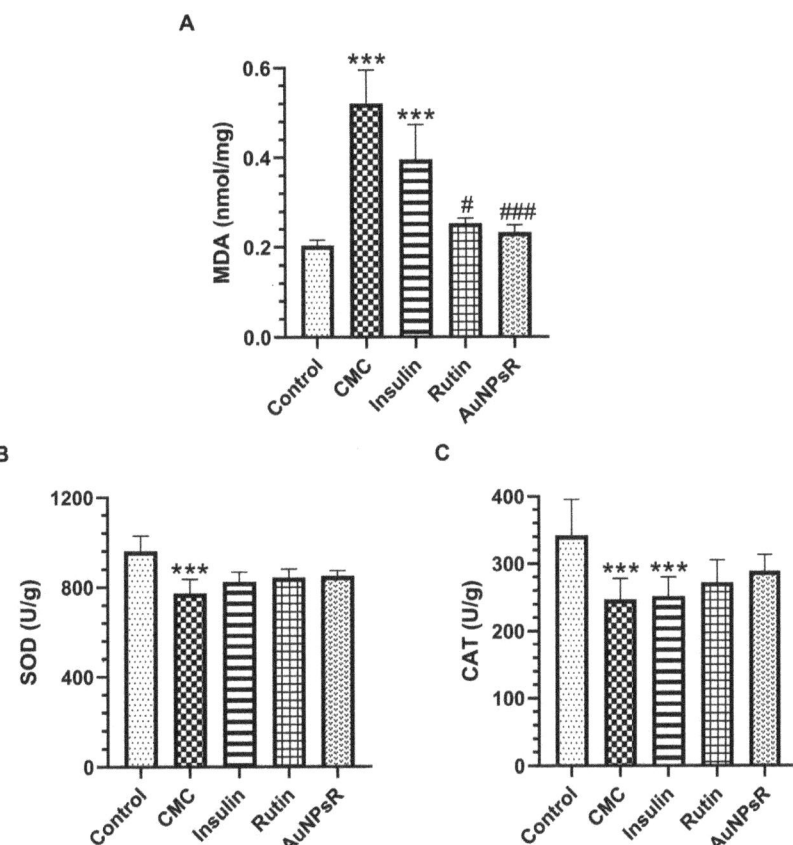

Figure 11. Oxidative stress parameters in eye tissues homogenates. (**A**) Malondialdehyde (MDA) levels, (**B**) superoxide dismutase (SOD), and (**C**) catalase (CAT) activities, in controls and in rats with DM (diabetes mellitus) and treated with CMC (carboxymethylcellulose), insulin, Rutin, and AuNPsR (gold nanoparticles phytoreduced with Rutin). The parameters are expressed as mean and standard deviation, with *** $p < 0.001$ compared to Control group; # $p < 0.05$, and ### $p < 0.001$ compared to CMC group.

3.5. Retina Histopathological Investigation

Images from the histopathological investigation of retina samples are illustrated in Figure 13.

In terms of global changes, a difference in average retinal thickness was observed. In comparison to the CMC group (115.2 ± 4.2 μ), all treatments increased this parameter: insulin (125 ± 1.2 μ), Rutin (179.4 ± 2.6 μ), and AuNPsR (204.4 ± 2.4 μ). In terms of neural-related changes, the width of the individual retinal layers was measured. Our target treatments, Rutin and AuNPsR, showed a higher width in all cell body layers, when compared to CMC: ganglion cell layer (CMC, 7.4 ± 0.8 μ; Rutin, 7.9 ± 0.2 μ; AuNPsR, 10.9 ± 0.1 μ), inner nuclear layer (CMC, 18.5 ± 0.4 μ; Rutin, 29.2 ± 0.4 μ; AuNPsR, 32.1 ± 0.3 μ), outer nuclear layer (CMC, 30.7 ± 0.2 μ; Rutin, 39 ± 0.7 μ; AuNPsR, 45.1 ± 0.5 μ), bacillary layer (CMC, 20.2 ± 0.1 μ; Rutin, 25.5 ± 0.1 μ; AuNPsR, 34.6 ± 0.2 μ). Insulin administration increased the width (8.2 ± 0.2 μ) of the ganglion cell layer compared to both CMC and Rutin, together with a slightly higher value (20.1 ± 0.1 μ) in the inner nuclear layer, when compared to CMC. In the remaining nuclear layers, when compared to CMC group, subjects treated with insulin showed a decrease in width: outer nuclear layer, 26.4 ± 0.8 μ; bacillary layer, 17.6 ± 0.2 µ. As per the synaptic layers, all substances administered increased the width, when compared to CMC specimens: inner plexiform layer (CMC, 30 ± 0.2 µ; insulin, 40 ± 0.5 µ; Rutin, 61.4 µ ± 0.2 µ; AuNPsR, 56.5 µ ± 0.2 µ), outer plexiform layer (CMC, 5 µ ± 0.1 µ; insulin, 5.8 µ ± 0.3 µ; Rutin, 6.8 µ ± 0.1 µ; AuNPsR, 8.9 µ ± 0.7 µ). Additionally, edema formation was observed in all treatment groups, as follows: minimal for insulin, moderate for Rutin, and advanced for AuNPsR.

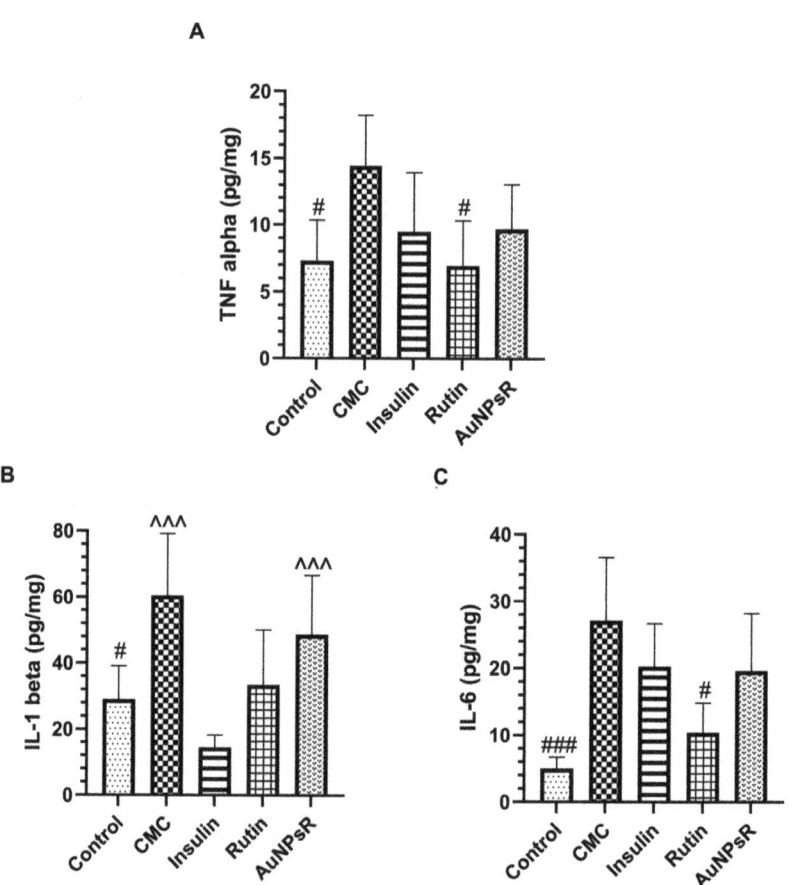

Figure 12. Proinflammatory cytokines levels in eye homogenates, (**A**) TNF alpha, (**B**) IL-1 beta, and (**C**) IL-6, in controls and in rats with DM and treated with CMC (carboxymethylcellulose), insulin, Rutin, and AuNPsR (gold nanoparticles phytoreduced with Rutin). Parameters are expressed as mean and standard deviation, with # $p < 0.05$, ### $p < 0.001$ compared to CMC group; ^^^ $p < 0.001$ compared to Insulin group.

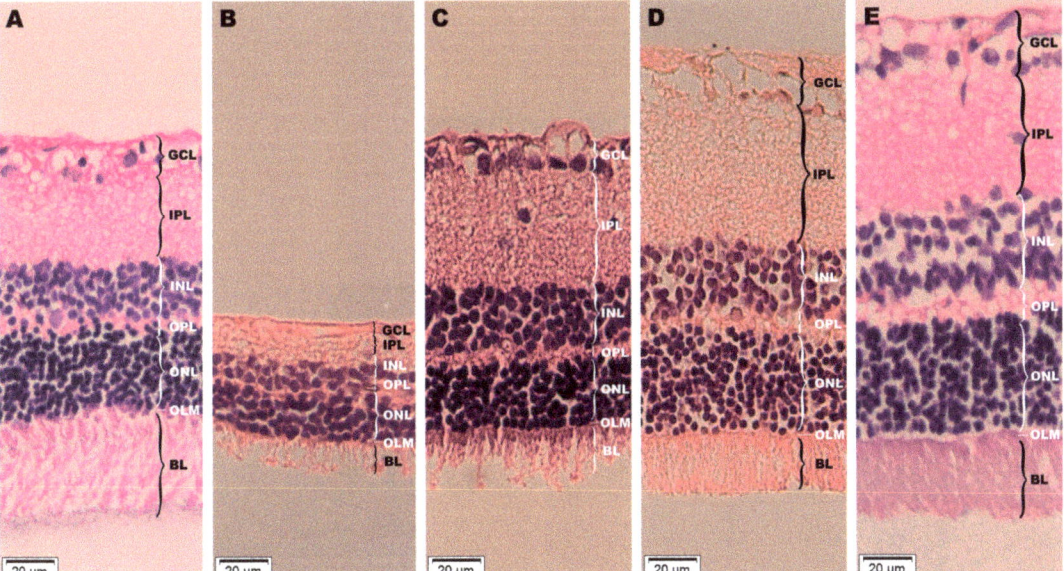

Figure 13. Histopathological investigation of retinas from (**A**) healthy specimens, and from six-week diabetic animals, with a subsequent one week of the following treatments: (**B**) CMC (carboxymethyl-cellulose), (**C**) insulin, (**D**) Rutin, (**E**) AuNPsR (gold nanoparticles phytoreduced with Rutin); a significant difference in overall retinal thickness is visible, with varying width for each individual layer; increasing levels of edema are perceptible, minimal for insulin (**C**), moderate for Rutin (**D**), and advanced for AuNPsR (**E**); layers of retinas from each group are delineated: GCL (ganglion cell layer), IPL (inner plexiform layer), INL (inner nuclear layer), OPL (outer plexiform layer), ONL (outer nuclear layer), OLM (outer limiting membrane), and BL (bacillary layer).

3.6. Eye Lens TEM Investigation

3.6.1. Morphology Investigation

The TEM morphological investigation of eye lenses is depicted in Figure 14. Examination of eye lenses from the Control group demonstrated a conventional ultrastructure. As such, upon inspection of randomly sampled sections, two components of higher interest can be described: primarily, tightly packed lens fibres (Lf), with a finely granular cytoplasm, and secondly, the notable delineations between them, consisting of thin, homogeneous electron lucent spaces. Regarding the areas of Lf, in CMC group, as well as in the Insulin group, most areas studied were of clear superior electron density, compared to controls. In diabetics treated with AuNPsR or Rutin, the general aspect of the tissue was comparable to that of the Control group. Additionally, a particular aspect was observed for animals with diabetes that received AuNPsR, focal Lf disorganisation. Subsequently, an enlargement of the spaces between Lf was noted in certain areas of lenses sampled from diabetic animals treated with insulin. A similar phenomenon was observed in the CMC group, and in the group treated with Rutin. Notably, in these two groups, spaces were less wide but more dispersed.

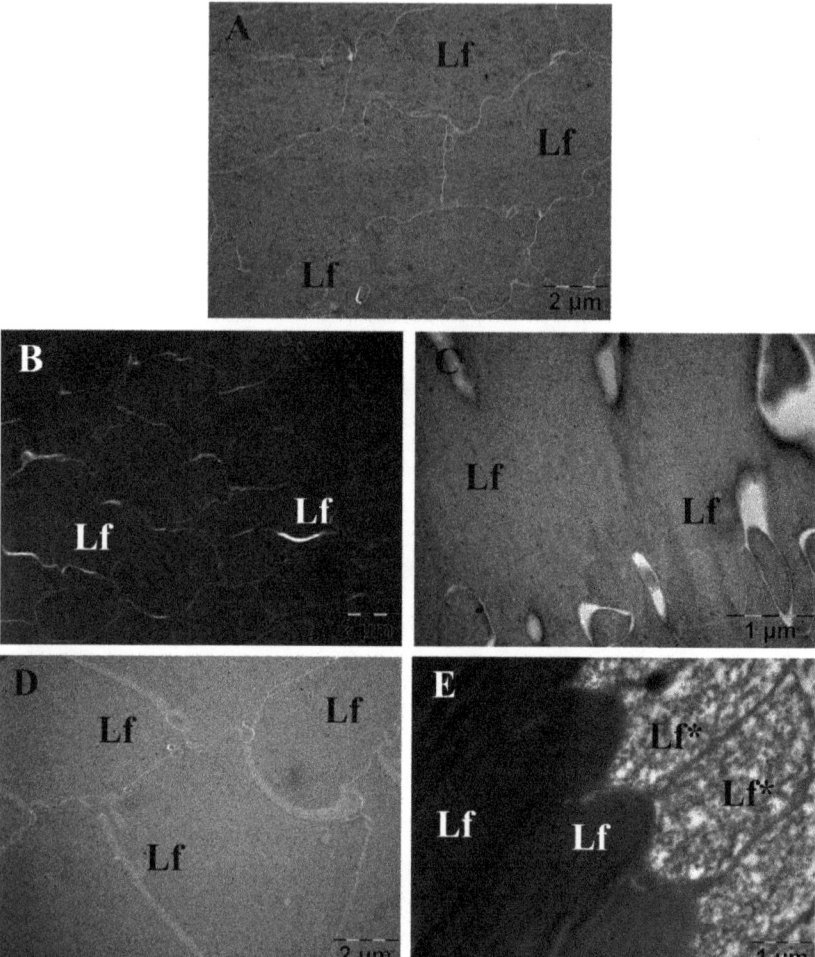

Figure 14. Transmission electron microscopy investigation of eye lenses from (**A**) age-matched controls, and from six-week diabetic specimens, followed by one week administration of treatments: (**B**) CMC (carboxymethylcellulose), (**C**) insulin, (**D**) Rutin, (**E**) AuNPsR (gold nanoparticles phytoreduced with Rutin); a superior electron density was observed in diabetic specimens from CMC group (**B**) and in diabetic subjects treated with insulin (**C**); diabetic animals treated with AuNPsR (**E**) showed focal lens fibre disorganisation; arrowhead points towards enlarged interfibrillar spaces (Lf, lens fibres; Lf* disorganised lens fibres).

3.6.2. Opacity Investigation

The Kruskal–Wallis test for not-normally distributed data was employed to assess variations in lens opacity between groups. Graphed results are depicted in Figure 15. Diabetic specimens that received CMC showed a statistically significant increase in lens opacity compared to controls ($p < 0.001$). Furthermore, statistical evidence supports that in diabetic animals, the administration of insulin had similar effects to CMC, increasing opacity in the eye lens ($p > 0.05$). Rutin statistically decreased opacity compared to CMC ($p < 0.01$), while AuNPsR yielded the most favourable outcomes ($p < 0.001$). In comparison to insulin treatment of diabetics, our experiment returned a statistically stable decrease in lens opacity for rodents treated with AuNPsR ($p < 0.001$). Moreover, AuNPsR proved to have a statistical difference when compared with Rutin ($p < 0.05$).

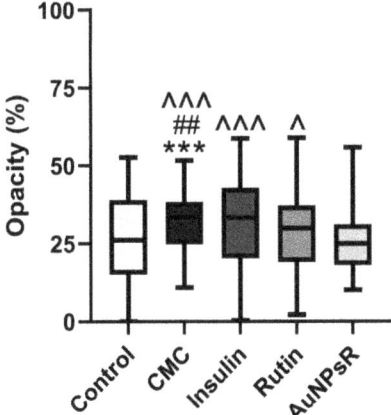

Figure 15. Lens opacity variation assessed on transmission electron microscopy micrographs, in controls and in rats with diabetes and treated with CMC (carboxymethylcellulose), insulin, Rutin, and AuNPsR (gold nanoparticles phytoreduced with Rutin). Parameters are expressed as minimum and maximum values, median, and interquartile range (Q1–Q3, the range between the 25th percentile and the 75th percentile), with *** $p < 0.001$ compared to Control group; ## $p < 0.01$ compared to Rutin group; ^ $p < 0.05$, ^^^ $p < 0.001$ compared to AuNPsR group.

4. Discussion

Diabetes is a chronic metabolic disorder associated with endothelial dysfunction and altered vascular contractility. Its various complications, which are of clinical importance, include diabetic retinopathy and cataracts. The underlying pathophysiology is related to hyperglycaemia, oxidative stress imbalance, and inflammation of the vascular wall, with the accompanying activation of the major pathways responsible for diabetes-related damage. The present study demonstrated that DM induced the vasoconstriction of retinal arterioles, with a marked reduction in diameter. Additionally, DM increased the lipid peroxidation in eye tissues and in serum, decreased the antioxidant defence, and triggered an inflammatory response. These findings were also associated with a decrease in retinal wall thickness, and a reduction in the width of retinal layers. Additionally, DM increased lens opacity and caused marked lens fibre disorganisation. Treatment with Rutin improved the retinal arteriolar diameter, increased the antioxidant enzymatic activity and reduced the ocular levels of TNF alpha and IL-6. Consequently, Rutin administration reduced the retinal edema and preserved eye lens structure. The administration of AuNPsR improved the appearance of retinal vessels upon fundus examination, decreased MDA formation and increased the overall antioxidant capacity. However, retinal edema and a degree of disorganisation in the eye lens fibres were still observed.

This study brings a new perspective regarding the early detection and treatment of ocular complications in DM. Additionally, this work proposed a solution to the gap in research delineated in previous articles—namely, that despite its beneficial effects in diabetic microvascular complications, Rutin has poor bioavailability and delivery, and thus lowered potency. Therefore, it was hypothesized that using gold nanoparticles as a delivery system would yield, together with an increase in systemic concentration and better ocular uptake, superior antihyperglycemic, antioxidant, and anti-inflammatory effects.

Diabetes was induced via the administration of STZ, a substance widely used due to its time and dose-dependent induction of apoptosis in pancreatic beta-cells [35]. The early development of CA and DR were closely monitored through serial examination of eye structures, using relevant studies from the literature as a guide.

Firstly, CA was considered to be in an incipient stage at the six-week mark, when, according to Muranov et al. [25], peripheral opacities were observed on anterior segment evaluation. Similarly, Aung et al. evaluated the development of CA in a rat model of post-STZ-induced diabetes and found that subcapsular CA, with characteristic spoke-like lesions, was developed only after six weeks of hyperglycaemia [36]. Moreover, they noted a gradual decline in visual acuity even before statistically significant CA formation; however, contrast sensitivity only began to decrease after nine weeks of diabetes. Thus, the studied hypothesis is further delineated, with a significant need for therapeutic strategies aimed at early-stage CA, before evident vision loss. Additionally, incipient CA development was evaluated by TEM analysis at the six-week mark, to reassure anterior segment examination findings. Similarly to our results, Majaw et al. observed a more severe disorder of lens fibres in four-week diabetic mice, compared to healthy controls, upon TEM examination [37].

The development of DR was monitored in parallel. Therefore, weekly fundus examination was used to compare diabetic subjects and healthy animals. Arteriole diameter modifications, indicative of early DR, were noted at the six-week mark. Accordingly, Lai et al. described a reduction in blood flow through the retinal arterioles between the fourth and sixth week of hyperglycaemia, in a Goto–Kakizaki rat model, a strain derived from the Wistar strain [38].

Furthermore, the therapeutic agent was chosen based on the pathophysiology of ocular diabetic complications. The mechanisms involved in incipient CA are related to lipid peroxidation, a process significantly increased in diabetes due to the imbalance between prooxidant and antioxidant systems [39]. This pathophysiological substrate justifies the use of TEM micrographs to study lens opacity. The compounds that form in the eye lens due to lipid peroxidation include dienes, a subclass of alkenes, chemical group readily reacted with OsO_4, the employed TEM fixative, and contrasting agent [40,41].

Early DR has been associated with reduced retinal blood flow, as observed in an experimental model by Muir et al. [42]. This mechanism is currently explained through the hyperactivation of retinal glia by diabetes caused oxidative stress [12], which then triggers the synthesis of Ang II by the intraocular RAS, which in turn leads to a decrease in retinal blood flow by acting on AT1 microglial receptors. Additionally, the same study found that Ang II increases the production of proinflammatory cytokines through its binding to AT1 microglial receptors. This pathophysiological explanation of incipient DR is further supported by Eshaq et al. [43]. Their study demonstrated that the administration of candesartan, an AT1 receptor blocker, to diabetic Wistar rats, decreased the angiotensin converting enzyme (ACE) level, and increased the retinal blood flow. Moreover, they concluded that candesartan reduced ROS production through a decrease in p22phox levels.

In terms of treatment, insulin was utilised as a positive control because STZ destroys pancreatic beta-cells and induces type 1 diabetes (T1D). On fundoscopy examination of retinal arteriole diameter, insulin showed favourable results, restoring normal width parameters. This is an accepted action of insulin, a known vasodilator agent [44]. However, vessel diameter could be altered immediately after treatment administration, and swiftly reverted. On TEM investigation of lens opacity induced by diabetes, insulin returned results that require a more in-depth discussion, as it increased the opacity in eye lenses, similarly to vehicle administration. The discrepancy between the worsening of CA with insulin administration and its beneficial effects upon fundus examination require further detailed investigations.

The mechanism through which insulin might worsen early CA is not well known. However, Papadimitriou et al. highlighted a possible direction of research, presenting a T1D patient under an intense insulin regime, that had an elevated insulin autoantibody count at the time of bilateral CA formation [45]. Additionally, a widely accepted hypothesis is related to early worsening of DR by severe insulin therapy. Meng et al. explained this phenomenon through the overexpression of NADPH oxidase 4 enzyme activity, and thus, through the overproduction of ROS, as a result of high doses of insulin [46]. Furthermore, a possible link could exist between the early worsening of DR and early lens opacification, based on the reasoning that both CA and DR develop in the same intraocular medium, frequently *in tandem* [47]. The early worsening of DR can be explained by the osmotic force theory, which states that a forceful reduction in glucose, an osmotically active molecule, by insulin use, can lead to a shift in intraocular pressure [48]. Okamoto et al. correlated this process to an aggravated eye lens state, where a series of patients developed hyperopia because of a rapid decrease in glycaemia after insulin administration [49]. This latter explanation was consistent with the changes seen in the present study upon TEM analysis and histopathological examination. Thus, the increased interfibrillar space observed through TEM, after insulin treatment, could be caused by an alteration of intraocular pressure. This could also be correlated with the edema observed upon the retinal histopathological investigation of diabetic rats treated with insulin. Moreover, the histopathological examination yielded a smaller width of both outer nuclear and photoreceptor layers, findings which have not been previously reported, as to our knowledge. An alternative explanation for edema formation in insulin-treated rats could be related to the increased production of IL-6. It is known that IL6 mediates retinal inflammation and vascular leakage, with significant in vivo effects as early as four weeks of hyperglycaemia, as shown by Rojas et al. in a DR model of IL-6 deficient mice [50]. In addition to this, anti-IL-6 antibodies have been demonstrated to have beneficial effects in the treatment of diabetic macular edema [51].

In terms of the target therapeutic agent, an evident pattern that supports the initial claim can be observed. Regarding CA, results confirmed the present hypothesis as the best outcomes were attributed to AuNPsR treatment. On TEM investigation of lens opacity induced by diabetes, AuNPsR restored the transparency and improved the arteriolar diameter in fundoscopy. This outcome was similar to that obtained by Rutin administration alone. In fact, it can be concluded that all treatments induced vasodilation and restored the retinal arteriole diameter in DM. Moreover, Rutin and AuNPsR showed a wide range of beneficial effects, additional to those produced by insulin. Thus, upon histopathological investigation, AuNPsR restored the width of all retinal layers, lowered MDA levels and increased SOD and CAT activities.

To our knowledge, no previous study has described the benefits of AuNPsR on DR and CA. However, a similar compound, resveratrol, from the same dietary polyphenol family has been examined. Chen et al. demonstrated a statistically significant in vitro eye lens epithelial cell uptake of gold nanoparticles functionalised with resveratrol (AuNPsRes) with high biocompatibility and reduced cytotoxicity [21]. Furthermore, this study showcased the anticataractogen abilities of AuNPsRes, as it delayed the eye lens opacification upon slit-lamp examination of the studied rats. In terms of restoring transparency, the present study results are consistent with those described by Chen et al., the AuNPsR treatment showing promising benefits. This can be correlated to the favourable antioxidant effect observed in both serum and homogenised eye tissue, where AuNPsR significantly decreased MDA formation, a factor responsible for early CA onset. However, an additional focal disarray of Lf was observed upon TEM structural examination. To our knowledge, no previous study highlighted this modification after administration of gold nanoparticles. Additionally, Cosert et al. underlined the significant discrepancies between in vivo and in vitro effects of gold engineered nanomaterials, offering supplementary reasoning for the conflicting results [52]. Nonetheless, Zhang et al. reported vacuolisation of eye lenses in developing zebrafish embryos after silver nanoparticles administration, which could imply a lens deterioration by a metal-based drug delivery system [53]. Notably, this study underlined no morphological modifications in the retinas of the same specimens. Subsequently, Dong et al. highlighted the implications of AuNPsRes in treatment of DR in a Wistar albino rat model [22]. They noticed a decrease in retinal vessels permeability compared to vehicle-treated diabetic rats. This would be physiologically correlated to the effect of gold nanoparticles on arteriolar vasoconstriction. Notably, they associated these findings with low levels of vascular endothelial growth factor (VEGF), a molecule that, when targeted in early DR, yielded no significant results in restoring vision, in a recently published clinical trial [54]. Probably, the involvement of VEGF in early DR is limited, and there are multiple other factors with a vasodilator role in the retina. It is worth noting that Dong et al. evaluated retinal changes after 14 weeks of hyperglycaemia, compared to the 7 weeks in our study. Thus, VEGF-related mechanisms may be characteristic for more advanced DR. This supposition is further supported by Shi et al. and Xiao et al., who found that retinal vessel permeability was significantly increased only after the eighth week of diabetes [55,56]. Furthermore, upon histopathological examination of the retina, a characteristic of early DR was noticed, neural degeneration [57]. Retinal layers showed a decrease in width in rats with DM treated with CMC in alignment with the existing literature. Thus, Lai et al. reported lowered cellularity in both the ganglion cell layer and outer nuclear layer, coupled with a reduction in total retinal width [38]. The retinal thickness and width of all individual layers were most significantly restored in the rats treated with AuNPsR. This could be explained by the levels of ocular IL-1 beta, which were highest in the AuNPsR group. Baptista and Alveleira et al. found that IL-1 beta plays a significant role in the proliferation of retinal microglia [58]. The size of the nanoparticles studied in the present work was 15 nm, therefore, a high penetrability in the ocular tissues was obtained. Despite their benefits against neural deterioration, administration of AuNPsR induced the accumulation of retinal edema, more severe than the other treatments administered. This finding could be correlated to an IL-6-induced edema formation.

Based on the presented data, further toxicological studies are needed in order to assess the safe use of gold nanoparticles and the real benefits for the management of early ocular diabetes complications. The present study investigated the effects of a lower dose, so as to maintain feasibility to human treatment extrapolation. However, varying doses should be examined in order to obtain the ideal therapeutic cutoff.

5. Conclusions

Our study demonstrated that STZ administered in two doses induced DM in rats and caused the development of ocular complications after six weeks of hyperglycaemia. These pathological changes were observed both macroscopically, upon anterior segment and fundus examination, and microscopically through TEM and histopathological investigation. These changes were triggered by an oxidative stress imbalance, together with a proinflammatory status. Rutin had beneficial effects on the incipient form of cataracts and diabetic retinopathy. After one week of treatment with AuNPsR, there were noticeable antioxidant as well as anti-inflammatory effects. Morphologically, AuNPsR restored the retinal arteriole diameter, previously constricted due to hyperglycaemia. Moreover, this therapeutic agent favoured the neural restoration of the retina, alongside a reduction in eye lens opacity.

Author Contributions: Conceptualization, M.M. (Mădălina Moldovan) and G.A.F.; methodology, M.M. (Mădălina Moldovan) and G.A.F.; software, M.M. (Mădălina Moldovan) and A.-M.P.; validation, M.M. (Mădălina Moldovan), M.M. (Mara Muntean), R.M.B., B.M. and G.K.; formal analysis, M.M. (Mădălina Moldovan) and A.-M.P.; investigation, M.M. (Mădălina Moldovan), A.-M.P., M.M. (Mara Muntean), R.M.B., D.G., B.M., G.K. and L.D.; resources, D.G., L.D. and G.A.F.; data curation, M.M. (Mădălina Moldovan) and A.-M.P.; writing—original draft preparation, M.M. (Mădălina Moldovan); writing—review and editing, G.A.F.; visualization, M.M. (Mădălina Moldovan) and A.-M.P.; supervision, G.A.F.; project administration, M.M. (Mădălina Moldovan); funding acquisition, M.M. (Mădălina Moldovan) and G.A.F. All authors have read and agreed to the published version of the manuscript.

Funding: This research was funded by Iuliu Hatieganu University of Medicine and Pharmacy in Cluj-Napoca, Romania, grant number 35178/17.12.2021.

Institutional Review Board Statement: The animal study protocol was approved by the Ethics Committee of Iuliu Hatieganu University of Medicine and Pharmacy in Cluj-Napoca, Romania and the Ethical Committee on Animal Welfare (No. 294/09.03.2022) of A.N.S.V.S.A. (The National Sanitary Veterinary and Food Safety Authority).

Informed Consent Statement: Not applicable.

Data Availability Statement: Data are contained within the article.

Acknowledgments: We express our appreciation for the insightful dialogues held with Adrian Florea and the guidance provided pertaining to the processing of ocular lenses for Transmission Electron Microscopy (TEM). Additionally, we extend our gratitude to Ophthalmologist Lăcrămioara Samoilă for her invaluable contributions in upholding the rigour of this article. Her expertise and guidance have been instrumental in ensuring the scholarly integrity and methodological precision of our work in the field of ophthalmology. Furthermore, we would like to extend our heartfelt gratitude to Gabriel Sergiu Macavei for his invaluable aid in enhancing our understanding of the structural properties of the studied nanoparticles through X-ray diffraction.

Conflicts of Interest: The authors declare no conflict of interest.

References

1. Xiao, L.; Yang, Y.J.; Liu, Q.; Peng, J.; Yan, J.F.; Peng, Q.H. Visualizing the intellectual structure and recent research trends of diabetic retinopathy. *Int. J. Ophthalmol.* **2021**, *14*, 1248–1259. [CrossRef]
2. Bixler, J.E. Cataracts and Their Treatment in People with Diabetes. In *Prevention and Management of Diabetes-Related Eye Disease*; American Diabetes Association: Arlington, TX, USA, 2019; pp. 6–10.
3. Yan, W.; Wang, W.; van Wijngaarden, P.; Mueller, A.; He, M. Longitudinal changes in global cataract surgery rate inequality and associations with socioeconomic indices. *Clin. Exp. Ophthalmol.* **2019**, *47*, 453–460. [CrossRef] [PubMed]
4. Denadai, L.; Mozetic, V.; Moore, R.A.; Yamada, V.H.; Riera, R. Pain control during panretinal photocoagulation for diabetic retinopathy. *Cochrane Database Syst. Rev.* **2022**, *2022*, CD014927. [CrossRef]
5. Jeng, C.J.; Hsieh, Y.T.; Yang, C.M.; Yang, C.H.; Lin, C.L.; Wang, I.J. Development of diabetic retinopathy after cataract surgery. *PLoS ONE* **2018**, *13*, e0202347. [CrossRef] [PubMed]
6. Wong, T.Y.; Sabanayagam, C. The War on Diabetic Retinopathy: Where Are We Now? *Asia Pac. J. Ophthalmol.* **2019**, *8*, 448–456. [CrossRef]
7. Manasvi, P.; Panimalar, V.; Veeramani, A.; Divya, N.; Bindu, B. Analysis of Cataract in Diabetic and Non-Diabetic Patients. *Int. J. Curr. Res. Rev.* **2021**, *13*, 67–71. [CrossRef]
8. Vujosevic, S.; Toma, C.; Villani, E.; Gatti, V.; Brambilla, M.; Muraca, A.; Ponziani, M.C.; Aimaretti, G.; Nuzzo, A.; Nucci, P.; et al. Early Detection of Microvascular Changes in Patients with Diabetes Mellitus without and with Diabetic Retinopathy: Comparison between Different Swept-Source OCT-A Instruments. *J. Diabetes Res.* **2019**, *2019*, 2547216. [CrossRef]
9. Rodriguez-Gutierrez, R.; Montori, V.M. Glycemic Control for Patients With Type 2 Diabetes Mellitus: Our Evolving Faith in the Face of Evidence. *Circ. Cardiovasc. Qual. Outcomes* **2016**, *9*, 504–512. [CrossRef]
10. Brownlee, M. The pathobiology of diabetic complications: A unifying mechanism. *Diabetes* **2005**, *54*, 1615–1625. [CrossRef]
11. Gomulka, K.; Ruta, M. The Role of Inflammation and Therapeutic Concepts in Diabetic Retinopathy—A Short Review. *Int. J. Mol. Sci.* **2023**, *24*, 24. [CrossRef]
12. Phipps, J.A.; Vessey, K.A.; Brandli, A.; Nag, N.; Tran, M.X.; Jobling, A.I.; Fletcher, E.L. The Role of Angiotensin II/AT1 Receptor Signaling in Regulating Retinal Microglial Activation. *Investig. Ophthalmol. Vis. Sci.* **2018**, *59*, 487–498. [CrossRef] [PubMed]
13. Mills, S.A.; Jobling, A.I.; Dixon, M.A.; Bui, B.V.; Vessey, K.A.; Phipps, J.A.; Greferath, U.; Venables, G.; Wong, V.H.Y.; Wong, C.H.Y.; et al. Fractalkine-induced microglial vasoregulation occurs within the retina and is altered early in diabetic retinopathy. *Proc. Natl. Acad. Sci. USA* **2021**, *118*, e2112561118. [CrossRef] [PubMed]
14. Shree, J.; Choudhary, R.; Bodakhe, S.H. Losartan delays the progression of streptozotocin-induced diabetic cataracts in albino rats. *J. Biochem. Mol. Toxicol.* **2019**, *33*, e22342. [CrossRef] [PubMed]
15. Ghorbani, A. Mechanisms of antidiabetic effects of flavonoid rutin. *Biomed. Pharmacother.* **2017**, *96*, 305–312. [CrossRef]
16. Oyagbemi, A.A.; Bolaji-Alabi, F.B.; Ajibade, T.O.; Adejumobi, O.A.; Ajani, O.S.; Jarikre, T.A.; Omobowale, T.O.; Ola-Davies, O.E.; Soetan, K.O.; Aro, A.O.; et al. Novel antihypertensive action of rutin is mediated via inhibition of angiotensin converting enzyme/mineralocorticoid receptor/angiotensin 2 type 1 receptor (ATR1) signaling pathways in uninephrectomized hypertensive rats. *J. Food. Biochem.* **2020**, *44*, e13534. [CrossRef]
17. Truzzi, F.; Tibaldi, C.; Zhang, Y.; Dinelli, G.; Eros, D.A. An Overview on Dietary Polyphenols and Their Biopharmaceutical Classification System (BCS). *Int. J. Mol. Sci.* **2021**, *22*, 5514. [CrossRef]
18. Frutos-Rincon, L.; Gomez-Sanchez, J.A.; Inigo-Portugues, A.; Acosta, M.C.; Gallar, J. An Experimental Model of Neuro-Immune Interactions in the Eye: Corneal Sensory Nerves and Resident Dendritic Cells. *Int. J. Mol. Sci.* **2022**, *23*, 2997. [CrossRef]
19. Addo, R.T. *Ocular Drug Delivery: Advances, Challenges and Applications*; Springer: Berlin/Heidelberg, Germany, 2016; pp. 53–74.

20. Rocha, S.; Lucas, M.; Ribeiro, D.; Corvo, M.L.; Fernandes, E.; Freitas, M. Nano-based drug delivery systems used as vehicles to enhance polyphenols therapeutic effect for diabetes mellitus treatment. *Pharmacol. Res.* **2021**, *169*, 105604. [CrossRef]
21. Chen, Q.; Gu, P.; Liu, X.; Hu, S.; Zheng, H.; Liu, T.; Li, C. Gold Nanoparticles Encapsulated Resveratrol as an Anti-Aging Agent to Delay Cataract Development. *Pharmaceuticals* **2022**, *16*, 26. [CrossRef]
22. Dong, Y.; Wan, G.; Yan, P.; Qian, C.; Li, F.; Peng, G. Fabrication of resveratrol coated gold nanoparticles and investigation of their effect on diabetic retinopathy in streptozotocin induced diabetic rats. *J. Photochem. Photobiol. B* **2019**, *195*, 51–57. [CrossRef]
23. Chockalingam, S.; Thada, R.; Dhandapani, R.K.; Panchamoorthy, R. Biogenesis, characterization, and the effect of vicenin-gold nanoparticles on glucose utilization in 3T3-L1 adipocytes: A bioinformatic approach to illuminate its interaction with PTP 1B and AMPK. *Biotechnol. Prog.* **2015**, *31*, 1096–1106. [CrossRef] [PubMed]
24. Schneider, C.A.; Rasband, W.S.; Eliceiri, K.W. NIH Image to ImageJ: 25 years of image analysis. *Nat. Methods* **2012**, *9*, 671–675. [CrossRef] [PubMed]
25. Muranov, K.; Poliansky, N.; Winkler, R.; Rieger, G.; Schmut, O.; Horwath-Winter, J. Protection by iodide of lens from selenite-induced cataract. *Graefes. Arch. Clin. Exp. Ophthalmol.* **2004**, *242*, 146–151. [CrossRef] [PubMed]
26. McLenachan, S.; Magno, A.L.; Ramos, D.; Catita, J.; McMenamin, P.G.; Chen, F.K.; Rakoczy, E.P.; Ruberte, J. Angiography reveals novel features of the retinal vasculature in healthy and diabetic mice. *Exp. Eye Res.* **2015**, *138*, 6–21. [CrossRef] [PubMed]
27. Miri, M.; Amini, Z.; Rabbani, H.; Kafieh, R. A Comprehensive Study of Retinal Vessel Classification Methods in Fundus Images. *J. Med. Signals Sens.* **2017**, *7*, 59–70. [PubMed]
28. Conti, M.; Morand, P.C.; Levillain, P.; Lemonnier, A. Improved fluorometric determination of malonaldehyde. *Clin. Chem.* **1991**, *37*, 1273–1275. [CrossRef]
29. Pippenger, C.E.; Browne, R.W.; Armstrong, D. Regulatory antioxidant enzymes. *Methods. Mol. Biol.* **1998**, *108*, 299–313. [CrossRef]
30. Beauchamp, C.; Fridovich, I. Superoxide dismutase: Improved assays and an assay applicable to acrylamide gels. *Anal. Biochem.* **1971**, *44*, 276–287. [CrossRef]
31. Wirahadikesuma, I.; Santoso, K.; Maheshwari, H.; Akhiruddin, M. Determining Image Opacity in Broiler Respiratory Radiographic Using ImageJ and Ansel Adam's Zone System. *J. Indones. Vet. Res.* **2020**, *4*, 22–35. [CrossRef]
32. Guzman-Hernandez, D.S.; Palomar-Pardave, M.; Sanchez-Perez, F.; Juarez-Gomez, J.; Corona-Avendano, S.; Romero-Romo, M.; Ramirez-Silva, M.T. Spectro-electrochemical characterization and quantification of Rutin in aqueous media. *Spectrochim. Acta. A Mol. Biomol. Spectrosc.* **2020**, *228*, 117814. [CrossRef]
33. Clichici, S.; David, L.; Moldovan, B.; Baldea, I.; Olteanu, D.; Filip, M.; Nagy, A.; Luca, V.; Crivii, C.; Mircea, P.; et al. Hepatoprotective effects of silymarin coated gold nanoparticles in experimental cholestasis. *Mater. Sci. Eng. C Mater. Biol. Appl.* **2020**, *115*, 111117. [CrossRef] [PubMed]
34. Tasca, F.; Antiochia, R. Biocide Activity of Green Quercetin-Mediated Synthesized Silver Nanoparticles. *Nanomaterials* **2020**, *10*, 909. [CrossRef] [PubMed]
35. Nahdi, A.; John, A.; Raza, H. Elucidation of Molecular Mechanisms of Streptozotocin-Induced Oxidative Stress, Apoptosis, and Mitochondrial Dysfunction in Rin-5F Pancreatic beta-Cells. *Oxid. Med. Cell. Longev.* **2017**, *2017*, 7054272. [CrossRef]
36. Aung, M.H.; Kim, M.K.; Olson, D.E.; Thule, P.M.; Pardue, M.T. Early visual deficits in streptozotocin-induced diabetic long evans rats. *Investig. Ophthalmol. Vis. Sci.* **2013**, *54*, 1370–1377. [CrossRef] [PubMed]
37. Majaw, S.; Challam, S.K.; Syiem, D. Effect of Potentilla fulgens L. onselected enzyme activities and altered tissue morphology in diabetic mice. *J. Morphol. Sci.* **2018**, *35*, 153–160. [CrossRef]
38. Lai, A.K.; Lo, A.C. Animal models of diabetic retinopathy: Summary and comparison. *J. Diabetes Res.* **2013**, *2013*, 106594. [CrossRef] [PubMed]
39. Hsueh, Y.J.; Chen, Y.N.; Tsao, Y.T.; Cheng, C.M.; Wu, W.C.; Chen, H.C. The Pathomechanism, Antioxidant Biomarkers, and Treatment of Oxidative Stress-Related Eye Diseases. *Int. J. Mol. Sci.* **2022**, *23*, 1255. [CrossRef]
40. Kisic, B.; Miric, D.; Zoric, L.; Ilic, A.; Dragojevic, I. Antioxidant capacity of lenses with age-related cataract. *Oxid. Med. Cell. Longev.* **2012**, *2012*, 467130. [CrossRef] [PubMed]
41. Mushtaq, A.; Zahoor, A.F.; Bilal, M.; Hussain, S.M.; Irfan, M.; Akhtar, R.; Irfan, A.; Kotwica-Mojzych, K.; Mojzych, M. Sharpless Asymmetric Dihydroxylation: An Impressive Gadget for the Synthesis of Natural Products: A Review. *Molecules* **2023**, *28*, 2722. [CrossRef]
42. Muir, E.R.; Renteria, R.C.; Duong, T.Q. Reduced ocular blood flow as an early indicator of diabetic retinopathy in a mouse model of diabetes. *Investig. Ophthalmol. Vis. Sci.* **2012**, *53*, 6488–6494. [CrossRef]
43. Eshaq, R.S.; Watts, M.N.; Carter, P.R.; Leskova, W.; Aw, T.Y.; Alexander, J.S.; Harris, N.R. Candesartan Normalizes Changes in Retinal Blood Flow and p22phox in the Diabetic Rat Retina. *Pathophysiology* **2021**, *28*, 86–97. [CrossRef]
44. Manrique, C.; Lastra, G.; Sowers, J.R. New insights into insulin action and resistance in the vasculature. *Ann. N. Y. Acad. Sci.* **2014**, *1311*, 138–150. [CrossRef] [PubMed]
45. Papadimitriou, D.T.; Bothou, C.; Skarmoutsos, F.; Papaevangelou, V.; Papadimitriou, A. Acute Bilateral Cataract in Type 1 Diabetes Mellitus. *Ann. Pediatr. Child. Health* **2015**, *3*, 1080. [CrossRef]
46. Meng, D.; Mei, A.; Liu, J.; Kang, X.; Shi, X.; Qian, R.; Chen, S. NADPH oxidase 4 mediates insulin-stimulated HIF-1alpha and VEGF expression, and angiogenesis in vitro. *PLoS ONE* **2012**, *7*, e48393. [CrossRef]

47. Nien, C.W.; Lee, C.Y.; Chen, H.C.; Chao, S.C.; Hsu, H.J.; Tzeng, S.H.; Yang, S.J.; Huang, J.Y.; Yang, S.F.; Lin, H.Y. The elevated risk of sight-threatening cataract in diabetes with retinopathy: A retrospective population-based cohort study. *BMC Ophthalmol.* **2021**, *21*, 349. [CrossRef] [PubMed]
48. Bain, S.C.; Klufas, M.A.; Ho, A.; Matthews, D.R. Worsening of diabetic retinopathy with rapid improvement in systemic glucose control: A review. *Diabetes Obes. Metab.* **2019**, *21*, 454–466. [CrossRef] [PubMed]
49. Okamoto, F.; Sone, H.; Nonoyama, T.; Hommura, S. Refractive changes in diabetic patients during intensive glycaemic control. *Br. J. Ophthalmol.* **2000**, *84*, 1097–1102. [CrossRef]
50. Rojas, M.A.; Zhang, W.; Xu, Z.; Nguyen, D.T.; Caldwell, R.W.; Caldwell, R.B. Interleukin 6 has a Critical Role in Diabetes-induced Retinal Vascular Inflammation and Permeability. *Investig. Ophthalmol. Vis. Sci.* **2011**, *52*, 1003.
51. Schmidt, M.; Matsumoto, Y.; Tisdale, A.; Lowden, P.; Kovalchin, J.; Wu, P.; Golden, K.; Dombrowski, C.; Lain, B.; Furfine, E.S. Optimized intravitreal IL-6 antagonist for the treatment of diabetic macular edema. *Investig. Ophthalmol. Vis. Sci.* **2015**, *56*, 3488.
52. Cosert, K.M.; Kim, S.; Jalilian, I.; Chang, M.; Gates, B.L.; Pinkerton, K.E.; Van Winkle, L.S.; Raghunathan, V.K.; Leonard, B.C.; Thomasy, S.M. Metallic Engineered Nanomaterials and Ocular Toxicity: A Current Perspective. *Pharmaceutics* **2022**, *14*, 981. [CrossRef]
53. Zhang, Y.; Wang, Z.; Zhao, G.; Liu, J.X. Silver nanoparticles affect lens rather than retina development in zebrafish embryos. *Ecotoxicol. Environ. Saf.* **2018**, *163*, 279–288. [CrossRef] [PubMed]
54. Maturi, R.K.; Glassman, A.R.; Josic, K.; Antoszyk, A.N.; Blodi, B.A.; Jampol, L.M.; Marcus, D.M.; Martin, D.F.; Melia, M.; Salehi-Had, H.; et al. Effect of Intravitreous Anti-Vascular Endothelial Growth Factor vs Sham Treatment for Prevention of Vision-Threatening Complications of Diabetic Retinopathy: The Protocol W Randomized Clinical Trial. *JAMA Ophthalmol.* **2021**, *139*, 701–712. [CrossRef] [PubMed]
55. Shi, K.P.; Li, Y.T.; Huang, C.X.; Cai, C.S.; Zhu, Y.J.; Wang, L.; Zhu, X.B. Evans blue staining to detect deep blood vessels in peripheral retina for observing retinal pathology in early-stage diabetic rats. *Int. J. Ophthalmol.* **2021**, *14*, 1501–1507. [CrossRef] [PubMed]
56. Xiao, A.; Zhong, H.; Xiong, L.; Yang, L.; Xu, Y.; Wen, S.; Shao, Y.; Zhou, Q. Sequential and Dynamic Variations of IL-6, CD18, ICAM, TNF-alpha, and Microstructure in the Early Stage of Diabetic Retinopathy. *Dis. Markers* **2022**, *2022*, 1946104. [CrossRef] [PubMed]
57. Sachdeva, M.M. Retinal Neurodegeneration in Diabetes: An Emerging Concept in Diabetic Retinopathy. *Curr. Diab. Rep.* **2021**, *21*, 65. [CrossRef]
58. Baptista, F.I.; Aveleira, C.A.; Castilho, A.F.; Ambrosio, A.F. Elevated Glucose and Interleukin-1beta Differentially Affect Retinal Microglial Cell Proliferation. *Mediat. Inflamm.* **2017**, *2017*, 4316316. [CrossRef]

Disclaimer/Publisher's Note: The statements, opinions and data contained in all publications are solely those of the individual author(s) and contributor(s) and not of MDPI and/or the editor(s). MDPI and/or the editor(s) disclaim responsibility for any injury to people or property resulting from any ideas, methods, instructions or products referred to in the content.

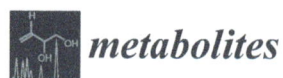

Article

Comparative Antihyperglycemic and Antihyperlipidemic Effects of Lawsone Methyl Ether and Lawsone in Nicotinamide-Streptozotocin-Induced Diabetic Rats

Muhammad Khan [1,2], Muhammad Ajmal Shah [3,*], Mustafa Kamal [4], Mohammad Shamsul Ola [5], Mehboob Ali [6] and Pharkphoom Panichayupakaranant [1,7,*]

1. Department of Pharmacognosy and Pharmaceutical Botany, Faculty of Pharmaceutical Sciences, Prince of Songkla University, Hat-Yai 90112, Thailand; 6210730010@email.psu.ac.th
2. Department of Pharmacology, Federal Urdu University of Arts, Science and Technology, Karachi 75300, Pakistan
3. Department of Pharmacy, Hazara University, Mansehra 21300, Pakistan
4. Department of Zoology, Abdul Wali Khan University Mardan, Mardan 23200, Pakistan; mustafakamal@awkum.edu.pk
5. Department of Biochemistry, College of Science, King Saud University, Riyadh 11451, Saudi Arabia; mola@ksu.edu.sa
6. Senior Scientist Toxicology Invivotek Nexus, a Genesis Biotech Group LLC Company, 17 Black Forest RD, Hamilton, NJ 08690, USA; mali@invivotek.com
7. Phytomedicine and Pharmaceutical Biotechnology Excellence Center, Faculty of Pharmaceutical Sciences, Prince of Songkla University, Hat-Yai 90112, Thailand
* Correspondence: ajmalshah@hu.edu.pk (M.A.S.); pharkphoom.p@psu.ac.th (P.P.); Tel.: +66-74-288980 (P.P.)

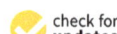

Citation: Khan, M.; Shah, M.A.; Kamal, M.; Ola, M.S.; Ali, M.; Panichayupakaranant, P. Comparative Antihyperglycemic and Antihyperlipidemic Effects of Lawsone Methyl Ether and Lawsone in Nicotinamide-Streptozotocin-Induced Diabetic Rats. *Metabolites* **2023**, *13*, 863. https://doi.org/10.3390/metabo13070863

Academic Editors: Cosmin Mihai Vesa and Dana Zaha

Received: 26 June 2023
Revised: 13 July 2023
Accepted: 16 July 2023
Published: 20 July 2023

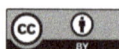

Copyright: © 2023 by the authors. Licensee MDPI, Basel, Switzerland. This article is an open access article distributed under the terms and conditions of the Creative Commons Attribution (CC BY) license (https://creativecommons.org/licenses/by/4.0/).

Abstract: Our previous study uncovered potent inhibitory effects of two naphthoquinones from *Impatiens balsamina*, namely lawsone methyl ether (2-methoxy-1,4-naphthoquinone, LME) and lawsone (2-hydroxy-1,4-naphthoquinone), against α-glucosidase. This gave us the insight to compare the hypoglycemic and hypolipidemic effects of LME and lawsone in high-fat/high-fructose-diet- and nicotinamide-streptozotocin-induced diabetic rats for 28 days. LME and lawsone at the doses of 15, 30, and 45 mg/kg, respectively, produced a substantial and dose-dependent reduction in the levels of fasting blood glucose (FBG), HbA1c, and food/water intake while boosting the insulin levels and body weights of diabetic rats. Additionally, the levels of total cholesterol (TC), triglycerides (TGs), high-density lipoproteins (HDLs), low-density lipoproteins (LDLs), aspartate transaminase (AST), alanine transaminase (ALT), creatinine, and blood urea nitrogen (BUN) in diabetic rats were significantly normalized by LME and lawsone, without affecting the normal rats. LME at a dose of 45 mg/kg exhibited the most potent antihyperglycemic and antihyperlipidemic effects, which were significantly comparable to glibenclamide but higher than those of lawsone. Furthermore, the toxicity evaluation indicated that both naphthoquinones were entirely safe for use in rodent models at doses ≤ 50 mg/kg. Therefore, the remarkable antihyperglycemic and antihyperlipidemic potentials of LME make it a promising option for future drug development.

Keywords: diabetes mellitus; hyperglycemic; hyperlipidemia; lawsone; lawsone methyl ether

1. Introduction

Diabetes mellitus (DM) is a chronic metabolic disorder characterized by hyperglycemia and disturbances of carbohydrate, fat, and protein metabolism resulting from defects in insulin secretion, insulin action, or both. Insulin is a hormone produced by the pancreas, and it plays a crucial role in regulating the uptake and utilization of glucose in the body. In type 1 diabetes, the pancreas does not produce enough insulin, while in type 2 diabetes, the body is unable to effectively utilize the insulin it produces [1]. DM is indeed the most prevalent metabolic disease of the contemporary age. Therefore, it is termed a "modern-day epidemic". It is a growing global public health issue that compromises living standards and places an undue financial burden on the healthcare systems. Based on the International Diabetes Federation (IDF), DM has affected around 463 million individuals in 2019. Of these, 4.2 million patients succumbed to death, costing a total of USD 760 billion in diabetes-related medical expenses [2].

Aside from glucose metabolism, insulin also regulates lipid metabolism. Hence, diabetic patients with poorly controlled glycemic levels frequently develop dyslipidemias. This implies that any fluctuations in insulin level or action may disrupt the body's lipid profiles, which usually leads to cardiovascular diseases [3]. Although controlling glycemic levels is a fundamental approach to managing DM, normalizing elevated lipid levels in diabetic individuals should also be a therapeutic necessity. For this purpose, a plethora of conventional antihyperglycemic and antihyperlipidemic medications are commercially available.

Insulin analogs, biguanides, sulfonylureas, thiazolidinedione (TZD), dipeptidyl peptidase-4 (DPP-4) inhibitors, sodium-glucose cotransporter (SGLT-2) inhibitors, and glucagon-like peptide-1 (GLP-1) receptor agonists are the major classes of antidiabetic medications [4]. On the other hand, statins, fibric acid derivatives, nicotinic acid derivatives, bile acid binding resins, and cholesterol absorption inhibitors are the commonly used antihyperlipidemic agents [5,6]. Although these conventional antihyperglycemic and antihyperlipidemic drugs are commonly prescribed, they are expensive, less efficacious, produce tolerance, and have undesirable side effects [7–9]. Biguanides (metformin) can cause anemia and neuropathy. DPP-4 inhibitors (sitagliptin) and sulfonylureas (glipizide) have the potential to cause hypoglycemia, weight gain, nausea, vomiting, headache, and dizziness. Similarly, insulin analogs and GLP-1 agonists (liraglutide), apart from being expensive, can cause hypoglycemia, allergy, and injection site reactions [10]. Statins, which are the most commonly used antihyperlipidemic drugs, can cause severe side effects like myopathy, rhabdomyolysis, nephrotoxicity, cardiomyopathy, and elevated serum transaminases. Recent clinical trials have linked statin use with an increase in the incidence of type 2 DM [11]. Ezetimibe is also associated with unwanted effects in the form of headaches, abdominal pain, and diarrhea. Moreover, it elevates the functional markers of the liver, namely alanine transaminase and aspartate transaminase [12].

The aforementioned limitations associated with conventional antihyperglycemic and antihyperlipidemic medications emphasize the necessity for novel drugs that offer improved efficacy and safety in lowering blood sugar and lipid levels. The World Health Organization (WHO) has also recommended the use of traditional plants for the treatment of DM, due to their effectiveness, non-toxic nature, and minimal or no side effects. These plant-based treatments are considered excellent options for oral therapy in the management of DM [13]. This research impetus led to the discovery of phytochemicals with remarkable antihyperglycemic potentials including berberine, curcumin, resveratrol, quercetin, epigallocatechin gallate (EGCG), etc. [14]. Plumbagin, shikonin, and rhinacanthin-C are noteworthy among these phytochemicals. They are the naphthoquinones, which not only demonstrate marvelous antihyperglycemic effects but also exhibit promising antihyperlipidemic activities [15–17]. Likewise, lawsone methyl ether (LME) and lawsone are naphthoquinones found in *Impatiens balsamina* L. [18]. Our previous in silico and in vitro studies uncovered potent inhibitory actions of LME and lawsone against α-glucosidase with excellent in silico ADMET (absorption, distribution, metabolism, excretion, and toxicity) profiles, revealing no toxicity in terms of tumorigenic, irritant, and reproductive effects [19]. This increased our interest in validating the in silico and in vitro results using animal models. Therefore, the present study aimed to investigate the antihyperglycemic and antihyperlipidemic effects of LME and lawsone in high-fat/high-fructose diet (HFFD)- and nicotinamide-streptozotocin (NA-STZ)-induced diabetic rats. Currently, LME can be semi-synthesized from lawsone with a high yield and low cost of production [20]. Thus, it might be a promising option for future drug development. Notably, this is a comprehensive and comparative study to discover new antidiabetic candidates that possess hypoglycemic and hypolipidemic potentials for further drug development.

2. Materials and Methods

2.1. Drugs and Chemicals

Lawsone, glibenclamide, streptozotocin (STZ), nicotinamide, cholesterol, and fructose were obtained from Sigma-Aldrich Chemie GmbH, Steinheim, Germany. LME was semi-synthesized by methylating lawsone using a method previously reported [20]. All the other chemicals and reagents were preferably of analytical grade.

2.2. Experimental Animals

A total of 90 adult male Wistar rats (6 weeks old), weighing approximately 130 ± 10 g, were obtained from the Pakistan Council of Scientific & Industrial Research (PCSIR) Laboratories Complex, Karachi. Before experimentation, the animals were allowed to acclimatize in the laboratory for almost one week and fed on a normal chow diet. The animals were provided with free access to food and water under standard environmental conditions at a room temperature of 24 ± 2 °C, humidity of $55 \pm 10\%$, and 12 h/12 h of light/darkness. All experimental protocols were approved by the Institutional Animal Care and Use Committee, PCSIR Laboratories Complex, Karachi, Pakistan (Ref. PCSIR–KLC/IEC/2022/02).

2.3. Induction of Obesity, Hyperlipidemia, and Insulin Resistance

After acclimatization, the animals were randomly split into two groups. Their body weights along with various biochemical indices, including fasting blood glucose (FBG), total cholesterol (TC), triglyceride (TG), high-density lipoprotein (HDL), low-density lipoprotein (LDL), and insulin levels were determined before the commencement of diet interventions. One group was fed a normal chow diet, while another group was fed a high-fat/high-fructose diet (HFFD). This diet was formulated indigenously in our laboratory in accordance with the method described earlier [21], with a few modifications. HFFD contained high-calorie meals by adding Banaspati ghee (hydrogenated oil), coconut oil, and raw cholesterol to the normal chow diet. It also included an additional 30% of refined coarse fructose in the drinking water ad libitum. The given diet plans were followed for each group of rats for 10 weeks (and continued during the treatment period). At the end of the 10th week, blood samples were collected from the tail veins of both groups. Their body weights along with the relevant biochemical indices were measured to evaluate the induction of obesity, hyperlipidemia, and insulin resistance.

2.4. Standardization of STZ Dose for the Induction of DM

After the 10th week of dietary intervention, the rats manifesting obesity and dyslipidemia were fasting overnight. Subsequently, a pilot study was conducted using various concentrations of STZ (35, 40, and 45 mg/kg) to determine its optimal dose for inducing diabetes. Based on the results, a single intraperitoneal dose of STZ (40 mg/kg) diluted in 0.1 M cold citrate buffer (pH 4.5) with a pre-nicotinamide (100 mg/kg) injection to minimize pancreatic damage was standardized to induce DM [22]. After 72 h of NA-STZ injection, the animal's tail vein was pricked to collect blood for the FBG determination using a glucometer (Accu-Chek, Roche, Burgdorf, Switzerland). Animals with an FBG level above 400 mg/dL and having symptoms of polyphagia, polydipsia, and polyuria were marked as diabetic.

According to the results of an acute toxicity investigation, the no observed adverse effect level (NOAEL) for LME and lawsone was 50 mg/kg. Furthermore, several previous studies reported varying doses of 1,4-napthoquinones that were therapeutically active in rodent models [15–17]. Based on these reports, three doses of LME and lawsone (15, 30, and 45 mg/kg) were selected for this experiment. In the present study, the antihyperglycemic and antihyperlipidemic effects of LME and lawsone were compared with the standard drug, glibenclamide. Its well-established mechanisms of action and widespread use in clinical practice make it a valuable drug for evaluating the antihyperglycemic effects of other compounds in rat models of diabetes. In addition, the ability of glibenclamide to reduce the elevated biomarkers of oxidative stress, liver function, kidney function, and lipid peroxidation during DM makes it a suitable choice to be used as a reference drug in antihyperglycemic and antihyperlipidemic assays [23,24].

Treatments with LME, lawsone, and glibenclamide (0.6 mg/kg) were started after 72 h of NA-STZ injection and were recorded as the first day. LME and lawsone were dissolved in a cosolvent system consisting of propylene glycol, Tween 80, and water (4:1:4). The required amounts of the drugs in a solution not exceeding 1 mL were administered once daily to the rats via feeding tubes for 28 days.

2.5. Experimental Design

The rats were experimentally assigned into 15 groups with six (6) rats per group as described below.

Group 1: normal control rats receiving cosolvent only.
Groups 2, 3, and 4: normal control rats receiving 15, 30, and 45 mg/kg of LME, respectively.
Groups 5,6, and 7: normal control rats receiving 15, 30, and 45 mg/kg of lawsone, respectively.
Group 8: diabetic control rats receiving cosolvent only.
Groups 9, 10, and 11: diabetic rats receiving 15, 30, and 45 mg/kg of LME, respectively.
Groups 12, 13, and 14: diabetic rats receiving 15, 30, and 45 mg/kg of lawsone, respectively.
Group 15: diabetic rats receiving 0.6 mg/kg of glibenclamide.

2.6. Determination of Body Weight, Food and Water Intake, and FBG

All animals' initial and final body weights as well as their daily food and water consumption were recorded. The FBG was determined on days 0, 7, 14, 21, and 28 with the help of a glucometer using the blood drawn from the animals' tails. On the final day of the experiment (the 28th day), the rats were fasted overnight and were euthanized with an intraperitoneal dose of phenobarbital ranging from 100 to 150 mg/kg. After performing a cardiac puncture, blood was collected from each rat and centrifuged at 4 °C and $800 \times g$ for 15 min. The collected serum was then utilized for various biochemical examinations.

2.7. Measurement of HbA1c and Insulin Levels

The iChroma™ HbA1c self-analyzer (Boditech Med Inc., Gangwon-do, Republic of Korea) was used to test HbA1c levels of whole blood samples. The electro-chemiluminescence technique with a Roche kit and a Cobas 6000 (Roche Diagnostics, Rotkreuz, Switzerland) was employed to detect insulin levels in serum.

2.8. Determination of Insulin Resistance and β-Cell Functioning Indices

Based on the fasting levels of insulin and blood glucose, the insulin resistance index (HOMA-IR) and β cell functioning index (HOMA-β) of all animals were calculated with the help of homoeostatic model assessment (HOMA) [25].

2.9. Measurement of Biochemical Indices for Lipid Profiles, Liver, and Kidney Functions

The levels of various biochemical indices, including total cholesterol (TC), triglycerides (TG), high-density lipoprotein (HDL), low-density lipoprotein (LDL), aspartate aminotransferase (AST), alanine aminotransferase (ALT), blood urea nitrogen (BUN), and creatinine were measured using standard kits (Martin Dow, Meymac, France) with the help of a hematology analyzer (Stat Fax 3300, Awareness Technology, FL, US). The following formulae were used to determine the atherogenic index (AI), atherogenic coefficient (AC), and cardiovascular risk index (CRI) [26].

$$AI = TC - HDL/HDL$$

$$AC = LDL/HDL$$

$$CRI = TC/HDL$$

2.10. Histopathological Findings of Pancreas

After blood sampling, the pancreases from euthanized rats were preserved in 10% neutral buffered formalin for 24 h. The specimens were washed in tap water, dehydrated using a graded alcohol series, cleared with xylene, and embedded in paraffin. Tissue blocks were prepared, and sections of 3–5 µm thickness were obtained using a microtome. The sections were mounted on glass slides, deparaffinized, and stained with hematoxylin-eosin (HE). Histopathological examination was performed at 10× magnification using a light microscope (Optika, Bergamo, Italy), and images were captured with a digital camera (Model B9, Optika, Bergamo, Italy) attached to the microscope at the microscopy unit of the Department of Pharmacy, COMSATS University Islamabad, Abbottabad Campus, Pakistan.

2.11. Statistical Analysis

The statistical analyses were performed using version 25 of the statistical software SPSS (SPSS Inc., Chicago, IL, USA). The analyses were conducted by using one-way ANOVA followed by Duncan's multiple comparison test. The statistical significance was declared at $p < 0.05$. In accordance with Duncan's multiple comparison test, all groups within the same parameter (e.g., food intake, ALT, or insulin levels) were compared not only with the control group but also with every other group within that parameter. The values obtained were expressed as means of six replicate determinations ($n = 6$) ± S.E.M.

3. Results and Discussion

3.1. Determination of a Non-Toxic Dose for LME and Lawsone

Prior to evaluating hypoglycemic and hypolipidemic activities, LME and lawsone were comprehensively evaluated for their possible hazardous effects using acute and sub-acute oral toxicity assays. Acute oral toxicity was conducted in mice according to the Organization of Economic Cooperation and Development (OECD) 423 guidelines [27]. In this study, animals were given a single oral dosage of LME (50, 300, and 2000 mg/kg) and lawsone (50 and 300 mg/kg) and monitored for 14 days to determine their acute toxic effects. In addition, a sub-acute toxicity study was carried out in Wistar rats by following the OECD 407 guidelines [28], with a few modifications. Based on previous reports, a 28-day repeated-dose oral toxicity study was performed using 15, 30, and 45 mg/kg of LME and lawsone [15–17]. The results of acute and sub-acute toxicity studies concluded that LME and lawsone were entirely safe for use in rodent models at doses ≤50 mg/kg.

3.2. Induction of Obesity, Hyperlipidemia, and Insulin Resistance

Obesity is a significant risk factor for type 2 DM. It contributes to the development of insulin resistance, which can progress to type 2 DM over the long run. High-calorie meals, particularly those rich in fats and carbohydrates, are the main contributors to obesity [29]. Using a high-fat (45% fat by energy) and high-fructose (30% fructose in drinking water ad libitum) diet in conjunction with NA-STZ injections was the focal point of the current study. This produced a perfect model of type 2 DM in adult male Wistar rats. This rat model precisely replicated the human stages of obesity, insulin resistance, prediabetes, and hyperlipidemias [30,31].

The effects of HFFD and a normal fat diet (NFD) on body weights, TC, TG, HDL, LDL, FBG, and insulin levels of rats fed for 10 weeks are illustrated in Table 1. Obesity was readily apparent in the rats fed an HFFD, which gained up to 45% more weight than the rats fed an NFD. Similarly, increased levels of TC, TG, and LDL but decreased levels of HDL were observed in HFFD-fed rats. However, no significant impact was found on the lipid profiles of rats given an NFD. In addition, FBG levels of rats given an HFFD were found to be considerably higher when compared to those rats fed a regular diet. In contrast, no marked difference was found in the insulin levels of the two groups. The overall results clearly indicated that rats fed an HFFD had developed obesity, hyperlipidemia, and insulin resistance, characteristics of prediabetes.

Table 1. Body weight changes and serum biochemical indices of rats fed on NFD and HFFD.

Parameters	Before Diet Intervention		After 10 Weeks of Diet Intervention	
	NFD	HFFD	NFD	HFFD
Weight (g)	132.8 ± 3.9 [a]	125.7 ± 4.3 [a]	193.9 ± 6.2 [b]	214.1 ± 6.0 [c]
BWG (g)	N/A	N/A	61.7 ± 6.0	88.6 ± 6.9
TC (mg/dL)	78.6 ± 5.1 [a]	84.3 ± 5.9 [a]	89.1 ± 4.3 [a]	113.3 ± 7.8 [b]
TG (mg/dL)	57.9 ± 3.7 [a]	60.6 ± 5.5 [a]	68.4 ± 6.0 [a]	97.1 ± 6.2 [b]
HDL (mg/dL)	28.3 ± 2.6 [ab]	32.9 ± 3.0 [b]	34.8 ± 3.3 [b]	21.4 ± 1.9 [a]
LDL (mg/dL)	8.5 ± 1.0 [a]	11.9 ± 0.9 [a]	12.3 ± 1.3 [a]	18.9 ± 2.1 [b]
FBG (mg/dL)	82.8 ± 4.6 [a]	89.6 ± 4.1 [ab]	91.4 ± 5.1 [ab]	103 ± 5.6 [b]
Insulin (μIU/mL)	9.9 ± 0.7 [a]	11.3 ± 0.4 [a]	12.0 ± 0.8 [a]	10.8 ± 1.2 [a]

NFD: Normal fat diet, HFFD: High-fat/high-fructose diet, BWG: Body weight gain, N/A: Not available. Data are expressed as mean ± S.E.M. (n = 6). Based on Duncan's multiple range test, the values with different letters of the alphabet or superscripts (a–c) indicate significant differences from one another at a significance level of $p < 0.05$. However, the values labeled with the same letters of the alphabet or superscripts indicate no significant differences.

3.3. Effects of LME and Lawsone on Body Weights, Food, and Water Consumptions

Hyperglycemia, a typical characteristic of DM, frequently appears as a range of symptoms, such as polydipsia (unusual thirst), polyphagia (extreme hunger), polyuria (frequent urination), and unexplained weight loss [32]. Insulin deficiency primarily results in two major clinical outcomes: hyperglycemia and protein catabolism. Hyperglycemia manifests itself in the form of increased hunger, unusual thirst, and frequent urination. Conversely, protein catabolism leads to muscle atrophy and weight loss. These symptoms are the characteristics of the metabolic imbalances caused by insufficient insulin levels in the body [33]. In this study, diabetic rats exhibited the aforementioned symptoms of DM after receiving NA-STZ for 72 h. Diabetic control rats consumed more food and water and lost weight faster than normal rats (Table 2). Interestingly, body weight and water/food intake in diabetic rats were markedly normalized in a dose-dependent manner after oral administration of LME and lawsone, with no effect on normal rats. These findings suggest that LME and lawsone possess therapeutic benefits in managing weight and regulating water and food intake in diabetic conditions. Although glibenclamide (0.6 mg/kg) generated the most potent effects, they were statistically equivalent to the effects of LME and lawsone given at 45 mg/kg. The results indicated that hypoglycemic effects of LME and lawsone were demonstrated by their restoration of normal body weight, water intake, and food consumption in diabetic rats.

3.4. Effects of LME and Lawsone on FBG, HbA1c, and Insulin Levels

Insulin is a hormone of utmost importance in regulating the body's metabolism. That is why any glitch in its action or production results in DM. In the current study, we firstly induced insulin resistance in rats by manipulating their diet. Subsequently, they received injections of NA-STZ, causing partial damage to the pancreatic ß-cells [34]. After 72 h of STZ injection, all of the rats showing elevated levels of FBG (above 400 mg/dL) and having symptoms of polyuria, polyphagia, polydipsia, and also weight loss were declared as diabetic.

Figures 1 and 2A indicated that nondiabetic rats receiving cosolvent, LME, and lawsone presented normal FBG and insulin levels over the course of the 28 days. However, diabetic rats treated with 15, 30, and 45 mg/kg of LME and lawsone showed a significant drop in FBG and a marked rise in insulin levels in a dose-dependent manner (Figures 1 and 2A). Glibenclamide (0.6 mg/kg) exhibited the most potent hypoglycemic effect, which was almost identical to the effect generated by LME at its maximal dose (45 mg/kg). However, lawsone's therapeutic impact on FBG at 45 mg/kg was markedly weaker when compared to the effect of LME at a similar dosage. In fact, lawsone at 45 mg/kg was able to create a hypoglycemic effect that was statistically comparable to LME at 30 mg/kg. This discrepancy in the hypoglycemic potentials of two naphthoquinones is consistent with our previous in vitro study, which found that

LME exhibited a higher inhibitory activity on α-glucosidase than lawsone. The hypoglycemic effects of LME and lawsone were correlated with the histopathological images of the pancreas, as depicted in Figure 3. These images apparently illustrated that the islets of Langerhans in the diabetic control group were noticeably shrunk with marked loss of its cells as compared to the normal control group. However, the repeated oral administration of LME and lawsone at doses of 15, 30, and 45 mg/kg resulted in a gradual increase in the size of the islets in the diabetic rats. In addition, both LME and lawsone exhibit pancreatic protective effects, as they have previously been reported to possess promising antioxidant and anti-inflammatory characteristics [35]. These properties suggest that LME and lawsone can mitigate oxidative stress and inflammation within the pancreas, potentially contributing to the preservation and improved function of pancreatic tissues. Moreover, significant hypoglycemic actions have been documented for several other 1,4-naphthoquinones, such as plumbagin, shikonin, and rhinacanthin-C. These compounds, like LME and lawsone, exhibit notable antihyperglycemic effects. The shared hypoglycemic actions among these 1,4-naphthoquinones highlight their potential as a class of compounds for the management of hyperglycemia and related metabolic disorders [15–17].

Table 2. Effects of LME and lawsone on body weight, food, and water intake in rats.

Group	Compound Dose	Parameters				
		Initial BW (g)	Final BW (g)	BWG (g)	Food/day (g)	H$_2$O/day (mL)
Normal	Control	197.6 ± 5.1 [b]	233.7 ± 7.7 [bc]	36.1	31.1 ± 3.1 [ab]	22.1 ± 1.9 [a]
	LME—15 mg/kg	189.4 ± 4.6 [ab]	216.9 ± 7.5 [ab]	27.5	28.6 ± 2.7 [a]	19.9 ± 1.5 [a]
	LME—30 mg/kg	189.5 ± 5.0 [ab]	221.3 ± 6.6 [b]	31.8	31.9 ± 3.4 [ab]	21.2 ± 1.4 [a]
	LME—45 mg/kg	199.6 ± 5.6 [b]	238.4 ± 8.1 [bc]	38.8	38.1 ± 4.2 [b]	24.2 ± 1.8 [ab]
	Lawsone—15 mg/kg	198.8 ± 4.9 [b]	225.1 ± 6.7 [b]	26.2	30.1 ± 2.9 [ab]	20.3 ± 1.6 [a]
	Lawsone—30 mg/kg	178.5 ± 3.6 [a]	211.7 ± 6.1 [ab]	33.2	33.4 ± 3.3 [ab]	23.1 ± 2.1 [ab]
	Lawsone—45 mg/kg	203.9 ± 6.1 [abc]	241.3 ± 8.7 [bc]	37.4	37 ± 3.9 [b]	24.9 ± 2.0 [ab]
Diabetic	Control	218.9 ± 6.3 [c]	194.1 ± 6.1 [a]	−24.8	64.9 ± 4.8 [d]	40.9 ± 3.7 [c]
	LME—15 mg/kg	213.3 ± 7.0 [bc]	227.9 ± 7.3 [b]	14.6	50.1 ± 4.5 [cd]	35.3 ± 2.9 [bc]
	LME—30 mg/kg	208.4 ± 4.5 [bc]	234.5 ± 7.9 [bc]	26.1	45.3 ± 3.9 [c]	30.8 ± 3.3 [abc]
	LME—45 mg/kg	221.1 ± 7.1 [c]	257.8 ± 8.9 [c]	36.7	40.8 ± 3.4 [bc]	29.9 ± 2.7 [abc]
	Lawsone—15 mg/kg	209.4 ± 5.1 [bc]	222.3 ± 4.9 [b]	12.9	53.7 ± 4.2 [cd]	39.1 ± 3.5 [c]
	Lawsone—30 mg/kg	217.1 ± 6.5 [bc]	239.2 ± 8.1 [bc]	22.1	46.9 ± 4.5 [bc]	38.2 ± 2.9 [c]
	Lawsone—45 mg/kg	205.7 ± 5.6 [bc]	238.1 ± 7.3 [bc]	32.4	41.3 ± 3.0 [bc]	30.8 ± 3.1 [abc]
	Glb—0.6 mg/kg	219.2 ± 6.9 [c]	257.1 ± 9.1 [c]	37.9	39.9 ± 3.6 [bc]	29.7 ± 2.8 [abc]

LME: Lawsone methyl ether, BW: Body weight, BWG: Body weight gain, Glb: Glibenclamide. Data are expressed as mean ± S.E.M. (n = 6). Based on Duncan's multiple range test, the values with different letters of the alphabet or superscripts (a–d) indicate significant differences from one another at a significance level of $p < 0.05$. However, the values labeled with the same letters of the alphabet or superscripts indicate no significant differences.

HbA1c is a clinical marker that indicates persistent hyperglycemia. It is widely regarded as the most reliable index for evaluating the long-term effectiveness of antidiabetic medications. HbA1c provides valuable insights into overall glycemic control and serves as an important tool for assessing the long-term efficacy of these drugs in managing diabetes [36]. As shown in Figure 2B, LME and lawsone substantially and dose-dependently decreased the elevated levels of HbA1c in diabetic rats. The most prominent reduction in HbA1c level was observed with 45 mg/kg of LME (6.9 ± 0.5%), which was equivalent to the standard drug, glibenclamide (6.95 ± 0.6%), but likely higher than lawsone (7.2 ± 0.5%) at its maximal dose. In contrast, both LME and lawsone exhibited no effect on the HbA1c levels of normal rats. These results are in line with those of previous studies, which have revealed that different plant-derived phenolics may exert their hypoglycemic effects via antioxidant and anti-glycation mechanisms [37].

The remarkable hypoglycemic effects induced by LME or lawsone are justified through multiple mechanisms. These mechanisms may include enhanced insulin secretion or synthesis, regeneration of pancreatic β-cells, improved insulin sensitivity, and potential modulation of glucose metabolism pathways. In the present study, both LME and lawsone are found to act as insulin secretagogues. This mechanism is supported by a substantial rise in the insulin levels of diabetic rats treated with LME or lawsone (Figure 2A). Both of these compounds may exhibit a mechanism of action similar to glibenclamide by blocking ATP-sensitive potassium channels. This action results in the depolarization of pancreatic β-cells, subsequently leading to the release of insulin [38].

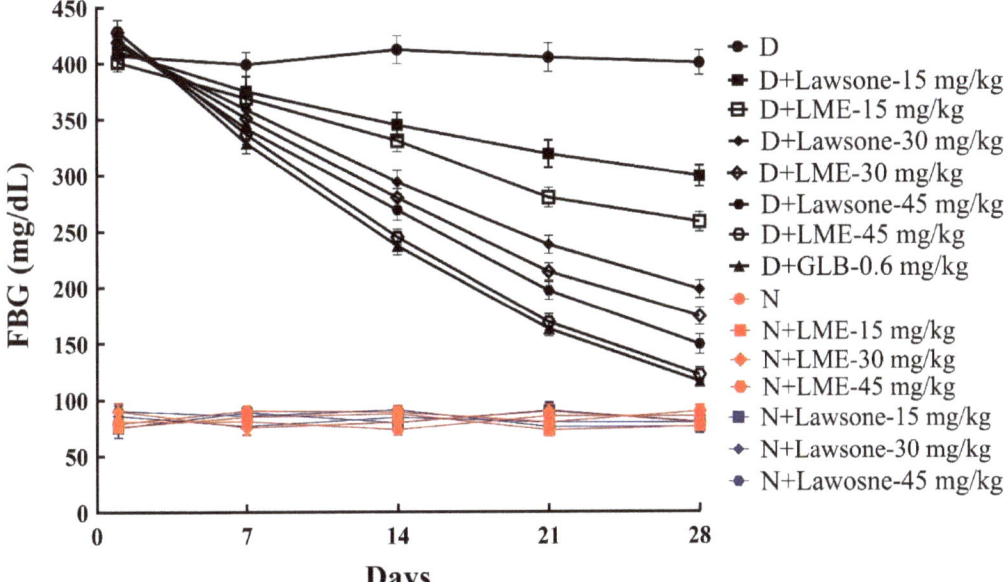

Figure 1. Comparative effects of LME and lawsone at weekly intervals on FBG levels. N: Nondiabetic control; D: Diabetic-control; N + LME or lawsone: nondiabetic receiving lawsone methyl ether or lawsone; D + LME or lawsone: Diabetic receiving lawsone methyl ether or lawsone; and D + GLB: Diabetic receiving glibenclamide.

Another mechanism that supports the antihyperglycemic effects of LME and lawsone is their potential to promote the regeneration of pancreatic β-cells. This regenerative action contributes to increased insulin production and secretion. Many antidiabetic drugs including GLP-1 receptor agonists and DPP-4 inhibitors are incretin-based therapies that have shown the potential to enhance β-cell function by promoting their proliferation [39]. The histopathological images of the pancreas from the current study provide apparent support for the aforementioned phenomenon (Figure 3). Observations revealed that the Islets of Langerhans in the diabetic control group were noticeably shrunk with marked loss of its cells as compared to the normal control group. However, the repeated oral administration of LME and lawsone at doses of 15, 30, and 45 mg/kg resulted in a gradual increase in the size of the islets in the diabetic rats. Furthermore, no significant effect was observed on the Islets of Langerhans in normal rats treated with different dosages of LME and lawsone. These findings suggest that LME and lawsone exhibit a potential role in promoting the regeneration or preservation of pancreatic β-cells in diabetic conditions. Nonetheless, it is important to note that β-cell regeneration is a complex process, and more research is needed to fully understand the antidiabetic mechanisms of LME and lawsone in terms of β-cell proliferation.

Additionally, our prior in vitro study showed that LME and lawsone have strong α-glucosidase inhibitory effects. Their hypoglycemic effects can be explained, in part, by the fact that they slow the digestion and absorption of dietary carbohydrates in the gut. Slowing the process of gluconeogenesis or enhancing the uptake and utilization of glucose in adipose tissues, skeletal muscles, and the liver are proposed mechanisms of action for LME and lawsone that warrant further investigation [40]. Additionally, activating peroxisome proliferator-activated receptor gamma (PPARγ) and inhibiting DPP-4 or SGLT-2 can also be the potential antidiabetic mechanisms of LME and lawsone that require further exploration [41]. These mechanisms, if confirmed, could contribute to the overall understanding of the multifaceted therapeutic potentials of LME and lawsone in the management of DM.

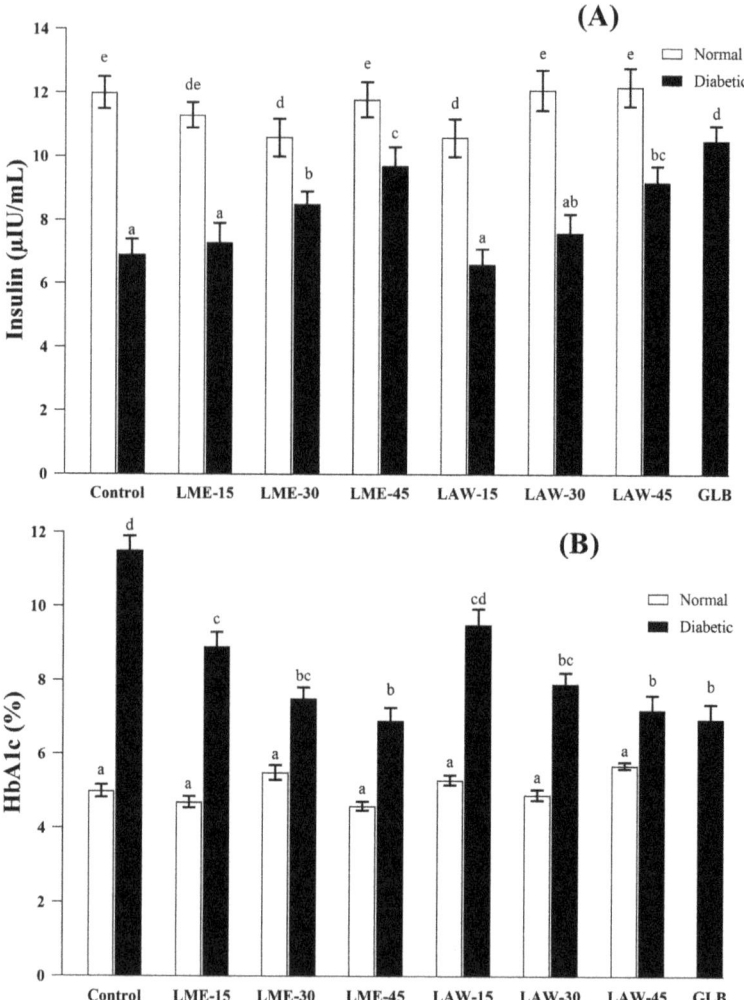

Figure 2. Effects of LME, lawsone (LAW), and glibenclamide (GLB) on insulin (A) and HbA1c (B) levels. White bars: Normal rats and black-colored bars: Diabetic rats. LME–15, LME–30, and LME–45: 15, 30, and 45 mg/kg of LME, respectively; LAW–15, LAW–30, and LAW–45: 15, 30, and 45 mg/kg of lawsone, respectively; and GLB: 0.6 mg/kg of Glibenclamide. Data are expressed as mean ± S.E.M. (n = 6). Based on Duncan's multiple range test, the values with different letters of the alphabet or superscripts (a–e) indicate significant differences from one another at a significance level of $p < 0.05$. However, the values labeled with the same letters of the alphabet or superscripts indicate no significant differences.

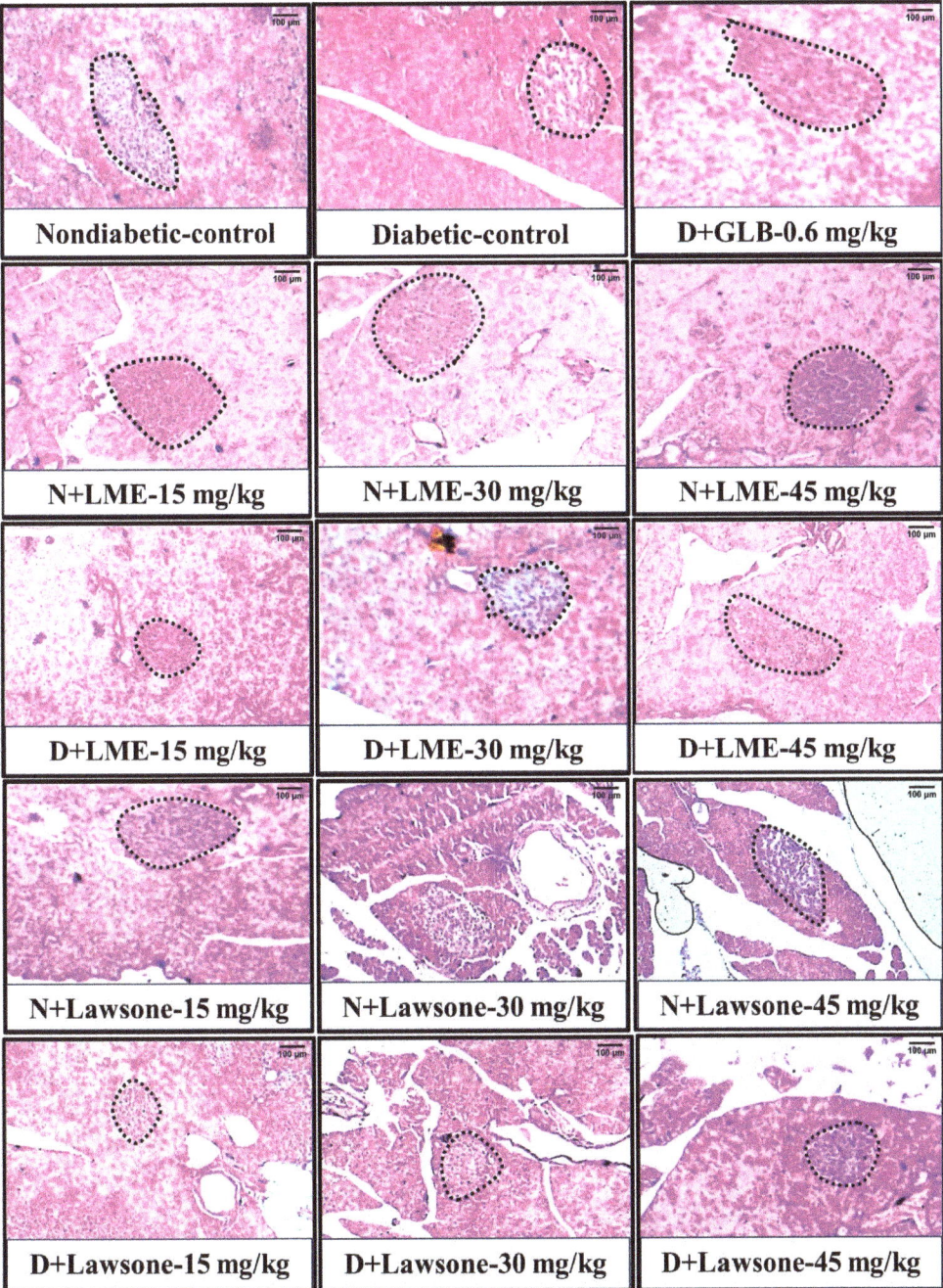

Figure 3. Effects of LME, lawsone, and glibenclamide (GLB) on the apparent size of the islets of Langerhans. Black dashes outline the islets of Langerhans. N + LME or lawsone: Normal rats receiving lawsone methyl ether or lawsone; D + LME or lawsone: Diabetic rats receiving lawsone methyl ether or lawsone; and D + GLB: Diabetic rats receiving glibenclamide. Scale bar = 100 μm.

3.5. Effects of LME and Lawsone on HOMA-IR and HOMA-β

In type 2 DM, two primary characteristics are observed: insulin resistance in peripheral tissues and inadequate insulin production from pancreatic β-cells. These factors, insulin resistance and insulin secretion, are commonly quantified using HOMA-IR and HOMA-β, respectively. Both HOMA indicators are clinically related to one another and have been carefully linked to the etiology, progression, and complications of DM [42]. HFFD- and NA-STZ-induced diabetic control rats exhibited a fivefold increase in insulin resistance (HOMA-IR) and a ninefold decrease in β-cell function (HOMA-β) as compared to the normal control rats (Table 3). The oral administration of LME and lawsone for 28 days showed a dose-dependent decrease in HOMA-IR and a dose-dependent increase in HOMA-β. However, there was no significant alteration in the HOMA indices for the normal rats treated with the same doses of LME and lawsone. The significant normalization of HOMA indicators (HOMA-IR and HOMA-β) observed after the administration of LME and lawsone suggests an improvement in glucose homeostasis. This normalization indicates an enhancement in insulin action, leading to increased insulin sensitivity, as well as an improvement in β-cell function. These findings imply that LME and lawsone may have the potential to improve the overall regulation of glucose levels by enhancing both insulin action and β-cell function.

Table 3. Effects of LME and lawsone on HOMA indices of adult male Wistar rats.

Group	Compound Dose	Parameters	
		HOMA Insulin Resistance	HOMA β-Cells Function
Normal	Control	2.7 ± 0.1 [a]	126.1 ± 7.5 [f]
	LME—15 mg/kg	2.2 ± 0.2 [a]	172.3 ± 5.6 [h]
	LME—30 mg/kg	2.1 ± 0.2 [a]	164.9 ± 4.8 [g]
	LME—45 mg/kg	2.5 ± 0.1 [a]	137.3 ± 4.6 [f]
	Lawsone—15 mg/kg	2.4 ± 0.3 [a]	125.4 ± 7.9 [f]
	Lawsone—30 mg/kg	2.5 ± 0.1 [a]	144.4 ± 8.6 [g]
	Lawsone—45 mg/kg	2.4 ± 0.2 [a]	184.6 ± 6.9 [h]
Diabetic	Control	9.9 ± 0.5 [d]	13.9 ± 0.9 [a]
	LME—15 mg/kg	4.5 ± 0.6 [c]	21.1 ± 1.0 [ab]
	LME—30 mg/kg	3.5 ± 0.3 [bc]	40.8 ± 5.3 [c]
	LME—45 mg/kg	2.9 ± 0.3 [b]	67.6 ± 4.1 [e]
	Lawsone—15 mg/kg	4.9 ± 0.6 [c]	17.5 ± 1.4 [a]
	Lawsone—30 mg/kg	3.8 ± 0.5 [bc]	31.9 ± 2.9 [b]
	Lawsone—45 mg/kg	3.2 ± 0.1 [bc]	51.5 ± 3.4 [cd]
	Glb—0.6 mg/kg	3.0 ± 0.4 [b]	69.4 ± 3.9 [e]

LME: Lawsone methyl ether, Glb: Glibenclamide. Data are expressed as mean ± S.E.M. ($n = 6$). Based on Duncan's multiple range test, the values with different letters of the alphabet or superscripts (a–h) indicate significant differences from one another at a significance level of $p < 0.05$. However, the values labeled with the same letters of the alphabet or superscripts indicate no significant differences.

3.6. Effects of LME and Lawsone on Lipid Profiles

DM has an intimate link with hyperlipidemia. This often leads to cardiomyopathy, a major cause of mortality among diabetics [43]. In the present study, a similar positive correlation was observed between hyperglycemia and hyperlipidemia. An ideal animal model of diabetic hyperlipidemia should closely resemble the human condition. One approach to achieve this is by inducing obesity/hyperlipidemia through dietary intervention and causing pancreatic damage via nicotinamide-streptozotocin. This combination better reflects the human scenario and provides a more suitable representation of diabetic hyperlipidemia in rats. Similarly, in the present study, an ideal model of diabetic hyperlipidemia was created in rats using NA-STZ injection in conjunction with a high-fat (45% fat by energy) and high-fructose (30% fructose in drinking water ad libitum) diet. Insulin deficiency is primarily responsible for diabetic hyperlipidemia. It instigates hormone-sensitive lipase that promotes lipolysis and boosts the release of free fatty acids [44]. Excessive fatty acids enhance the production of TC, TG, and LDL while decreasing HDL biosynthesis, as observed in untreated diabetic rats of the current study.

Regular oral administration of LME and lawsone (15, 30, and 45 mg/kg) for 28 days delivered a substantial and dose-dependent amelioration of deteriorated effects on TC, TG, LDL, and HDL (Table 4). However, normal rats, which were given similar doses of LME and lawsone, showed no discernible change in their lipid profiles. LME at 45 mg/kg seemed to be the most effective in normalizing TC, HDL, and LDL levels in diabetic rats, which were better than the standard drug, glibenclamide. These findings suggest that LME has potent therapeutic benefits in improving lipid profiles in diabetic conditions, surpassing the efficacy of glibenclamide in this particular study. Lawsone at 45 mg/kg was the most potent in lowering the TG level without any distinguishable impact on other lipid parameters. The hypolipidemic effects of LME and lawsone are attributed to their potential for stimulation of residual β-cells. This stimulation could result in increased insulin synthesis, secretion, or sensitivity. The precise mechanism underlying these effects requires further investigation. However, it is hypothesized that the improvement in lipid profiles seen with LME and lawsone could be related to their impact on β-cell function and insulin-related pathways, which ultimately contribute to the regulation of lipid metabolism in the body. The findings of this study align with previous research that has demonstrated the hypolipidemic properties of other 1,4-naphthoquinones, including plumbagin, shikonin, and rhinacanthin-C [15–17].

Table 4. Effects of LME and lawsone on lipid profiles in adult male Wistar rats.

Group	Compound Dose	Parameters (mg/dL)			
		TC	TG	HDL	LDL
Normal	Control	92.6 ± 5.2 [ab]	76.2 ± 6.1 [ab]	50.8 ± 6.1 [bc]	11.2 ± 1.2 [a]
	LME—15 mg/kg	94.8 ± 5.9 [ab]	68.6 ± 5.0 [a]	48.6 ± 5.0 [bc]	10.6 ± 1.4 [a]
	LME—30 mg/kg	97.8 ± 6.9 [ab]	71.6 ± 5.4 [a]	50.6 ± 4.8 [bc]	10.7 ± 0.8 [a]
	LME—45 mg/kg	88.9 ± 4.3 [a]	78.2 ± 4.9 [ab]	49.8 ± 5.1 [bc]	11.9 ± 1.1 [a]
	Lawsone—15 mg/kg	94.9 ± 4.8 [ab]	74.8 ± 4.2 [ab]	47.9 ± 4.0 [bc]	11.5 ± 1.4 [a]
	Lawsone—30 mg/kg	101.2 ± 6.8 [ab]	81.2 ± 5.1 [ab]	54.7 ± 3.9 [c]	12.1 ± 0.9 [a]
	Lawsone—45 mg/kg	89.0 ± 6.5 [a]	80 ± 6.9 [ab]	45.9 ± 3.8 [abc]	10.3 ± 1.2 [a]
Diabetic	Control	201 ± 11.1 [f]	168.4 ± 8.2 [e]	28.6 ± 4.7 [a]	71.8 ± 5.9 [g]
	LME—15 mg/kg	167.8 ± 9.5 [de]	147.2 ± 7.4 [e]	35.1 ± 4.2 [ab]	50.8 ± 5.6 [ef]
	LME—30 mg/kg	122.6 ± 7.9 [bc]	113.2 ± 5.4 [cd]	42.2 ± 3.8 [abc]	31.6 ± 3.4 [cd]
	LME—45 mg/kg	109 ± 5.7 [ab]	95.4 ± 4.9 [bc]	50.5 ± 5.7 [bc]	16.5 ± 2.2 [ab]
	Lawsone—15 mg/kg	184.4 ± 8.9 [ef]	145.9 ± 6.9 [e]	34.8 ± 3.9 [ab]	57.8 ± 4.4 [f]
	Lawsone—30 mg/kg	151.8 ± 7.1 [cd]	119.4 ± 6.3 [d]	40.8 ± 5.0 [abc]	38.9 ± 4.3 [de]
	Lawsone—45 mg/kg	121.2 ± 6.4 [b]	89.4 ± 4.9 [ab]	45.4 ± 4.7 [abc]	27.6 ± 2.2 [bcd]
	Glb—0.6 mg/kg	116.2 ± 5.1 [ab]	96.2 ± 5.4 [bc]	48.6 ± 5.1 [bc]	19.8 ± 1.6 [abc]

LME: Lawsone methyl ether, Glb: Glibenclamide. Data are expressed as mean ± S.E.M. ($n = 6$). Based on Duncan's multiple range test, the values with different letters of the alphabet or superscripts (a–f) indicate significant differences from one another at a significance level of $p < 0.05$. However, the values labeled with the same letters of the alphabet or superscripts indicate no significant differences.

Dyslipidemia is associated with an increased risk of cardiovascular pathology, which is quantified by measuring atherogenicity indicators, such as the AI, AC, and CRI. As illustrated in Table 5, the diabetic control rats had noticeably higher atherogenicity risk indicators compared to the normal control rats. A substantial and dose-dependent reduction in atherogenicity indicators was observed in diabetic rats treated with LME/lawsone (15, 30, and 45 mg/kg) for 28 days. LME at 45 mg/kg caused the most potent decline in atherogenic indicators, followed by glibenclamide (0.6 mg/kg) and lawsone (45 mg/kg). The most striking impact of LME (45 mg/kg) was found on CRI, decreasing it to a level of 2.1 ± 0.2, which was significantly comparable with that of the normal level (1.78 ± 0.2). Indeed, numerous studies have reported that antioxidant and anti-inflammatory agents derived from plants have the ability to protect against the formation and progression of atherosclerosis, which is the underlying cause of atherogenicity [45]. Thus, lowering of the aforesaid markers is an indication of the cardioprotective potential of LME and lawsone due to their antioxidant, anti-inflammatory, and antihyperlipidemic potentials. By targeting these mechanisms, LME and lawsone demonstrate potential as therapeutic agents for promoting heart health and reducing the risk of cardiovascular complications in diabetic patients.

Table 5. Effects of LME and lawsone on atherogenicity indicators for adult male Wistar rats.

Group	Compound Dose	Atherogenicity Indicators		
		AI	AC	CRI
Normal	Control	0.82 ± 0.1 [a]	0.22 ± 0.02 [a]	1.82 ± 0.2 [a]
	LME—15 mg/kg	0.95 ± 0.1 [a]	0.21 ± 0.03 [a]	1.95 ± 0.1 [a]
	LME—30 mg/kg	0.93 ± 0.2 [a]	0.2 ± 0.01 [a]	1.93 ± 0.2 [a]
	LME—45 mg/kg	0.81 ± 0.1 [a]	0.23 ± 0.02 [a]	1.78 ± 0.2 [a]
	LAW—15 mg/kg	0.98 ± 0.2 [a]	0.24 ± 0.03 [a]	1.98 ± 0.3 [a]
	LAW—30 mg/kg	0.85 ± 0.09 [a]	0.18 ± 0.01 [a]	1.85 ± 0.2 [a]
	LAW—45 mg/kg	0.93 ± 0.1 [a]	0.22 ± 0.03 [a]	1.93 ± 0.1 [a]
Diabetic	Control	6.1 ± 0.9 [e]	2.51 ± 0.3 [e]	7.02 ± 1.0 [d]
	LME—15 mg/kg	3.8 ± 0.4 [cd]	1.44 ± 0.1 [d]	4.78 ± 0.3 [c]
	LME—30 mg/kg	1.9 ± 0.2 [ab]	0.74 ± 0.05 [bc]	2.9 ± 0.3 [ab]
	LME—45 mg/kg	1.15 ± 0.1 [ab]	0.32 ± 0.04 [ab]	2.1 ± 0.2 [a]
	LAW—15 mg/kg	4.3 ± 0.5 [d]	1.66 ± 0.2 [d]	5.29 ± 0.5 [c]
	LAW—30 mg/kg	2.7 ± 0.3 [bc]	0.95 ± 0.1 [c]	3.72 ± 0.4 [bc]
	LAW—45 mg/kg	1.66 ± 0.2 [ab]	0.6 ± 0.07 [abc]	2.66 ± 0.2 [ab]
	GLB—0.6 mg/kg	1.39 ± 0.2 [ab]	0.4 ± 0.06 [ab]	2.39 ± 0.3 [ab]

LME: Lawsone methyl ether, Glb: Glibenclamide. Data are expressed as mean $\pm$ S.E.M. (n = 6). Based on Duncan's multiple range test, the values with different letters of the alphabet or superscripts (a–e) indicate significant differences from one another at a significance level of $p < 0.05$. However, the values labeled with the same letters of the alphabet or superscripts indicate no significant differences.

3.7. Effects of LME and Lawsone on Liver and Kidney Function Parameters

The liver maintains healthy blood glucose levels by performing various metabolic processes, including glycogenesis, glycogenolysis, and gluconeogenesis. AST and ALT are the enzymes, which are the indicative markers of liver health. Due to a liver injury, they may seep into the bloodstream, leading to their increased levels [46]. In the current study, increases in levels of AST and ALT were observed in the untreated diabetic rats, indicating an altered liver function that can be linked to hyperglycemia. The higher levels of AST and ALT in diabetic rats were significantly reduced by LME/lawsone (15, 30, and 45 mg/kg) in a dose-dependent manner (Table 6). Amongst these, lawsone at 45 mg/kg caused the maximum reduction in AST and ALT levels in diabetic livers, followed by LME (45 mg/kg) and glibenclamide (0.6 mg/kg). On the other hand, LME and lawsone did not significantly alter the liver biomarkers in normal rats. In the present study, lawsone demonstrated the most significant reduction in liver functional markers. These findings align with previous reports highlighting the hepatoprotective effects of lawsone [47]. Moreover, the prior studies on lawsone and LME have provided additional evidence supporting their hepatoprotective effects, specifically due to their promising antioxidant and anti-inflammatory activities [35].

Long-term uncontrolled hyperglycemia may result in diabetic nephropathy, which is one of the serious complications of DM. It develops from undue oxidative stress that is induced by an excess of free radicals [48]. In nephropathic conditions, serum creatinine and BUN levels are useful markers to assess the functional efficiency of kidneys [49]. In this study, elevated levels of creatinine and BUN were observed in untreated diabetic rats, indicating impaired renal function resulting from hyperglycemia. The elevated levels of creatinine and BUN in diabetic rats were significantly reduced by LME/lawsone (15, 30, and 45 mg/kg) in a dose-dependent manner (Table 6). The highest decline in the renal biomarkers of diabetic rats was observed with LME at a dose of 45 mg/kg, followed by glibenclamide at 0.6 mg/kg and lawsone at 45 mg/kg. Neither LME nor lawsone significantly altered the renal biomarkers in normal rats. These findings are consistent with the antioxidant and anti-inflammatory properties of LME and lawsone [34]. These results suggest that LME and lawsone not only demonstrate efficacy as hypoglycemic agents but also have the potential to ameliorate diabetic nephropathy. These effects of LME and lawsone are similar to those observed with another 1,4-naphthoquinone compound, rhinacanthin-C [50]. The ability of LME, lawsone, and rhinacanthin-C to exhibit hypoglycemic and nephroprotective properties further highlights the potential of 1,4-naphthoquinones in managing diabetes and its related complications.

Table 6. Effects of LME and lawsone on liver and kidney functions in adult male Wistar rats.

Group	Compound Dose	Parameters (mg/dL)			
		AST (IU/dL)	ALT (IU/dL)	Cr (mg/dL)	BUN (mg/dL)
Normal	Control	88.6 ± 6.0^a	44.0 ± 3.6^{ab}	0.39 ± 0.06^a	28.1 ± 3.2^a
	LME—15 mg/kg	90.9 ± 5.7^{ab}	39.8 ± 3.0^a	0.38 ± 0.04^a	26.9 ± 3.0^a
	LME—30 mg/kg	88.4 ± 6.6^a	41.8 ± 5.1^{ab}	0.40 ± 0.06^a	30.9 ± 3.7^{abc}
	LME—45 mg/kg	92.3 ± 5.4^{ab}	38.6 ± 4.1^a	0.41 ± 0.05^a	31.6 ± 4.3^{abc}
	Lawsone—15 mg/kg	89.3 ± 6.1^a	47.9 ± 4.7^{ab}	0.45 ± 0.06^{ab}	28.6 ± 3.2^{ab}
	Lawsone—30 mg/kg	99.0 ± 7.6^{abc}	51.1 ± 4.3^{ab}	0.37 ± 0.03^a	33.8 ± 2.9^{abc}
	Lawsone—45 mg/kg	100.8 ± 7.3^{abc}	40.3 ± 63.5^a	0.40 ± 0.05^{ab}	30.8 ± 4.0^{abc}
Diabetic	Control	169.8 ± 11.1^f	98.4 ± 6.0^g	1.1 ± 0.09^e	61.9 ± 5.1^e
	LME—15 mg/kg	157.8 ± 7.3^{ef}	89.1 ± 5.4^{fg}	0.85 ± 0.06^{cd}	53.4 ± 4.3^{de}
	LME—30 mg/kg	136.6 ± 5.3^{de}	75.6 ± 6.0^{cdef}	0.61 ± 0.03^{abc}	45.6 ± 4.0^{cde}
	LME—45 mg/kg	118.9 ± 5.7^{bcd}	60.1 ± 3.6^{abcd}	0.39 ± 0.04^a	33.8 ± 3.0^{abc}
	Lawsone—15 mg/kg	153.9 ± 7.6^{ef}	85.3 ± 4.6^{efg}	0.86 ± 0.09^d	54.9 ± 5.1^{de}
	Lawsone—30 mg/kg	139.6 ± 5.3^{de}	79.9 ± 5.4^{defg}	0.73 ± 0.07^{bcd}	45.0 ± 4.3^{bcd}
	Lawsone—45 mg/kg	117.8 ± 7.5^{bcd}	54.2 ± 4.5^{abc}	0.51 ± 0.05^{ab}	41.9 ± 3.7^{abcd}
	Glb—0.6 mg/kg	120.2 ± 6.5^{cd}	63.6 ± 5.5^{bcde}	0.42 ± 0.04^a	35.1 ± 4.1^{abc}

LME: Lawsone methyl ether, Cr: Creatinine, Glb: Glibenclamide. Data are expressed as mean $\pm$ S.E.M. ($n = 6$). Based on Duncan's multiple range test, the values with different letters of the alphabet or superscripts (a–g) indicate significant differences from one another at a significance level of $p < 0.05$. However, the values labeled with the same letters of the alphabet or superscripts indicate no significant differences.

4. Conclusions

The present study supports that LME is a potent antidiabetic drug. Furthermore, the study suggests that LME is also a potential compound to mitigate the lethal complications associated with DM due to its promising antihyperlipidemic, hepatoprotective, and nephroprotective properties. The optimum dose of LME possessing maximum efficacy and safety was found to be 45 mg/kg. Interestingly, LME was found to be more potent and safer than lawsone. Various mechanisms could define the antidiabetic potential of LME; however, in the present study, LME was found to act via α-glucosidase inhibition and pancreatic β-cell regeneration. These findings highlight the multifaceted therapeutic potential of LME in managing DM along with its complications, thereby emphasizing its significance as a potential treatment option. Nevertheless, further research is warranted to explore the antidiabetic mechanisms of LME using various pathways and targets involved in glucose regulation, such as gluconeogenesis, glucose transportation, ATP-sensitive potassium channels, incretin hormones, and ghrelin.

Author Contributions: M.K. (Muhammad Khan), M.A.S. and P.P. conceived and designed the research study. M.K. (Muhammad Khan) conducted the experiments. M.K. (Mustafa Kamal) and M.S.O. helped in hematological evaluation. M.S.O. and M.A. carried out histopathological analysis. All authors analyzed the data, discussed the findings, and prepared the manuscript. All authors have read and agreed to the published version of the manuscript.

Funding: This research was financially supported by the Ph.D. Award 2020–2022 from the Discipline of Excellence, Faculty of Pharmaceutical Sciences, Prince of Songkla University, Thailand. Additionally, a Research Grant for the Thesis in the Fiscal Year 2022 was allocated by the Graduate School, Prince of Songkla University, Thailand. The authors would also like to thank the funding of Researchers Supporting Project number (RSPD2023R710) from King Saud University, Riyadh, Saudi Arabia.

Institutional Review Board Statement: The animal study protocol was approved by the Institutional Animal Care and Use Committee, PCSIR Laboratories Complex, Karachi, Pakistan (Ref. PCSIR–KLC/IEC/2022/02).

Informed Consent Statement: Not applicable.

Data Availability Statement: The data presented in this study are available in article.

Acknowledgments: The authors would also like to thank the Pakistan Council of Scientific & Industrial Research (PCSIR) Laboratories Complex, Karachi, for providing the housing facility for animals. The authors are also grateful to Saffanah Mohd Ab Azid for her assistance with English editing. The authors would also like to thank the funding of Researchers Supporting Project Number (RSPD2023R710) from King Saud University, Riyadh, Saudi Arabia.

Conflicts of Interest: The authors declared that they have no conflicts of interest. There is no connection between Invivotek Ltd. and the subject of this manuscript.

References

1. World Health Organization (WHO). Available online: https://www.who.int (accessed on 8 July 2023).
2. Saeedi, P.; Salpea, P.; Karuranga, S.; Petersohn, I.; Malanda, B.; Gregg, E.W.; Unwin, N.; Wild, S.H.; Williams, R. Mortality Attributable to Diabetes in 20–79 Years Old Adults, 2019 Estimates: Results from the International Diabetes Federation Diabetes Atlas. *Diabetes Res. Clin. Pract.* **2020**, *162*, 108086. [CrossRef] [PubMed]
3. Ormazabal, V.; Nair, S.; Elfeky, O.; Aguayo, C.; Salomon, C.; Zuñiga, F.A. Association between Insulin Resistance and the Development of Cardiovascular Disease. *Cardiovasc. Diabetol.* **2018**, *17*, 122. [CrossRef] [PubMed]
4. Chamberlain, J.J.; Rhinehart, A.S.; Shaefer, C.F., Jr.; Neuman, A. Diagnosis and Management of Diabetes: Synopsis of the 2016 American Diabetes Association Standards of Medical Care in Diabetes. *Ann. Intern. Med.* **2016**, *164*, 542–552. [CrossRef]
5. Jeyabalan, S.; Palayan, M. Antihyperlipidemic Activity of Sapindus emarginatus in Triton WR-1339 Induced Albino Rats. *Res. J. Pharm. Technol.* **2009**, *2*, 319–323.
6. Sharma, A.; Khanijau, M.R.; Agarwal, M.R. Hyperlipidemia: A Review Article. *Soc. Sci. Rev.* **2019**, *5*, 11–22.
7. Hung, H.-Y.; Qian, K.; Morris-Natschke, S.L.; Hsu, C.-S.; Lee, K.-H. Recent Discovery of Plant-Derived Anti-Diabetic Natural Products. *Nat. Prod. Rep.* **2012**, *29*, 580–606. [CrossRef] [PubMed]
8. Ibrahim, S.R.; Mohamed, G.A.; Banjar, Z.M.; Kamal, H.K. Natural Antihyperlipidemic Agents: Current Status and Future Perspectives. *Phytopharmacology* **2013**, *4*, 492–531.
9. Arya, N.; Kharjul, M.D.; Shishoo, C.J.; Thakare, V.N.; Jain, K.S. Some Molecular Targets for Antihyperlipidemic Drug Research. *Eur. J. Med. Chem.* **2014**, *85*, 535–568. [CrossRef]
10. Chaudhury, A.; Duvoor, C.; Reddy Dendi, V.S.; Kraleti, S.; Chada, A.; Ravilla, R.; Marco, A.; Shekhawat, N.S.; Montales, M.T.; Kuriakose, K. Clinical Review of Antidiabetic Drugs: Implications for Type 2 Diabetes Mellitus Management. *Front. Endocrinol.* **2017**, *8*, 6. [CrossRef] [PubMed]
11. Mills, E.J.; Wu, P.; Chong, G.; Ghement, I.; Singh, S.; Akl, E.A.; Eyawo, O.; Guyatt, G.; Berwanger, O.; Briel, M. Efficacy and Safety of Statin Treatment for Cardiovascular Disease: A Network Meta-Analysis of 170 255 Patients from 76 Randomized Trials. *QJM Int. J. Med.* **2011**, *104*, 109–124. [CrossRef]
12. Pattis, P.; Wiedermann, C.J. Ezetimibe-Associated Immune Thrombocytopenia. *Ann. Pharmacother.* **2008**, *42*, 430–433. [CrossRef]
13. Navitha, A.; Helen Sheeba, D.A.; Ramesh, C.; Sartaj Banu, M. Hypoglycemic and Anti-Diabetic Activity of Ethanolic Extract of *Catharanthus pusillus* (Murray) G. Don. *IOSR J. Pharm.* **2012**, *2*, 17–21.
14. Ahangarpour, A.; Sayahi, M.; Sayahi, M. The Antidiabetic and Antioxidant Properties of Some Phenolic Phytochemicals: A Review Study. *Diabetes Metab. Syndr. Clin. Res. Rev.* **2019**, *13*, 854–857. [CrossRef]
15. Gwon, S.Y.; Ahn, J.Y.; Jung, C.H.; Moon, B.K.; Ha, T.Y. Shikonin Suppresses ERK 1/2 Phosphorylation during the Early Stages of Adipocyte Differentiation in 3T3-L1 Cells. *BMC Complement. Altern. Med.* **2013**, *13*, 207. [CrossRef]
16. Yong, R.; Chen, X.-M.; Shen, S.; Vijayaraj, S.; Ma, Q.; Pollock, C.A.; Saad, S. Plumbagin Ameliorates Diabetic Nephropathy via Interruption of Pathways That Include NOX4 Signalling. *PLoS ONE* **2013**, *8*, e73428. [CrossRef] [PubMed]
17. Shah, M.A.; Reanmongkol, W.; Radenahmad, N.; Khalil, R.; Ul-Haq, Z.; Panichayupakaranant, P. Anti-Hyperglycemic and Anti-Hyperlipidemic Effects of Rhinacanthins-Rich Extract from *Rhinacanthus nasutus* Leaves in Nicotinamide-Streptozotocin Induced Diabetic Rats. *Biomed. Pharmacother.* **2019**, *113*, 108702. [CrossRef]

18. Oda, Y.; Nakashima, S.; Kondo, E.; Nakamura, S.; Yano, M.; Kubota, C.; Masumoto, Y.; Hirao, M.; Ogawa, Y.; Matsuda, H. Comparison of Lawsone Contents among *Lawsonia inermis* Plant Parts and Neurite Outgrowth Accelerators from Branches. *J. Nat. Med.* **2018**, *72*, 890–896. [CrossRef]
19. Khan, M.; Shah, M.A.; Bibi, S.; Panichayupakaranant, P. Inhibitory effects of lawsone methyl ether and lawsone and their synergistic interactions with acarbose against α-glucosidase: In silico and in vitro studies. In Proceedings of the 7th Current Drug Development International Conference 2023 & 1st World Kratom Conference (CDD2023 & WKC2023), Phuket, Thailand, 22–25 August 2023.
20. Meah, M.S.; Lertcanawanichakul, M.; Pedpradab, P.; Lin, W.; Zhu, K.; Li, G.; Panichayupakaranant, P. Synergistic Effect on Anti-Methicillin-Resistant *Staphylococcus aureus* among Combinations of α-Mangostin-Rich Extract, Lawsone Methyl Ether and Ampicillin. *Lett. Appl. Microbiol.* **2020**, *71*, 510–519. [CrossRef] [PubMed]
21. Yoo, S.; Ahn, H.; Park, Y.K. High Dietary Fructose Intake on Cardiovascular Disease Related Parameters in Growing Rats. *Nutrients* **2016**, *9*, 11. [CrossRef]
22. Shirwaikar, A.; Rajendran, K.; Barik, R. Effect of Aqueous Bark Extract of *Garuga pinnata* Roxb. in Streptozotocin-Nicotinamide Induced Type-II Diabetes Mellitus. *J. Ethnopharmacol.* **2006**, *107*, 285–290. [CrossRef]
23. Alotaibi, M.R.; Fatani, A.J.; Almnaizel, A.T.; Ahmed, M.M.; Abuohashish, H.M.; Al-Rejaie, S.S. In Vivo Assessment of Combined Effects of Glibenclamide and Losartan in Diabetic Rats. *Med. Princ. Pract.* **2019**, *28*, 178–185. [CrossRef] [PubMed]
24. Elmalí, E.; Altan, N.; Bukan, N. Effect of the Sulphonylurea Glibenclamide on Liver and Kidney Antioxidant Enzymes in Streptozocin-Induced Diabetic Rats. *Drugs R D* **2004**, *5*, 203–208. [CrossRef]
25. Matthews, D.R.; Hosker, J.P.; Rudenski, A.S.; Naylor, B.A.; Treacher, D.F.; Turner, R.C. Homeostasis Model Assessment: Insulin Resistance and β-Cell Function from Fasting Plasma Glucose and Insulin Concentrations in Man. *Diabetologia* **1985**, *28*, 412–419. [CrossRef]
26. Elangovan, A.; Subramanian, A.; Durairaj, S.; Ramachandran, J.; Lakshmanan, D.K.; Ravichandran, G.; Nambirajan, G.; Thilagar, S. Antidiabetic and Hypolipidemic Efficacy of Skin and Seed Extracts of *Momordica cymbalaria* on Alloxan Induced Diabetic Model in Rats. *J. Ethnopharmacol.* **2019**, *241*, 111989. [CrossRef]
27. OECD Test No. 423; Acute Oral Toxicity—Acute Toxic Class Method. Organisation for Economic Co-Operation and Development: Paris, France, 2002.
28. Hartmann, E.; Strauss, V.; Eiben, R.; Freyberger, A.; Kaufmann, W.; Loof, I.; Reissmueller, E.; Rinke, M.; Ruehl-Fehlert, C.; Schorsch, F. ESTP Comments on the Draft Updated OECD Test Guideline 407. *Exp. Toxicol. Pathol.* **2008**, *59*, 297–300. [CrossRef] [PubMed]
29. Vessby, B.; Uusitupa, M.; Hermansen, K.; Riccardi, G.; Rivellese, A.A.; Tapsell, L.C.; Nälsén, C.; Berglund, L.; Louheranta, A.; Rasmussen, B.M. Substituting Dietary Saturated for Monounsaturated Fat Impairs Insulin Sensitivity in Healthy Men and Women: The KANWU Study. *Diabetologia* **2001**, *44*, 312–319. [CrossRef]
30. Risérus, U.; Willett, W.C.; Hu, F.B. Dietary Fats and Prevention of Type 2 Diabetes. *Prog. Lipid Res.* **2009**, *48*, 44–51. [CrossRef]
31. Isken, F.; Klaus, S.; Petzke, K.-J.; Loddenkemper, C.; Pfeiffer, A.F.; Weickert, M.O. Impairment of Fat Oxidation under High-vs. Low-Glycemic Index Diet Occurs before the Development of an Obese Phenotype. *Am. J. Physiol.-Endocrinol. Metab.* **2010**, *298*, E287–E295. [CrossRef] [PubMed]
32. Cloete, L. Diabetes Mellitus: An Overview of the Types, Symptoms, Complications and Management. *Nurs. Stand. R. Coll. Nurs. Great Br.* **2021**, *37*, 61–66. [CrossRef]
33. Frier, B.C.; Noble, E.G.; Locke, M. Diabetes-Induced Atrophy Is Associated with a Muscle-Specific Alteration in NF-κB Activation and Expression. *Cell Stress Chaperones* **2008**, *13*, 287–296. [CrossRef]
34. Lenzen, S. The Mechanisms of Alloxan-and Streptozotocin-Induced Diabetes. *Diabetologia* **2008**, *51*, 216–226. [CrossRef]
35. Reanmongkol, W.; Subhadhirasakul, S.; Panichayupakaranant, P.; Kim, K.-M. Anti-Allergic and Antioxidative Activities of Some Compounds from Thai Medicinal Plants. *Pharm. Biol.* **2003**, *41*, 592–597. [CrossRef]
36. Alqahtani, N.; Khan, W.; Alhumaidi, M.; Ahmed, Y.A. Use of Glycated Hemoglobin in the Diagnosis of Diabetes Mellitus and Pre-Diabetes and Role of Fasting Plasma Glucose, Oral Glucose Tolerance Test. *Int. J. Prev. Med.* **2013**, *4*, 1025.
37. Chinchansure, A.A.; Korwar, A.M.; Kulkarni, M.J.; Joshi, S.P. Recent Development of Plant Products with Anti-Glycation Activity: A Review. *RSC Adv.* **2015**, *5*, 31113–31138. [CrossRef]
38. Basit, A.; Riaz, M.; Fawwad, A. Glimepiride: Evidence-Based Facts, Trends, and Observations. *Vasc. Health Risk Manag.* **2012**, *8*, 463–472. [CrossRef] [PubMed]
39. Mahmood, N. A Review on Insulin-Producing Beta Cell: Regenerative Role of Drugs Acting on DYRK1A, GLP-1 and DPP-4 Receptors. Ph.D. Thesis, Brac University, Dhaka, Bangladesh, 2021.
40. Kaur, N.; Kishore, L.; Singh, R. Attenuating Diabetes: What Really Works? *Curr. Diabetes Rev.* **2016**, *12*, 259–278. [CrossRef] [PubMed]
41. Bosenberg, L.H.; Van Zyl, D.G. The Mechanism of Action of Oral Antidiabetic Drugs: A Review of Recent Literature. *J. Endocrinol. Metab. Diabetes S. Afr.* **2008**, *13*, 80–88. [CrossRef]
42. Ghasemi, A.; Tohidi, M.; Derakhshan, A.; Hasheminia, M.; Azizi, F.; Hadaegh, F. Cut-off Points of Homeostasis Model Assessment of Insulin Resistance, Beta-Cell Function, and Fasting Serum Insulin to Identify Future Type 2 Diabetes: Tehran Lipid and Glucose Study. *Acta Diabetol.* **2015**, *52*, 905–915. [CrossRef]

43. Paneni, F.; Costantino, S.; Cosentino, F. Insulin Resistance, Diabetes, and Cardiovascular Risk. *Curr. Atheroscler. Rep.* **2014**, *16*, 419. [CrossRef]
44. Schofield, J.D.; Liu, Y.; Rao-Balakrishna, P.; Malik, R.A.; Soran, H. Diabetes Dyslipidemia. *Diabetes Ther.* **2016**, *7*, 203–219. [CrossRef]
45. Rafieian-Kopaei, M.; Setorki, M.; Doudi, M.; Baradaran, A.; Nasri, H. Atherosclerosis: Process, Indicators, Risk Factors and New Hopes. *Int. J. Prev. Med.* **2014**, *5*, 927.
46. Eidi, A.; Mortazavi, P.; Bazargan, M.; Zaringhalam, J. Hepatoprotective Activity of Cinnamon Ethanolic Extract against CCl4-Induced Liver Injury in Rats. *Excli J.* **2012**, *11*, 495.
47. Darvin, S.S.; Esakkimuthu, S.; Toppo, E.; Balakrishna, K.; Paulraj, M.G.; Pandikumar, P.; Ignacimuthu, S.; Al-Dhabi, N.A. Hepatoprotective Effect of Lawsone on Rifampicin-Isoniazid Induced Hepatotoxicity in in vitro and in vivo Models. *Environ. Toxicol. Pharmacol.* **2018**, *61*, 87–94. [CrossRef]
48. Cade, W.T. Diabetes-Related Microvascular and Macrovascular Diseases in the Physical Therapy Setting. *Phys. Ther.* **2008**, *88*, 1322–1335. [CrossRef]
49. Ikewuchi, C.C.; Ikewuchi, J.C.; Ifeanacho, M.O. Restoration of Plasma Markers of Liver and Kidney Functions/Integrity in Alloxan-Induced Diabetic Rabbits by Aqueous Extract of *Pleurotus tuberregium* Sclerotia. *Biomed. Pharmacother.* **2017**, *95*, 1809–1814. [CrossRef] [PubMed]
50. Zhao, L.-L.; Makinde, E.A.; Shah, M.A.; Olatunji, O.J.; Panichayupakaranant, P. Rhinacanthins-Rich Extract and Rhinacanthin C Ameliorate Oxidative Stress and Inflammation in Streptozotocin-Nicotinamide-Induced Diabetic Nephropathy. *J. Food Biochem.* **2019**, *43*, e12812. [CrossRef] [PubMed]

Disclaimer/Publisher's Note: The statements, opinions and data contained in all publications are solely those of the individual author(s) and contributor(s) and not of MDPI and/or the editor(s). MDPI and/or the editor(s) disclaim responsibility for any injury to people or property resulting from any ideas, methods, instructions or products referred to in the content.

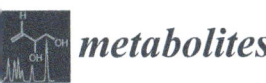

Article

The Beneficial Effect of Swimming Training Associated with Quercetin Administration on the Endothelial Nitric Oxide-Dependent Relaxation in the Aorta of Rats with Experimentally Induced Type 1 Diabetes Mellitus

Irina-Camelia Chis [1,†], Carmen-Maria Micu [2,†], Alina Toader [1], Remus Moldovan [1], Laura Lele [3], Simona Clichici [1,*] and Daniela-Rodica Mitrea [1]

1. Department of Physiology, Iuliu Hatieganu University of Medicine and Pharmacy, 1-3 Clinicilor Street, 400006 Cluj-Napoca, Cluj County, Romania; ichis@umfcluj.ro (I.-C.C.); toader.alina@umfcluj.ro (A.T.); moldovan.remus@umfcluj.ro (R.M.); rdmitrea@gmail.com (D.-R.M.)
2. Department of Anatomy and Embryology, Iuliu Hatieganu University of Medicine and Pharmacy, 3-5 Clinicilor Street, 400006 Cluj-Napoca, Cluj County, Romania; carmen.micu@umfcluj.ro
3. Department of Medical Disciplines, Faculty of Medicine and Pharmacy, University of Oradea, 10 1 Decembrie Street, 410073 Oradea, Bihor County, Romania; dr.laura.lele@gmail.com
* Correspondence: sclichici@umfcluj.ro
† These authors contributed equally to this work.

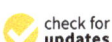

Citation: Chis, I.-C.; Micu, C.-M.; Toader, A.; Moldovan, R.; Lele, L.; Clichici, S.; Mitrea, D.-R. The Beneficial Effect of Swimming Training Associated with Quercetin Administration on the Endothelial Nitric Oxide-Dependent Relaxation in the Aorta of Rats with Experimentally Induced Type 1 Diabetes Mellitus. *Metabolites* **2023**, *13*, 586. https://doi.org/10.3390/metabo13050586

Academic Editors: Cosmin Mihai Vesa and Dana Zaha

Received: 2 April 2023
Revised: 19 April 2023
Accepted: 23 April 2023
Published: 24 April 2023

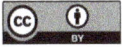

Copyright: © 2023 by the authors. Licensee MDPI, Basel, Switzerland. This article is an open access article distributed under the terms and conditions of the Creative Commons Attribution (CC BY) license (https://creativecommons.org/licenses/by/4.0/).

Abstract: Type 1 diabetes mellitus is related to the vascular oxidative and nitrosative stress, the trigger for atherosclerosis and cardiovascular complications. The effects of moderate swimming training associated with quercetin oral administration were evaluated in aorta of rats with experimentally induced type 1 diabetes mellitus (T1DM), by analysing the nitric oxide-endothelial dependent relaxation (NO-EDR). T1DM rats received daily quercetin 30 mg/kg and followed the protocol of 5-weeks swimming exercise (30 min/day; 5 days/week). Aorta relaxation to acetylcholine (Ach) and sodium nitroprusside (SNP) were measured at the end of the experiment. Ach-induced endothelial dependent relaxation was significantly decreased in phenylephrine (PE) pre-contracted aorta of diabetic rats. Swimming exercise with quercetin administration preserved Ach-induced EDR but did not have any impact on SNP-induced endothelium-independent relaxation in the diabetic aorta. These findings suggest that quercetin administration associated with moderate swimming exercise could improve the endothelial NO-dependent relaxation in the aorta of rats with experimentally induced type 1 diabetes mellitus, showing that this therapeutic combination may improve and even prevent the vascular complications that occur in diabetic patients.

Keywords: acetylcholine; endothelium; diabetes; quercetin; moderate swimming training; aorta

1. Introduction

The endothelial dysfunction (ED) that occurs in type 1 diabetes mellitus (T1DM) involves numerous and diverse pathogenetic mechanisms including inflammation, hyperglycaemia, production of reactive oxygen species (ROS) and of reactive nitrogen species (RNS), the decrease of nitric oxide (NO) availability or dyslipidemia [1–9]. Endothelial dysfunction is characterised by altered endothelial-dependent relaxation (EDR) produced by the decreased NO levels in the vessel wall [8–10], a process that leads to micro- and macrovascular complications, increasing significantly the morbidity and mortality in T1DM [1].

Endothelial dysfunction decreases the EDR to vasorelaxant substances like acetylcholine (Ach) and represents a preliminary phase in the development of vascular alterations. ED development is based on oxidative stress and ROS production, especially of the superoxide anion, which has an important role in NO scavenging.

The moderate training physical effort enhances the insulin sensitivity and the carbohydrates metabolism in T1DM. Several recent studies made on T1DM presented the ameliorated endothelial dysfunction and the improved EDR after moderate exercise training that decreased the inflammation, the ROS/RNS production, and increased NO levels in vessel walls [4,6,11–14]. The type of the performed physical effort and its duration were correlated with the training efficacy in T1DM [11], the favourable effects in EDR enhancement and on the oxidative/nitrosative stress being recorded only after moderate exercise training [15] while the strenuous training intensified the ROS production [11,15].

Numerous studies present the flavonoids like potent natural antioxidants in diabetes mellitus, preventing the cardiovascular complications [16,17].

Quercetin is a flavonol of plant origin found in numerous vegetables and fruits like onion, tea, grapes, apple, berries, etc. [18]. Quercetin presents beneficial effects: antioxidant, hypoglycaemic, vasodilator, anti-inflammatory, antiapoptotic, anti-atherogenic, hypolipidemic, etc. [18–24]. It is a flavonol that protects the function and the viability of β-pancreatic cells against oxidative stress and may stimulate the insulin secretion regenerating the islets of Langerhans [25]. Quercetin is an efficient antioxidant, being able to scavenge directly the ROS and to increase the endogenous antioxidants [18,21]; it may improve the endothelial function in hyperglycaemic conditions through its vasodilator endothelium-dependent effects, protecting the eNOS levels, decreasing the iNOS and enhancing the NO bioavailability [4,21,26].

In the present study, the effects on endothelium dysfunction of moderate exercise training associated with quercetin administration in an experimentally induced type 1 diabetes mellitus were investigated. Since the Ach-induced EDR was affected in aorta at 6 weeks after diabetes mellitus development, the authors hypothesised that moderate swimming training associated with oral administration of quercetin may restore the EDR.

2. Material and Methods

2.1. Drugs and Chemicals

Streptozotocin (STZ), phenylephrine (PE), indomethacin (IND), acetylcholine chloride (Ach), sodium nitroprusside (SNP), and quercetin (Que) were all obtained from Sigma-Aldrich Chemical Company Inc. (Gillingham, Dorset, UK). Streptozotocin was freshly dissolved in citrate sodium buffer (0.1 mol/L, pH 4.5) and maintained on ice before being used. Quercetin was suspended in 0.5% carboxymethyl cellulose (CMC) solution as a vehicle.

2.2. Equipment

Biopac MP150, modular tissue baths DA 100C, UgoBasile, Trappe, PA, USA was used to analyse the aorta rings responses at different solutions.

2.3. Procedure

The study was realised in the Physiology Department of Iuliu Hatieganu University of Medicine and Pharmacy Cluj-Napoca Romania, with the approval of Ethical Committee on Animal Welfare (No. 44/13.03.2017) of A.N.S.V.S.A. (The National Sanitary Veterinary and Food Safety Authority) and following the Guidelines in the Use of Animals in Toxicology.

2.3.1. Experimental Protocol

Male albino Wistar rats, with ages of three months, weights between 260 and 310 g, were purchased from the Biobase of Iuliu Hatieganu University of Medicine and Pharmacy, Cluj-Napoca, Romania. The animals were fed with a standard diet, water ad libitum, and were kept in standard conditions (22 ± 2 °C, 45–50% relative humidity) with a day–night cycle of 12 h.

For induction of type 1 diabetes mellitus, streptozotocin (STZ) 60 mg/kg intraperitoneal single injection was used. Carboxymethyl cellulose was used for streptozotocin solution [4,20,27]. After 96 h post-injection, all the rats developed T1DM which was confirmed through the fasting blood glucose levels that were above 250 mg/dL (13.89 mmol/L). After 7 days from the T1DM development, exercise training was started in association with quercetin (Que) administration (30 mg/kg body weight/day/5 weeks. The animals from the control group received carboxymethyl cellulose (CMC) 0.6 mL/day for 5 weeks.

The animals were randomly allocated into four control groups (N = 10): Group S-sedentary, untreated animals; Group T-trained, untreated animals; Group SQ-sedentary animals, treated with quercetin; Group TQ-trained animals, treated with quercetin (Figure 1); and into four experimental diabetic groups: Group DS-diabetic, sedentary, untreated animals; Group DT-diabetic, trained, untreated animals; Group DSQ-diabetic, sedentary animals, treated with quercetin; and Group DTQ-diabetic, trained animals, treated with quercetin (Figure 2).

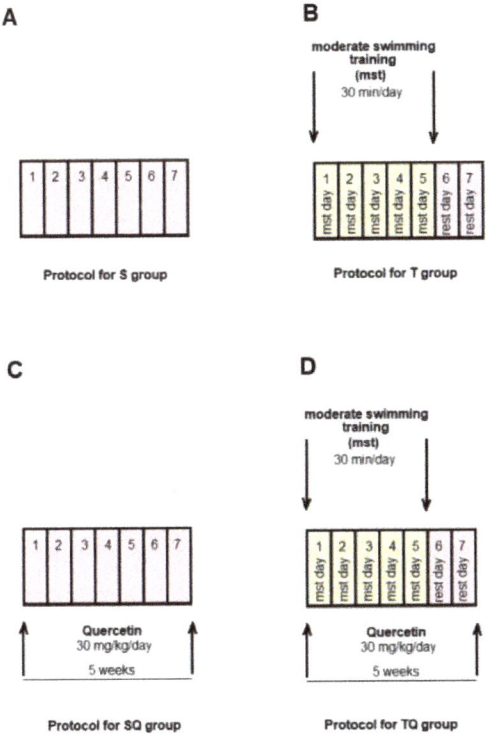

Figure 1. The time course of scheduled experiment for the groups of rats without T1DM: (**A**) healthy sedentary rats (S group); (**B**) healthy trained rats, 30 min/day, 5 days/week for 5 weeks (T group); (**C**) healthy sedentary rats treated with quercetin 30 mg/kg/day, for 5 weeks (SQ group); (**D**) healthy trained rats, 30 min/day, 5 days/week and treated with quercetin 30 mg/kg/day, for 5 weeks (TQ group).

At the end of the experiment, after the last night with food deprivation, the glycaemia was measured from retro-orbital venous plexus with the ACCU-CHEK Sensor System from Roche Diagnostics GmbH (Mannheim, Germany). Deep anaesthesia of all the rats was realised with ketamine 10% (5 mg/100 gbw) and xylazine hydroxychloride 2% (100 mg/100 gbw), to collect the samples of thoracic aorta while the connective tissue was removed.

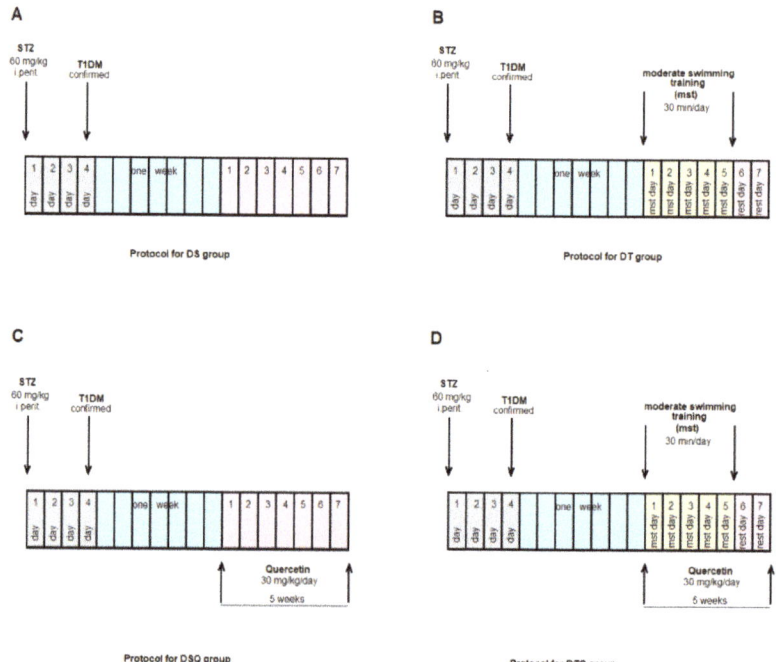

Figure 2. The time course of scheduled experiment for the groups of rats with T1DM: (**A**) diabetic sedentary rats (DS group); (**B**) diabetic trained rats, 30 min/day, 5 days/week for 5 weeks (DT group); (**C**) diabetic sedentary rats treated with quercetin 30 mg/kg/day, for 5 weeks (DSQ group); (**D**) diabetic trained rats, 30 min/day, 5 days/week and treated with quercetin 30 mg/kg/day, for 5 weeks (DTQ group).

2.3.2. Moderate Swimming Training Protocol

The rats were trained through a moderate swimming exercise inside a cylindrical tank (60/100/45 cm) at a temperature maintained constantly at 36 °C. The swimming exercise was performed for 30 min/day, 5 days/week, for 5 weeks [4,28–30].

2.3.3. Preparation of Aortic Tissue and Measurement of Isometric Force

Thoracic aorta fragments between aortic arch and diaphragm were taken and inserted in ice-cold, oxygenated, modified Krebs–Henseleit solution (KHS) that consisted of (in mM) 118 NaCl; 25.0 NaHCO$_3$; 4.7 KCl; 1.6 CaCl$_2$; 1.2 KH$_2$PO$_4$; 1.2 MgSO$_4$ and 11.1 Glucose. Thoracic aortas were segmented into fragments of 2–2.5 mm width. The aorta rings were placed between stainless steel triangles into individual tissue bath (Tissue Bath Station: for baths of 20 mL with MP150 Data Acquisition System-BIOPAC System Inc., Goleta, CA, USA), with oxygenated (95% O$_2$, 5% CO$_2$) modified KHS (37 °C, pH 7.4), one end connected to a tissue holder and the other to a force-displacement transducer (Isometric Force Transducers-BIOPAC System Inc., USA).

To evaluate the endothelial dysfunction, isolated vessel in tissue bath was performed using the experimental protocol for endothelial vasomotor response, and to analyse the vascular reactivity, cumulative doses of vasodilator agents were used. In the tissue bath, indomethacin (10^{-5} M) was added to inhibit the prostaglandin release. The aorta samples were maintained for 60 min at 1.5–2 g resting tension (the optimal tension obtained through prior experiments) with KHS solution changed every 20 min.

The viability of the aorta smooth muscle was evaluated before the beginning of the vessel reactivity test by achieving two similar contractile responses at KCl, 80 mM/L, the contraction to KCl representing the standard of maximum contraction. The response through contraction to PE must be 80–100% from the KCl contraction.

The vasodilator response to Ach (10^{-5} M) above 10–15% of the contraction produced by KCl ensures the viability of the endothelium.

2.3.4. Testing Phase: The Evaluation of Phenylephrine (PE), Acetylcholine (Ach), and Sodium Nitroprusside (SNP) Effects on Aorta Rings

The endothelial integrity was established, and then, the aorta rings were precontracted with phenylephrine (PE), an α_1-adrenergic agonist, in increasing concentrations (10^{-9} to 10^{-6} M) in organ bath, until a stable plateau of the vessel smooth muscle tension was obtained. For all the investigated aorta rings, vasoconstrictor substance was added in cumulative concentrations inside the organ bath. The percentage of the KCl contraction was used to express the contractile response to PE. This test was done to investigate the maximum contraction of the aorta rings.

To evaluate the maximum endothelium-dependent relaxation of rats' aortas, the aorta rings were pre-contracted with PE before being exposed to the cumulative concentrations of acetylcholine (10^{-9} to 10^{-5} M), an endothelium-dependent vasorelaxant. Subsequently, the aorta rings were washed with Krebs solution and then pre-contracted with a similar concentration of PE, before being treated with cumulative concentrations of SNP (10^{-11} to 10^{-6} M), an endothelium-independent vasorelaxant. This test was done to investigate the maximum endothelial-independent relaxation in the rats' thoracic aortas.

2.3.5. Statistical Analysis

The precontraction PE-induced was expressed as dose–response assessment calculated as percentage of contraction produced by high KCl solution/mg tissue weight against PE concentration (logarithmic scale). For the relaxation Ach-induced, the dose–response curves were obtained as a percentage of PE (0.1 µM) contraction/mg tissue weight against Ach concentration (logarithmic scale), while for the relaxation SNP-induced, the dose–response graphs were calculated as percentage of PE (0.1 µM) contraction/mg tissue weight against SNP concentration (logarithmic scale).

The relaxation, Ach- and SNP-induced, was calculated at every concentration as the percentage of relaxation from the maximum PE contraction. The contraction force was calculated as a percentage of maximum contraction at the highest dose of PE.

The statistical interpretation of the data was realised using Two-way ANOVA followed by the Post-test Bonferroni. The significance threshold was set at $p < 0.05$.

3. Results

3.1. Blood Glucose and Animal Body Weights in the Control and Experimental Groups

At the beginning of our study, all the rats had similar values of the fasting blood glucose (FBG) and of the body weights (BW). At 7 days after streptozotocin (STZ) administration, FBG levels increased significantly in diabetic groups (DS, DT, DSQ, DTQ), compared to the control groups (S, T, SQ, TQ). In comparison with DS group, moderate swimming training produced significant decreases of the FBG levels in DT group ($p < 0.05$), and when this type of exercise was associated with quercetin administration (DSQ group), a greater reduction ($p < 0.0001$) of this investigated parameter was recorded.

The body weights of rats did not present significant modifications among the groups, with one exception: sedentary diabetic rats (DS group) showed significant decreases ($p < 0.05$) compared to sedentary untreated control (S) group of rats (Table 1).

Table 1. The effects of moderate swimming training in association with quercetin on fasting blood glucose and body weights, in experimental groups.

Parameters	S	T	SQ	TQ	DS	DT	DSQ	DTQ
Initial FBG (mg/dL)	69.9 ± 2.23	68.4 ± 1.84	67.6.0 ± 4.6	67.4 ± 3.37	573.1 ± 45.35 aaa	542.8 ± 62.04 aaa	535.5 ± 35.63 aaa	523.0 ± 38.7 aaa
Final FBG (mg/dL)	72.0 ± 3.2	70.0 ± 2.6	69.8 ± 3.6	70.3 ± 2.75	583.1 ± 31.24 aaa	477.4 ± 44.2 b	380.5 ± 25.2 bbb	293.0 ± 38.0 bbb
Initial body weight (g)	271.5 ± 14.6	270.0 ± 16.9	281.4 ± 13.7	288.9 ± 12.9	273.5 ± 18.9	282.5 ± 18.49	279.8 ± 15.27	280.4 ± 18.3
Final body weight (g)	277.5 ± 13.9	265.5 ± 12.9	286.4 ± 11.8	290.0 ± 11.67	238.5 ± 10.34 a	270.9 ± 12.80	274.2 ± 11.03	276.4 ± 13.9

S = sedentary, untreated animals, T = trained, untreated animals, SQ = sedentary animals, treated with quercetin, TQ = trained animals, treated with quercetin, DS = diabetic, sedentary, untreated animals, DT = diabetic, trained, untreated animals, DSQ = diabetic, sedentary animals, treated with quercetin, DTQ = diabetic, trained animals, treated with quercetin. Results are mean ± SD of 10 rats per each group. Statistically significant differences are indicated by the symbols: [a] $p < 0.05$, [aaa] $p < 0.0001$ vs. S group; [b] $p < 0.05$, [bbb] $p < 0.0001$ vs. DS group.

3.2. Aortic Contractile Responses to Phenylephrine (PE) in Control and Experimental Groups

The responses of aorta rings to phenylephrine (PE) were investigated using cumulative doses (10^{-9} to 10^{-6} M). Sedentary diabetic rats (DS group) had significant increases of aorta rings contractile responses, compared to healthy sedentary (S group) or trained rats (T group) ($p < 0.001$), especially at PE between 3×10^{-7} and 10^{-6} M (not signalised in Figure 1 because of too many points of significance). The quercetin administration (DSQ group) or moderate swimming training associated with quercetin treatment (DTQ group) in diabetic rats decreased significantly ($p < 0.001$) the vessels' contraction, compared to sedentary diabetic rats (group DS), between the same concentrations of PE (3×10^{-7}–10^{-6} M) (Figure 3).

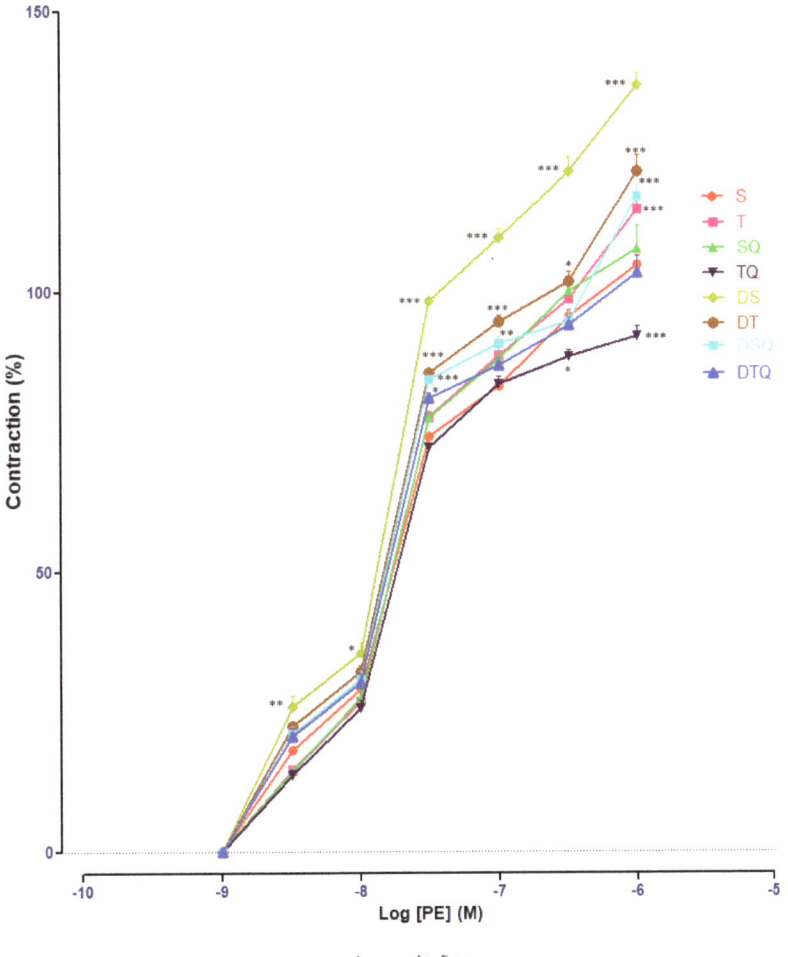

*compared to S group

Figure 3. The aorta rings contractile response to cumulative concentrations of phenylephrine (PE) (10^{-9}–10^{-6} M) in: sedentary, untreated animals (S); trained, untreated animals (T); sedentary animals, treated with quercetin (SQ); trained animals, treated with quercetin (TQ); diabetic, sedentary, untreated animals (DS); diabetic, trained, untreated animals (DT); diabetic, sedentary animals, treated with quercetin (DSQ) and in diabetic, trained animals, treated with quercetin (DTQ). Contraction was expressed as % of high KCl contraction. Values are expressed as mean ± SEM (* $p < 0.05$; ** $p < 0.01$; *** $p < 0.001$ compared to S group).

3.3. Aortic Relaxation Responses to Acetylcholine (Ach) in Control and Experimental Groups

To determine the effects of the moderate swimming training associated or not with quercetin administration on endothelium-dependent relaxation, acetylcholine (Ach) of different concentrations (10^{-9}–10^{-5} M) was used. The responses in the pre-contracted aorta rings of healthy and of diabetic rats were recorded. Figure 4 presents all the results of all the investigated groups; the numerous significant values are not marked on the graph but explained in the separated next images.

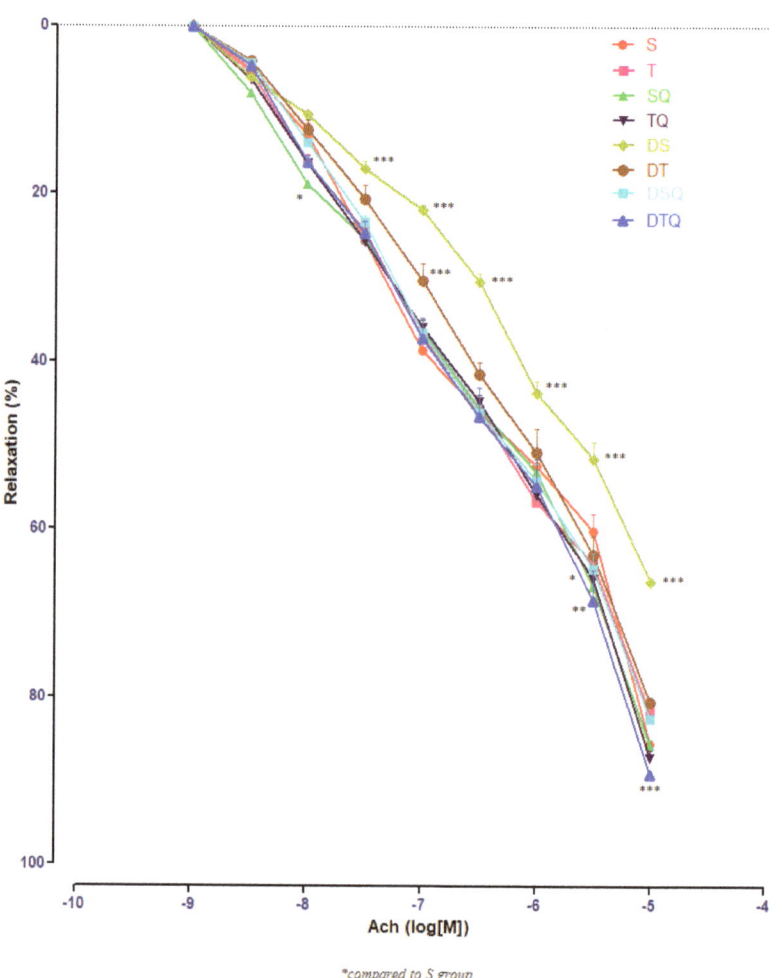

*compared to S group

Figure 4. The aorta rings relaxation responses to cumulative concentrations of acetylcholine (Ach) (10^{-9}–10^{-5} M) in: sedentary, untreated animals (S); trained, untreated animals (T); sedentary animals, treated with quercetin (SQ); trained animals, treated with quercetin (TQ); diabetic, sedentary, untreated animals (DS); diabetic, trained, untreated animals (DT); diabetic, sedentary animals, treated with quercetin (DSQ) and in diabetic, trained animals, treated with quercetin (DTQ). The relaxation responses are expressed as percentages of relaxation from an induced maximal contraction at PE. The values are expressed as mean ± SEM (* $p < 0.05$; ** $p < 0.01$; *** $p < 0.001$ compared to S group).

Sedentary diabetic rats (DS group) had the lowest relaxation along the experiment ($p < 0.001$), compared to the sedentary rats that received quercetin, healthy or with T1DM

(S, SQ and DSQ groups), especially at Ach concentrations between 3×10^{-7} and 10^{-5} M. Quercetin administration in healthy sedentary rats (SQ group) improved the vessel relaxation only at Ach concentration of 10^{-8} ($p < 0.01$) and of 3×10^{-5} M ($p < 0.001$), compared to the healthy rats that did not receive treatment (S group) (Figure 5).

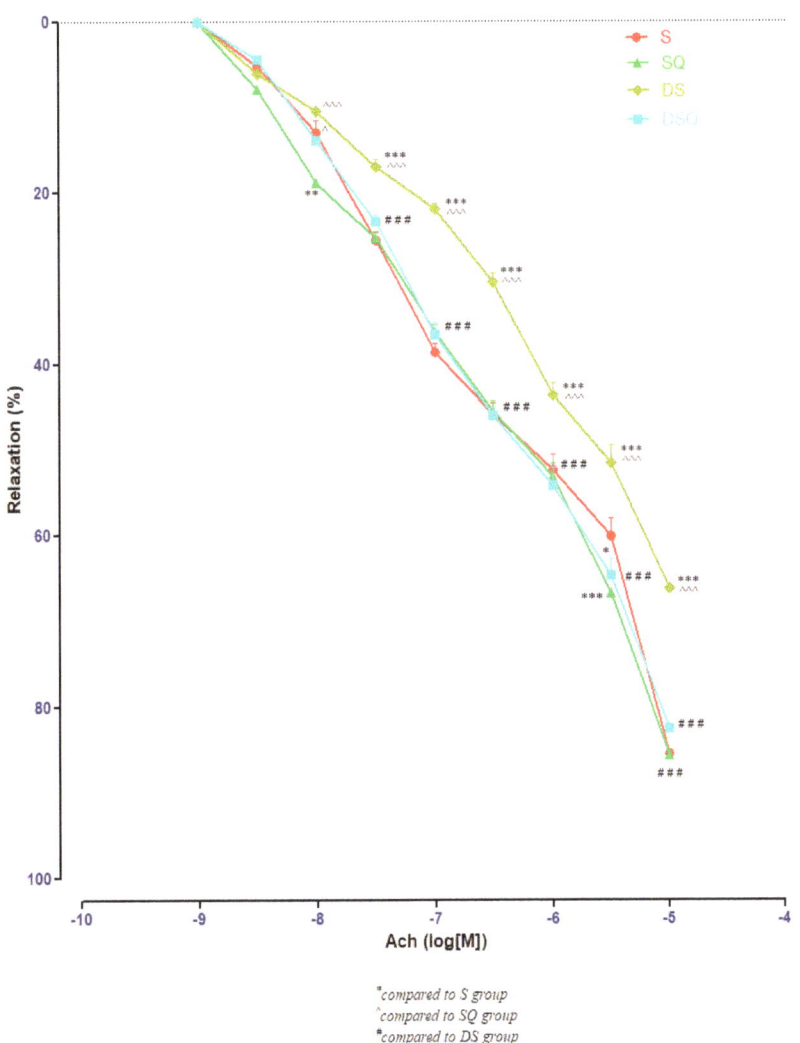

Figure 5. The aorta rings relaxation responses to cumulative concentrations of acetylcholine (Ach) (10^{-9}–10^{-5} M) in: sedentary, untreated animals (S); sedentary animals, treated with quercetin (SQ); diabetic, sedentary, untreated animals (DS); diabetic, sedentary animals, treated with quercetin (DSQ). The relaxation responses are expressed as percentages of relaxation from an induced maximal contraction at PE. The values are expressed as mean ± SEM (* $p < 0.05$, ** $p < 0.01$, *** $p < 0.001$ compared to S group; ^ $p < 0.05$, ^^^ $p < 0.001$ compared to SQ group; ### $p < 0.001$ compared to DS group).

Quercetin administration improved significantly the vessel relaxation in diabetic trained rats (DTQ group) at 10^{-7} M ($p < 0.05$) and at 10^{-5} M ($p < 0.001$) compared to diabetic trained animals (DT group), and at 10^{-5} M ($p < 0.01$) compared to the healthy trained rats (T group). In diabetic rats (DT group), moderate physical training produced similar aorta responses like in healthy animals (T group) with only one significant modification ($p < 0.05$) recorded at 10^{-7} M Ach concentration (Figure 6).

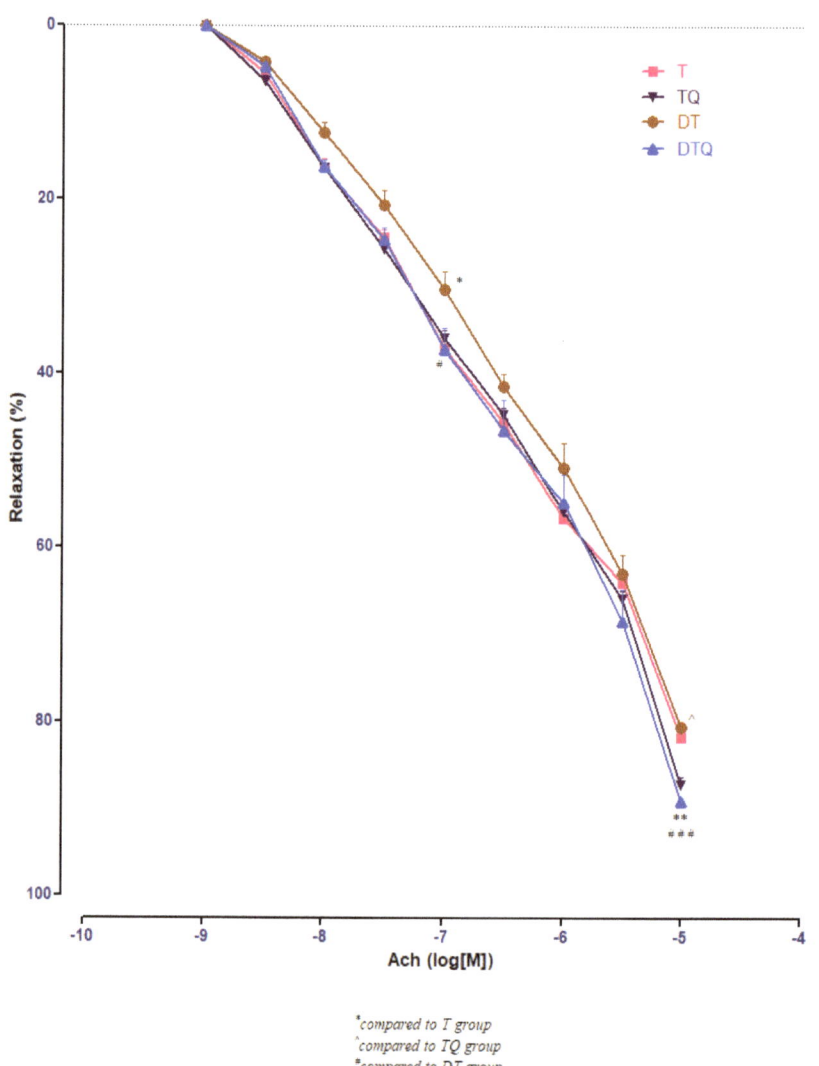

* compared to T group
^ compared to TQ group
# compared to DT group

Figure 6. The aorta rings relaxation responses to cumulative concentrations of acetylcholine (Ach) (10^{-9}–10^{-5} M) in: trained, untreated animals (T); trained animals, treated with quercetin (TQ); diabetic, trained, untreated animals (DT); diabetic, trained animals, treated with quercetin (DTQ). The relaxation responses are expressed as percentages of relaxation from an induced maximal contraction at PE. The values are expressed as mean ± SEM (* $p < 0.05$, ** $p < 0.01$ compared to T group; ^ $p < 0.05$ compared to TQ group; # $p < 0.05$; ### $p < 0.001$ compared to DT group).

In healthy rats, moderate swimming training did not modify significantly the aorta rings responses to Ach. In diabetic rats, compared to DS group, moderate physical training

(DT group) improved significantly ($p < 0.001$) the aorta relaxation at Ach, at concentrations between 10^{-7} and 10^{-5} M (Figure 7).

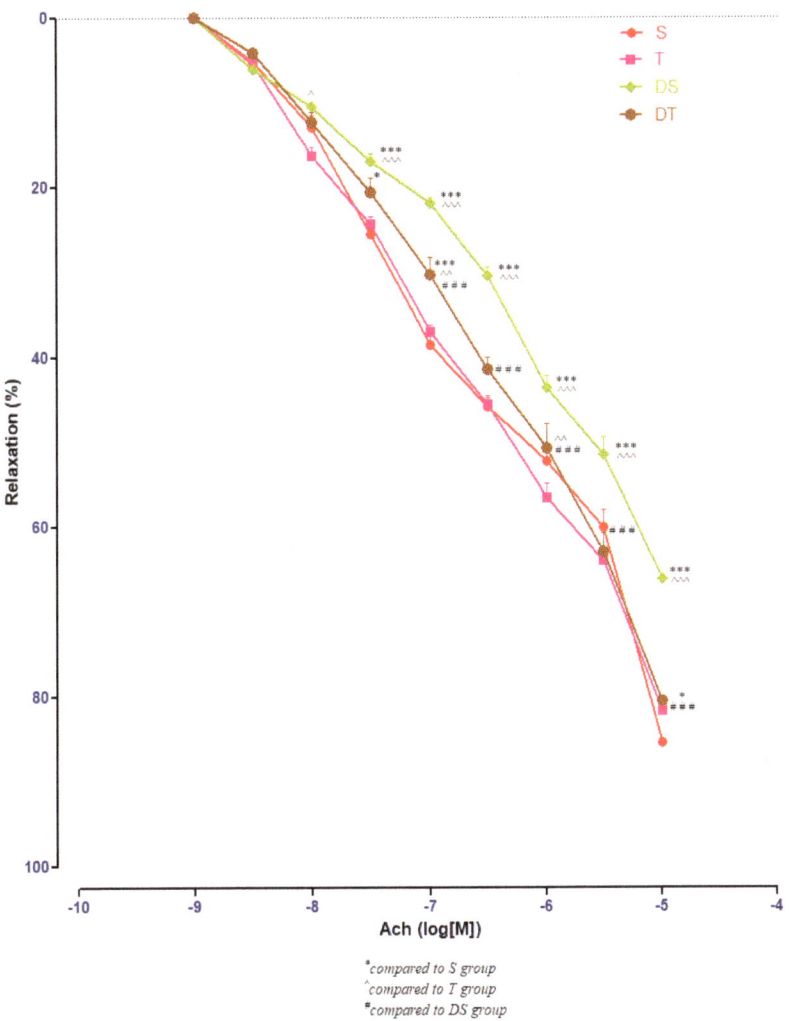

*compared to S group
^compared to T group
#compared to DS group

Figure 7. The aorta rings relaxation responses to cumulative concentrations of acetylcholine (Ach) (10^{-9}–10^{-5} M) in: sedentary, untreated animals (S); trained, untreated animals (T); diabetic, sedentary, untreated animals (DS); diabetic, trained, untreated animals (DT). The relaxation responses are expressed as percentages of relaxation from an induced maximal contraction at PE. The values are expressed as mean ± SEM (* $p < 0.05$, *** $p < 0.001$ compared to S group; ^ $p < 0.05$, ^^ $p < 0.01$, ^^^ $p < 0.001$ compared to T group; ### $p < 0.001$ compared to DS group).

3.4. Aortic Relaxation Responses to Sodium Nitroprusside (SNP) in Control and Experimental Groups

Moderate swimming training and quercetin effects were evaluated on endothelial-independent relaxation responses to sodium nitroprusside (SNP) (10^{-11} to 10^{-6} M), and not significant modifications were recorded among the investigated groups of rats (Figure 8).

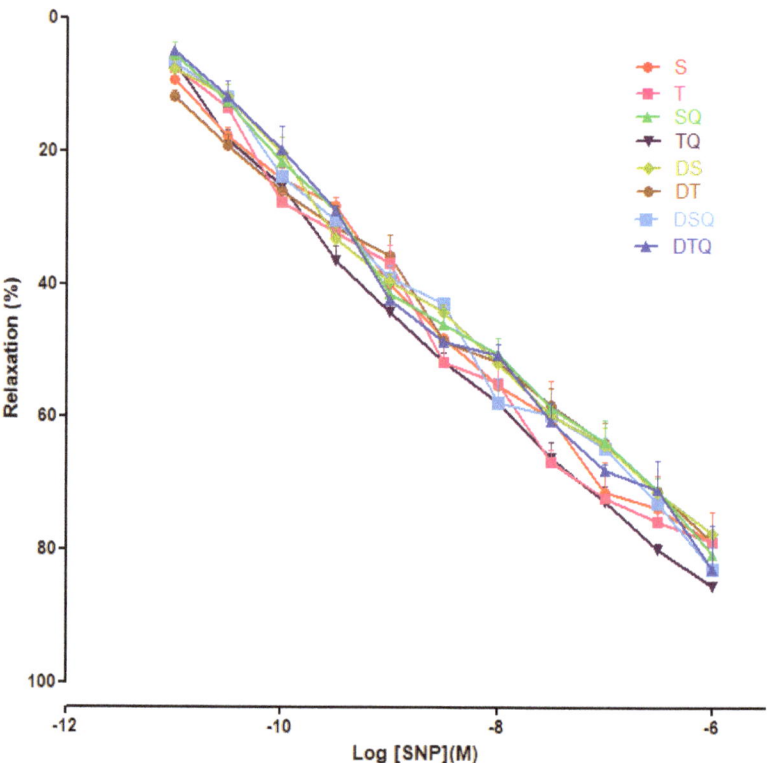

Figure 8. The relaxation responses of the aorta rings, precontracted with phenylephrine (PE), to cumulative concentrations of sodium nitroprusside (SNP 10^{-11} to 10^{-6} M) in: sedentary, untreated animals (S); trained, untreated animals (T); sedentary animals, treated with quercetin (SQ); trained animals, treated with quercetin (TQ); diabetic, sedentary, untreated animals (DS); diabetic, trained, untreated animals (DT); diabetic, sedentary animals, treated with quercetin (DSQ) and in diabetic, trained animals, treated with quercetin (DTQ). The relaxation responses are expressed as percentages of relaxation from an induced maximal contraction at PE. The values are expressed as mean ± SEM.

4. Discussion

Streptozotocin (STZ) intraperitoneal administration induces type 1 diabetes mellitus (T1DM), a metabolic disease characterised by significant increases of blood glucose levels associated with altered endothelial-dependent relaxation [31,32].

The present study showed that, in streptozotocin-induced diabetes mellitus rats, 5 weeks of moderate swimming training associated with quercetin administration significantly reduced the blood glucose levels and restored the endothelial function.

The patients with diabetes mellitus (DM) have a high risk of death because of cardiovascular diseases. The main risk factor involved in cardiovascular diseases development is represented by the endothelial dysfunction [1,7,33]. In T1DM, endothelial dysfunction may be produced by numerous factors including hyperglycaemia, dyslipidemia, decreases of NO bioavailability, insulin resistance or ROS increased synthesis [2,3,34]. Endothelial dysfunction is characterised by altered endothelial-dependent relaxation with satisfactory endothelial-independent vessel relaxation.

Hyperglycaemia produces endothelial dysfunction through NF-kB (nuclear factor-kB) activation. Therefore, the iNOS (inducible nitric oxide synthase) expression increases, leading to NO increased synthesis. Nitric oxide reacts with superoxide anion radical producing peroxynitrite, a strong oxidant with numerous noxious effects [7,33–35].

Streptozotocin is a natural compound produced by Streptomyces achromogenes that produces specific inflammation of pancreatic β-cells with the result of insulin absolute deficit [31,32]. In our experiment, fasting blood glucose (FBG) levels increased significantly after STZ administration. The results of our study showed that quercetin administration (30 mg/kg body weight/day/5 weeks) may produce significant decreases of glycaemia in T1DM. Recent studies revealed the mechanisms through which quercetin exerts its hypoglycaemic effects: it increases insulin sensitivity, inhibits α-glycosidase activity (in vitro), stimulates the hexokinase activity, increases the GLUT-4 (insulin-dependent glucose transporter) mRNA expression and this transporter translocation to the plasma membrane, and stimulates the glycogen production [21,36].

In the present study, the diabetic rats with moderate swimming training for 5 weeks showed significant decreased levels of FBG, in comparison with sedentary diabetic rats. These results are concordant to recent studies that presented the hypoglycaemic effects of moderate physical effort in diabetic rats [3,6,11,20,24,37]. The group of rats with DM and moderate swimming training treated with quercetin (DTQ group) showed a greater improvement of FBG levels, compared to the groups with only one approach: only training, or only quercetin treatment. Our results, in concordance with recent studies, may indicate the preservation of β-cells function and GLUT-4 expression as effects of quercetin and moderate swimming training which increase the glucose transport inside the cells [14,37].

In the present study, the vessel response to PE (α_1-adrenoreceptor agonist) in diabetic rats was investigated. The thoracic aorta rings were precontracted with PE in cumulative doses (10^{-9} to 10^{-6} M). The results of our study showed a significant increase of contractile response in aortas of sedentary diabetic rats, while the quercetin administration or moderate swimming training associated with quercetin treatment decreased significantly the vessels' contraction. These results may be the effects of endothelial impairment caused by hyperglycaemia, oxidative stress, NO decreased bioavailability, increased synthesis of superoxide anion and dyslipidemia. In our previous study [4], we observed the increased production of ROS, nitrites, and iNOS in diabetic rats' aortas. In the present study, quercetin administration decreased significantly the levels of mentioned parameters in aorta of diabetic rats while the association of quercetin treatment with moderate physical training had the best effects.

Acetylcholine produces the relaxation of the vessel smooth muscle layer through an endothelium-dependent mechanism by increasing the synthesis and release of vasodilator substances from this layer, including the NO and prostacyclin. Several studies showed the overreaction to Ach of the diabetic vessels in rats [33–36], but in our study the diabetic aortas' response to this neurotransmitter was decreased. The group of rats with DM and moderate swimming training had an improved vascular function. The sedentary and trained diabetic rats treated with quercetin presented an EDR restoring to acetylcholine. These results may be produced in diabetic rats by hyperglycaemia, reduced insulin level in plasma, and by the decrease of NO bioavailability from endothelial cells while the quercetin administration, with or without moderate physical effort training, blocked the NO oxidative inactivation by the superoxide anion. Our findings suggest that quercetin may have antioxidant properties, acting directly on ROS in aorta wall. Recent studies performed on diabetic thoracic aorta showed that endothelial dysfunction is partially determined by the decreased NO release and bioavailability, and by the altered signalling cascades post-NO release from the endothelial cells [36]. Hyperglycaemia induces vessel lesions through different mechanisms including the increase of ROS synthesis, production of advanced glycation end products (AGEs), activation of polyol pathway, and apoptosis. The high levels of plasma glucose increase significantly the ROS synthesis in endothelial cells but also in smooth muscle cells through glucose auto-oxidation, NO decreased synthesis, NO inactivation in a high rate and the increase of PCK activity [37].

The mechanisms through which the moderate physical training re-establish the endothelial function in T1DM are still not completely understood. It is presumed that the beneficial effects of moderate exercise training may be produced by the increase of blood flow that increases the shear stress on the endothelium leading to the increased NOS activity and NO bioavailability [4,38]. Moderate exercise training decreases the oxidative stress and the expression of the proinflammatory molecules [38], both mechanisms being considered trigger factors for the endothelial dysfunction, and it also re-establishes the function of the endothelial progenitor cells, promoting the endothelium repair and angiogenesis [38].

Quercetin, a flavonoid found in vegetables and fruits, has numerous favourable effects on health. In diabetes mellitus type 1, quercetin has hypoglycaemic effects through the increase of glucose intracellular transport and glycogen synthesis, decrease of insulin resistance, activation of enzymes involved in glucose metabolism, inhibition of apoptosis and damages through oxidative stress of the β-pancreatic cells, repair of these insulin secreting cells, etc. [39]. Quercetin has antioxidant effects in DM, scavenges the ROS, and also ensures anti-inflammatory and antiapoptotic protection participating in different protective mechanisms [36,39]. The results of the present study related to the quercetin properties in endothelial function recovery are concordant with recent literature data [4,6,36,39].

In our study, SNP (NO donor) did not modify significantly the aorta rings responses, among the groups.

5. Conclusions

Moderate swimming training associated with quercetin administration had hypoglycaemic effects and recovered the aorta reactivity to vasoconstrictor and vasodilator substances in streptozotocin-induced diabetes mellitus, this combination showing better results than their individual effects. The results of our study present the value of combined moderate physical training with quercetin administration in the management of diabetes mellitus type 1.

Author Contributions: Conceptualization, I.-C.C., C.-M.M., S.C. and D.-R.M.; methodology, I.-C.C., C.-M.M. and R.M.; software, D.-R.M.; validation, I.-C.C., C.-M.M. and D.-R.M.; formal analysis, I.-C.C., C.-M.M. and R.M.; investigation, A.T., R.M. and L.L.; resources, R.M. and S.C.; data curation, I.-C.C., C.-M.M., D.-R.M. and R.M; writing—original draft preparation, I.-C.C., C.-M.M. and D.-R.M.; writing—review and editing, I.-C.C., C.-M.M. and D-R.M; visualization, D.-R.M.; supervision, I.-C.C., C.-M.M., S.C. and D.-R.M.; project administration, A.T., R.M and L.L.; funding acquisition I.-C.C., C.-M.M. and S.C. All authors have read and agreed to the published version of the manuscript.

Funding: This research received no external funding.

Institutional Review Board Statement: The animal study protocol was approved by Ethical Committee on Animal Welfare (No.44/13.03.2017) of A.N.S.V.S.A. (The National Sanitary Veterinary and Food Safety Authority).

Informed Consent Statement: Not applicable.

Data Availability Statement: Data is contained within the article.

Conflicts of Interest: The authors declare no conflict of interest.

References

1. Paneni, F.; Beckman, J.A.; Creager, M.A.; Cosentino, F. Diabetes and vascular disease: Pathophysiology, clinical consequences, and medical therapy: Part I. *Eur. Heart J.* **2013**, *34*, 2436–2443. [CrossRef] [PubMed]
2. Tiwari, B.K.; Pandey, K.B.; Abidi, A.B.; Rizvi, S.I. Markers of Oxidative Stress during Diabetes Mellitus. *J. Biomarkers* **2013**, *2013*, 378790. [CrossRef] [PubMed]
3. Fiorentino, T.V.; Prioletta, A.; Zuo, P.; Folli, F. Hyperglycemia-induced Oxidative Stress and its Role in Diabetes Mellitus Related Cardiovascular Diseases. *Curr. Pharm. Des.* **2013**, *19*, 5695–5703. [CrossRef]
4. Chis, I.C.; Coseriu, A.; Simedrea, R.; Oros, A.; Nagy, A.L.; Clichici, S. In Vivo Effects of Quercetin in Association with Moderate Exercise Training in Improving Streptozotocin-Induced Aortic Tissue Injuries. *Molecules* **2015**, *20*, 21770–21786. [CrossRef] [PubMed]

5. Chiș, I.C.; Clichici, A.; Simedrea, R.; Moldovan, R.; Lazar, V.L.; Clichici, S.; Oniga, O.; Nastasă, C. The effects of a new chromenyl-methylenethiazolidine-2,4-dione in alleviating oxidative stress in a rat model of streptozotocin induced diabetes. *Stud. UBB Chem.* **2018**, *63*, 103–112. [CrossRef]
6. Chis, I.C.; Socaciu, M.; Moldovan, R.; Clichici, S. Vascular impact of quercetin administration in association with moderate exercise training in experimental type 1 diabetes. *Rev. Romana Med. Lab.* **2019**, *27*, 269–279. [CrossRef]
7. Avogaro, A.; Albiero, M.; Menegazzo, L.; de Kreutzenberg, S.; Fadini, G.P. Endothelial Dysfunction in Diabetes: The role of reparatory mechanisms. *Diabetes Care* **2011**, *34*, S285–S290. [CrossRef]
8. Sena, C.M.; Pereira, A.M.; Seiça, R. Endothelial dysfunction—A major mediator of diabetic vascular disease. *Biochim. Biophys. Acta* **2013**, *1832*, 2216–2231. [CrossRef]
9. Fowler, M.J. Microvascular and Macrovascular Complications of Diabetes. *Clin. Diabetes* **2008**, *26*, 77–82. [CrossRef]
10. Sundaram, B.; Singhal, K.; Sandhir, R. Anti-atherogenic effect of chromium picolinate in streptozotocin-induced experimental diabetes. *J. Diabetes* **2013**, *5*, 43–50. [CrossRef]
11. Zguira, M.S.; Vincent, S.; Le Douairon Lahaye, S.; Malarde, L.; Tabka, Z.; Saïag, B. Intense exercise training is not effective to restore the endothelial NO-dependent relaxation in STZ-diabetic rat aorta. *Cardiovasc. Diabetol.* **2013**, *12*, 32. [CrossRef] [PubMed]
12. Zhang, H.; Zhang, C. Vasoprotection by Dietary Supplements and Exercise: Role of TNFαSignaling. *Exp. Diabetes Res.* **2012**, *2012*, 972679. [CrossRef]
13. Lee, S.; Park, Y.; Dellsperger, K.C.; Zhang, C. Exercise training improves endothelial function via adiponectin-dependent and independent pathways in type 2 diabetic mice. *Am. J. Physiol. Circ. Physiol.* **2011**, *301*, H306–H314. [CrossRef] [PubMed]
14. Coskun, O.; Ocakci, A.; Bayraktaroglu, T.; Kanter, M. Exercise Training Prevents and Protects Streptozotocin-Induced Oxidative Stress and beta-Cell Damage in Rat Pancreas. *Tohoku J. Exp. Med.* **2004**, *203*, 145–154. [CrossRef] [PubMed]
15. Heylen, E.; Guerrero, F.; Mansourati, J.; Theron, M.; Thioub, S.; Saïag, B. Effect of training frequency on endothelium-dependent vasorelaxation in rats. *Eur. J. Cardiol. Prev. Rehabil.* **2008**, *15*, 52–58. [CrossRef] [PubMed]
16. Umeno, A.; Horie, M.; Murotomi, K.; Nakajima, Y.; Yoshida, Y. Antioxidative and Antidiabetic Effects of Natural Polyphenols and Isoflavones. *Molecules* **2016**, *21*, 708. [CrossRef]
17. Sevastre-Berghian, A.C.; Ielciu, I.; Mitre, A.O.; Filip, G.A.; Oniga, I.; Vlase, L.; Benedec, D.; Gheldiu, A.-M.; Toma, V.A.; Mihart, B.; et al. Targeting Oxidative Stress Reduction and Inhibition of HDAC1, MECP2, and NF-kB Pathways in Rats with Experimentally Induced Hyperglycemia by Administration of Thymus marshallianus Willd. Extracts. *Front. Pharmacol.* **2020**, *11*, 581470, eCollection 2020. [CrossRef]
18. Boots, A.W.; Haenen, G.R.; Bast, A. Health effects of quercetin: From antioxidant to nutraceutical. *Eur. J. Pharmacol.* **2008**, *585*, 325–337. [CrossRef]
19. Chiş, I.C.; Baltaru, D.; Dumitrovici, A.; Coseriu, A.; Radu, B.C.; Moldovan, R.; Mureşan, A. Protective effects of quercetin from oxidative/nitrosative stress under intermittent hypobaric hypoxia exposure in the rat's heart. *Physiol. Int.* **2018**, *105*, 233–246. [CrossRef]
20. Chiş, I.C.; Mureşan, A.; Oros, A.; Nagy, A.L.; Clichici, S. Protective effects of Quercetin and chronic moderate exercise (training) against oxidative stress in the liver tissue of streptozotocin-induced diabetic rats. *Acta Physiol. Hung.* **2016**, *103*, 49–64. [CrossRef]
21. Alam, M.M.; Meerza, D.; Naseem, I. Protective effect of quercetin on hyperglycemia, oxidative stress and DNA damage in alloxan induced type 2 diabetic mice. *Life Sci.* **2014**, *109*, 8–14. [CrossRef]
22. Pashevin, D.A.; Tumanovska, L.V.; Dosenko, V.E.; Nagibin, V.S.; Gurianova, V.L.; Moibenko, A.A. Antiatherogenic effect of quercetin is mediated by proteasome inhibition in the aorta and circulating leukocytes. *Pharmacol. Rep.* **2011**, *63*, 1009–1018. [CrossRef] [PubMed]
23. Larson, A.J.; Symons, J.D.; Jalili, T. Therapeutic Potential of Quercetin to Decrease Blood Pressure: Review of Efficacy and Mechanisms. *Adv. Nutr.* **2012**, *3*, 39–46. [CrossRef]
24. Jeong, S.-M.; Kang, M.-J.; Choi, H.-N.; Kim, J.-H.; Kim, J.I. Quercetin ameliorates hyperglycemia and dyslipidemia and improves antioxidant status in type 2 diabetic db/db mice. *Nutr. Res. Pract.* **2012**, *6*, 201–207. [CrossRef]
25. Kim, J.H.; Kang, M.-J.; Choi, H.-N.; Jeong, S.-M.; Lee, Y.-M.; Kim, J.I. Quercetin attenuates fasting and postprandial hyperglycemia in animal models of diabetes mellitus. *Nutr. Res. Pract.* **2011**, *5*, 107–111. [CrossRef] [PubMed]
26. Mahmoud, M.F.; Hassan, N.A.; El-Bassossy, H.M.; Fahmy, A. Quercetin Protects against Diabetes-Induced Exaggerated Vasoconstriction in Rats: Effect on Low Grade Inflammation. *PLoS ONE* **2013**, *8*, e63784. [CrossRef] [PubMed]
27. Chis, I.C.; Ungureanu, M.I.; Marton, A.; Simedrea, R.; Muresan, A.; Postescu, I.-D.; Decea, N. Antioxidant effects of a grape seed extract in a rat model of diabetes mellitus. *Diabetes Vasc. Dis. Res.* **2009**, *6*, 200–204. [CrossRef]
28. Chis, I.C.; Clichici, A.; Nagy, A.L.; Oros, A.; Catoi, C.; Clichici, S. Quercetin in association with moderate exercise training attenuates injuries induced by experimental diabetes in sciatic nerves. *J. Physiol. Pharmacol.* **2017**, *68*, 877–886.
29. Pyun, S.B.; Kwon, H.K.; Uhm, C.S. Effect of exercise on reinnervating soleus muscle after sciatic nerve injury in rats. *J. Korean Acad. Rehabil. Med.* **1999**, *23*, 1063–1075.
30. Teixeira de Lemos, E.; Pinto, R.; Oliveira, J.; Garrido, P.; Sereno, J.; Mascarenhas-Melo, F.; Páscoa-Pinheiro, J.; Teixeira, F.; Reis, F. Differential Effects of Acute (Extenuating) and Chronic (Training) Exercise on Inflammation and Oxidative Stress Status in an Animal Model of Type 2 Diabetes Mellitus. *Mediat. Inflamm.* **2011**, *2011*, 253061. [CrossRef]
31. Gajdosík, A.; Gajdosíková, A.; Stefek, M.; Navarová, J.; Hozová, R. Streptozotocin-induced experimental diabetes in male Wistar rats. *Gen. Physiol. Biophys.* **1999**, *18*, 54–62. [PubMed]

32. Prabakaran, D.; Ashokkumar, N. Protective effect of esculetin on hyperglycemia-mediated oxidative damage in the hepatic and renal tissues of experimental diabetic rats. *Biochimie* **2013**, *95*, 366–373. [CrossRef] [PubMed]
33. De Vriese, A.S.; Verbeurenm, T.J.; Van de Voorde, J.; Lameire, N.H.; Vanhoutte, P.M. Endothelial dysfunction in diabetes. *Br. J. Pharmacol.* **2000**, *130*, 963–974. [CrossRef] [PubMed]
34. Meza, C.A.; La Favor, J.D.; Kim, D.-H.; Hickner, R.C. Endothelial Dysfunction: Is There a Hyperglycemia-Induced Imbalance of NOX and NOS? *Int. J. Mol. Sci.* **2019**, *20*, 3775. [CrossRef]
35. Ji, B.; Yuan, K.; Li, J.; Ku, B.J.; Leung, P.S.; He, W. Protocatechualdehyde restores endothelial dysfunction in streptozotocin-induced diabetic rats. *Ann. Transl. Med.* **2021**, *9*, 711. [CrossRef]
36. Chellian, J.; Mak, K.-K.; Chellappan, D.K.; Krishnappa, P.; Pichika, M.R. Quercetin and metformin synergistically reverse endothelial dysfunction in the isolated aorta of streptozotocin-nicotinamide- induced diabetic rats. *Sci. Rep.* **2022**, *12*, 21393. [CrossRef]
37. Alkaabi, J.; Sharma, C.; Yasin, J.; Afandi, B.; Beshyah, S.A.; Almazrouei, R.; Alkaabi, A.; Al Hamad, S.; Ahmed, L.A.; Beiram, R.; et al. Relationship between lipid profile, inflammatory and endothelial dysfunction biomarkers, and type 1 diabetes mellitus: A case-control study. *Am. J. Transl. Res.* **2022**, *14*, 4838–4847.
38. McDonald, M.W.; Olver, T.D.; Dotzert, M.S.; Jurrissen, T.J.; Noble, E.G.; Padilla, J.; Melling, C.J. Aerobic exercise training improves insulin-induced vasorelaxation in a vessel-specific manner in rats with insulin-treated experimental diabetes. *Diabetes Vasc. Dis. Res.* **2019**, *16*, 77–86. [CrossRef]
39. Shi, G.-J.; Li, Y.; Cao, Q.-H.; Wu, H.-X.; Tang, X.-Y.; Gao, X.-H.; Yu, J.-Q.; Chen, Z.; Yang, Y. In vitro and in vivo evidence that quercetin protects against diabetes and its complications: A systematic review of the literature. *Biomed. Pharmacother.* **2019**, *109*, 1085–1099. [CrossRef]

Disclaimer/Publisher's Note: The statements, opinions and data contained in all publications are solely those of the individual author(s) and contributor(s) and not of MDPI and/or the editor(s). MDPI and/or the editor(s) disclaim responsibility for any injury to people or property resulting from any ideas, methods, instructions or products referred to in the content.

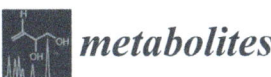

Article

Influence of Flavonoid-Rich Fraction of *Monodora tenuifolia* Seed Extract on Blood Biochemical Parameters in Streptozotocin-Induced Diabetes Mellitus in Male Wistar Rats

Samuel Nzekwe [1], Adetoun Morakinyo [1], Monde Ntwasa [2], Oluwafemi Oguntibeju [3], Oluboade Oyedapo [4] and Ademola Ayeleso [2,5,*]

1. Department of Biochemistry, Faculty of Science, Adeleke University, Ede 232101, Osun State, Nigeria
2. Department of Life and Consumer Sciences, University of South Africa, Florida Park, Johannesburg 1709, South Africa
3. Phytomedicine and Phytochemistry Group, Oxidative Stress Research Centre, Department of Biomedical Sciences, Faculty of Health and Wellness Sciences, Cape Peninsula University of Technology, Bellville 7535, South Africa
4. Department of Biochemistry, Obafemi Awolowo University, Ife 220282, Osun State, Nigeria
5. Biochemistry Programme, College of Agriculture, Engineering and Science, Bowen University, Iwo 232102, Osun State, Nigeria
* Correspondence: ademola.ayeleso@bowen.edu.ng; Tel.: +234-8144556529

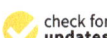

Citation: Nzekwe, S.; Morakinyo, A.; Ntwasa, M.; Oguntibeju, O.; Oyedapo, O.; Ayeleso, A. Influence of Flavonoid-Rich Fraction of *Monodora tenuifolia* Seed Extract on Blood Biochemical Parameters in Streptozotocin-Induced Diabetes Mellitus in Male Wistar Rats. *Metabolites* 2023, 13, 292. https://doi.org/10.3390/metabo13020292

Academic Editors: Cosmin Mihai Vesa and Dana Zaha

Received: 12 December 2022
Revised: 11 February 2023
Accepted: 13 February 2023
Published: 16 February 2023

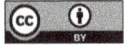

Copyright: © 2023 by the authors. Licensee MDPI, Basel, Switzerland. This article is an open access article distributed under the terms and conditions of the Creative Commons Attribution (CC BY) license (https://creativecommons.org/licenses/by/4.0/).

Abstract: Diabetes mellitus is a metabolic disorder caused by either the total destruction of the pancreatic beta cells that secrete insulin for the uptake of glucose from the circulation or as a result of the inability of body cells to respond to the presence of insulin in the blood. The present study investigated the effect of a flavonoid-rich fraction of *Monodora tenuifolia* seed extract (FFMTSE) on blood parameters in streptozotocin (STZ)-induced diabetic male Wistar rats. The rats were divided into seven groups ($n = 6$). Group 1: normal control rats, Group 2: rats + FFMTSE (25 mg/kgbwt), Group 3: rats + FFMTSE (50 mg/kgbwt), Group 4: diabetic control rats, Group 5: diabetic rats + FFMTSE (25 mg/kgbwt), Group 6: diabetic rats + FFMTSE (50 mg/kgbwt), and Group 7: diabetic rats + Metformin. The assessment of the lipid profile, kidney functions (urea and creatinine), and cardiac biomarkers (LDH and CK-MB) were carried out in the plasma using established protocols. The results showed a significant increase in the concentrations of triacylglycerol, cholesterol, LDL-cholesterol, VLDL-cholesterol, urea, and creatinine, as well as in cardiac enzyme activities in diabetic rats. However, the administration of the FFMTSE significantly improved the observed biochemical parameters. In addition, an increased concentration of HDL-cholesterol concentration was observed in the diabetic rats upon treatment with FFMTSE. These findings indicate that FFMTSE could be a potent anti-nephropathy and anti-cardiomyopathy agent in diabetic conditions.

Keywords: diabetes mellitus; *M. tenuifolia*; lipid profile; kidney functions; cardiac functions

1. Introduction

Diabetes mellitus is a global disease that results in substantial morbidity, mortality, and long-term complications, including retinopathy, nephropathy, peripheral nerve damage, and cardiovascular diseases [1]. It is characterized by chronic hyperglycemia and impaired metabolism of carbohydrates, fat, and protein associated with an absolute or relative deficiency in insulin secretion or insulin action [2]. Obesity, genetic disposition, sedentary lifestyle, and unhealthy diets are well-known risk factors associated with the development of type 2 diabetes mellitus (T2DM). The International Diabetes Federation (IDF) established that about 415 million adults between the ages of 20 to 79 years were living with diabetes mellitus as of 2015. In addition, diabetes mellitus has proven to be a global public health burden, and it has been projected that the number of diabetic patients will increase to 200 million by 2040 [3]. Diabetes mellitus is characterized by chronic hyperglycemia, which is in synergy with other metabolic aberrations, such as cardiovascular diseases (CVD), obesity, hypertension and fatty liver diseases. These metabolic disorders can cause damage to various organs or tissues, leading to the development of disabling and life-threatening health complications [4]. Medicinal plants contain potent substance(s) that can be used in the treatment of disease(s) or can be used as basic raw materials to produce synthetic drugs [5]. They are rich sources of phytochemicals and bioactive metabolites that can act in synergy as preventive or chemotherapeutics against different diseases or as complementary or alternative therapeutics to modern medicines [6,7]. Recently, there has been an upsurge of interest in the therapeutic potentials of medicinal plants as antioxidants against free radical-induced tissue injury. Besides, well-known and traditionally used natural antioxidants are derived from tea, wine, fruits, vegetables, and spices, while some natural antioxidants are exploited commercially either as antioxidant additives or as nutritional supplements [8]. These bioactive compounds, such as phenols, flavonoids, alkaloids, saponins, tannins, steroids, terpenoids, and stilbenes, in medicinal plants are involved in the management of different diseases [9]. The active ingredients of plants are also extracted and used as raw materials in pharmaceutical industries for the synthesis of drugs [10]. These bioactive compounds possess therapeutic effects, such as blood thinning, antibiotics, anti-malaria, anti-depression, laxative, and anticancer effects [11].

Monodora is a genus of plants in the family 'Annonacea.' The species of *Monodora* include *Monodora myristica* and *Monodora tenuifolia* Benth, which are widely used as spices [12]. It is a plant endowed with rich ethnobotanical history, and its medicinal properties have been reported [13,14]. In traditional medicine practice, it is widely used against toothache, dysentery, diarrhea, dermatitis, headache, and parasitic worms [15,16]. The seeds are aromatic and used as an ingredient in herbal medicines in Southern Nigeria. In the food industry, the seeds are used as spices in condiments and flavors; also, when roasted, the ground seeds are rubbed on the skin for skin diseases [17,18]. The present study investigated the effects of a flavonoid-rich fraction of *Monodora tenuifolia* seeds extract (FFMTSE) on some biochemical parameters in the blood of streptozotocin-induced diabetic male Wistar rats.

2. Materials and Methods

2.1. Collection of Plant Materials

The fruits of *Monodora tenuifolia* were collected from the Botanical Garden, Obafemi Awolowo University (OAU), Ile-Ife, Nigeria. It was identified by a botanist in the Department of Botany, Faculty of Science, Obafemi Awolowo University (OAU), Ile-Ife, and deposited at the IFE Herbarium with an identification number (IFE17979). The fruits were cut open to remove the hard-coated seeds and dried. Next, the dried seeds were deshelled to remove the seed coat, followed by the grinding of the seeds to fine powder with an electronic blender according to the method of Akinwunmi and Oyedapo [19]. The powdered seed was soaked in 80% (*v/v*) ethanol in the ratio of 1:5 (*w/v*) for 48 h and filtered using a clean cellophane material and white cotton wool, followed by concentration to a thick slurry in a rotary evaporator.

2.2. Reagents and Chemicals

All reagents used in the study were of analytical grade and obtained from various sources. Ethanol, n-hexane, and ethylacetate were from Fisher Scientific U.K, Merck KGaA, Germany, and Guandang Guanghan Chemical, China, respectively. D-fructose was from Mumbai, India, HCl was from Mumbai, India, and disodium hydrogen phosphate and monosodium dihydrogen phosphate were from Guandong, China. Other reagents, such as sodium citrate, trichloroacetic acid, hydrogen peroxide, aluminum chloride, and sodium nitrite, were all bought from BDH laboratories in Poole, UK. Diagnostic kits for plasma urea, plasma creatinine, and lipid profile were purchased from Randox Laboratories Ltd., UK. Diagnostic kits for CK-MB and LDH were purchased from Biorex diagnostics UK.

2.3. Preparation of Flavonoids-Rich Fraction of the Extract

Hydro-ethanolic extract of *Monodora tenuifolia* seeds was partitioned using a solvent-solvent extraction method according to Akinwunmi and Oyedapo [20] as reported by Chukwuma and Chiamaka [21] with slight modification.

The extract was dissolved in hot distilled water in a ratio of 1:5 (*w/v*). Next, the solution was hydrolyzed with 1% H_2SO_4 (1:4 *v/v*) by refluxing using a condensation assembly mounted on a magnetic stirrer for 5 min and filtered after cooling on an ice pack to obtain the filtrate. The filtrate was mixed thoroughly with ethylacetate (1:4 *v/v*) successively and poured into a separating funnel, and it was then allowed to settle. The ethylacetate fraction of the extract was then concentrated in a rotary evaporator and used as the flavonoid-rich fraction, according to the work of Gupta et al. [22] and Bala et al. [23].

2.4. Determination of Total Flavonoid Content

The total flavonoid concentration in the ethylacetate fraction of *M. tenuifolia* seed extract was determined using the method of Kostic et al. [24] with slight modifications, with rutin as the standard. Rutin (1 mg/mL) was prepared in methanol-distilled water (1:1 *v/v*) to form the stock solution, then further diluted into 6 serial dilutions of 0–1000 µL and made up to 1 mL with distilled water. The dilutions (200 µL) and sample (5 mg/mL) were pipetted separately and added to 300 µL of freshly prepared 5% $NaNO_3$, followed by the addition of 300 µL of 10% $AlCl_3$ and then 1 mL of 4% NaOH. After incubation at 25 °C for 10 min, the absorbance of the reaction mixture was read at 500 nm. The standard calibration graph was plotted, and the concentrations of flavonoids were determined and are expressed as mgRE/g extract.

where, RE = Rutin Equivalent.

2.5. Collection of Experimental Animals

Forty-two (42) male Wistar rats weighing 150–200 g were purchased from the Department of Anatomy, LAUTECH, Ogbomoso, Nigeria. The animals were acclimatized for 2 weeks in the animal House, Department of Biochemistry, Adeleke University and maintained under 12 h light/dark cycle in normal conditions of temperature and humidity. They were fed with standard pellets and water ad-libitum according to the method described by Hamid et al. [25].

2.6. Induction of Diabetes Using Streptozotocin (STZ)

Twenty-four (24) male Wistar rats were fed with 10% fructose in drinking water for 2 weeks before the intraperitoneal administration of a single dose of streptozotocin (STZ) (40 mg/kg bwt) injection [26]. Diabetes was confirmed using an Acu-check glucometer 72 h after induction, and the rats with ≥250 mg/dL glucose level were considered diabetic. The diabetes-induced groups were allowed to stabilize for 21 days with routine checks for glucose levels at 7-day intervals using an Acu-check glucometer.

2.7. Grouping and Treatment of Experimental Animals

The rats were divided into seven groups of six (6) rats in each group.
Group 1: Normal control rats
Group 2: Normal rats + 25 mg/kg FFMTSE
Group 3: Normal rats + 50 mg/kg FFMTSE
Group 4: Diabetic control rats
Group 5: Diabetic rats + 25 mg/kg FFMTSE
Group 6: Diabetic rats + 50 mg/kg FFMTSE
Group 7: Diabetic rats + 500 mg/kg Metformin

After 21 days of maintaining diabetes in the rats, plant extracts (25 mg/kg FFMTSE and 50 mg/kg FFMTSE) and standard drugs (metformin, 500 mg/kg) were administered in a single dose daily. Group 1 served as the control group taking water and feed only. Groups 2 and 3 were normal rats that received 25 mg/kg and 50 mg/kg FFMTSE, respectively.

Group 4 served as the untreated diabetic (diabetic control) group, while groups 5 and 6 were diabetic groups that were administered 25 mg/kg and 50 mg/kg FFMTSE, respectively. Group 7 was the diabetic group treated with 500 mg/kg metformin. The treatments were administered in single doses of the extract and metformin daily in 1ml for 14 days.

2.8. Sacrificing of Experimental Animals and Blood Collection

At the end of the experimental period, the rats were sacrificed after overnight fasting using diethylether anesthesia according to the method of Akinwunmi and Oyedapo [19]. The blood samples were collected through venous punctures using different anticoagulant (lithium heparin)-coated vials and kept on ice. The blood samples were then centrifuged at 4000 rpm in centrifuge 800D, and the plasma was separated and frozen at 20 °C for subsequent biochemical analysis.

2.9. Determination of Lipid Profile

2.9.1. Estimation of Total Cholesterol Concentration

Cholesterol concentration was determined according to the procedure described in the Randox manufacturer's instructional manual.

2.9.2. Estimation of Triglycerides Concentration

Triglyceride concentration was determined using a kit according to the procedure described in the Randox manufacturer's instructional manual.

2.9.3. Determination of High-Density Lipoprotein Cholesterol (HDL-c) Concentration

The concentration of HDL-cholesterol (HDL-c) concentration was determined according to the procedure described in the Randox manufacturer's instructional manual.

2.9.4. Estimation of Low-Density Lipoprotein Cholesterol (LDL-c) Concentration

The concentration of plasma low-density lipoprotein cholesterol (LDL-c) was evaluated using Friedewald's formula according to the expression below [27].

$$\text{LDL-c (mg/dL)} = \text{Total Cholesterol} - (\frac{\text{Triglycerides}}{5} + \text{HDL} - \text{cholesterol})$$

2.9.5. Estimation of Very Low-Density Lipoprotein Cholesterol (VLDL-c) Concentration

The plasma concentration of VLDL-cholesterol (VLDL-c) was calculated according to Friedewald's equation, expressed below [27]:

$$\text{VLDL-c (mg/dL)} = \frac{\text{Triglycerides}}{5}$$

2.10. Determination of the Concentrations of Renal Biomarkers

2.10.1. Estimation of Plasma Urea Nitrogen Concentration

Blood urea nitrogen (BUN) concentration was estimated by the method of Fawcett and Scott [28] using the commercially available kit. The absorbance of test and standard samples was measured spectrophotometrically against blank at 578 nm and expressed as mg/dL.

$$\text{Urea concentration (mg/dL)} = \frac{\text{Abs. of Sample} \times \text{Conc. of Standard (mg/dL)}}{\text{Abs. of Standard}}$$

2.10.2. Estimation of Plasma Creatinine Concentration

The creatinine concentration was estimated by the alkaline picrate method, as described by Bonsnes and Taussky [29], using a commercially available diagnostic kit. The absorbance was measured at 510 nm against distilled water and expressed as mg/dL.

$$\text{Creatinine concentration (mg/dL)} = \frac{\text{Abs. of Sample} \times \text{Conc. of Standard (mg/dL)}}{\text{Abs. of Standard}}$$

2.11. Determination of Cardiac Biomarkers in Plasma

2.11.1. Assay of Creatinine Kinase-Myocardial Band [CK-MB] Activity

The assay of CK-MB activity was carried out according to the method of Jansson and Sylvén [30]. Briefly, 1 mL of the working reagent was pipetted into test tubes containing 40 µL of plasma, followed by incubation at 37 °C for 3 min. The mixture was measured at 475 nm in intervals of 1 min for 5 min.

$$\text{CK-MB activity (mg/dL)} = \frac{\text{Abs. of Sample} \times \text{Conc. of Standard (mg/dL)}}{\text{Abs. of Standard}}$$

2.11.2. Assay of Lactate Dehydrogenase (LDH) Activity

The assay for the LDH activity was carried out according to the method of Bernstein [31] using a commercially available kit. The plasma (40 µL) was added to 1 mL of the working reagent and incubated at 37 °C for 3 min. The absorbance was measured at 340 nm within the interval of 30 s for 150 s. The activity was calculated as shown below, and the result was expressed in mmol/L.

$$\text{LDH activity (mmol/L)} = \frac{\text{Abs. of Sample} \times \text{Conc. of Standard (mmol/L)}}{\text{Abs. of StandAbs. of Standardard}} \quad (1)$$

2.12. Statistical Analysis

The data were expressed as mean ± standard deviation (SD) of triplicates. Statistical significance was determined by a 1-way analysis of variance (ANOVA), followed by Duncan's multiple comparisons between control and treated rats in all the groups.

3. Results

3.1. Total Flavonoid Concentration in FFMTSE

Table 1 shows the concentration of flavonoids present in 1 mg of the FFMTSE extracted with ethylacetate. One (1 mg) of the extract contained 0.078 mg of flavonoid expressed in standard rutin equivalent with a standard deviation of 0.001.

Table 1. Concentration of total flavonoid in FFMTSE.

Plant Sample	Concentration (mgRE/mg FFMTSE)
Flavonoid-rich fraction of *M. tenuifolia*	0.078 ± 0.001

3.2. Effect of FFMTSE on Lipid Profile

The concentration of plasma cholesterol was significantly higher ($p < 0.05$) in the diabetic control group (Figure 1a) than in the normal control group. However, when the diabetic groups were treated with the plant extracts (25 mg/kg FFMTSE and 50 mg/kg FFMTSE) and metformin, there was a significant reduction in cholesterol concentrations compared with that in the diabetic control group.

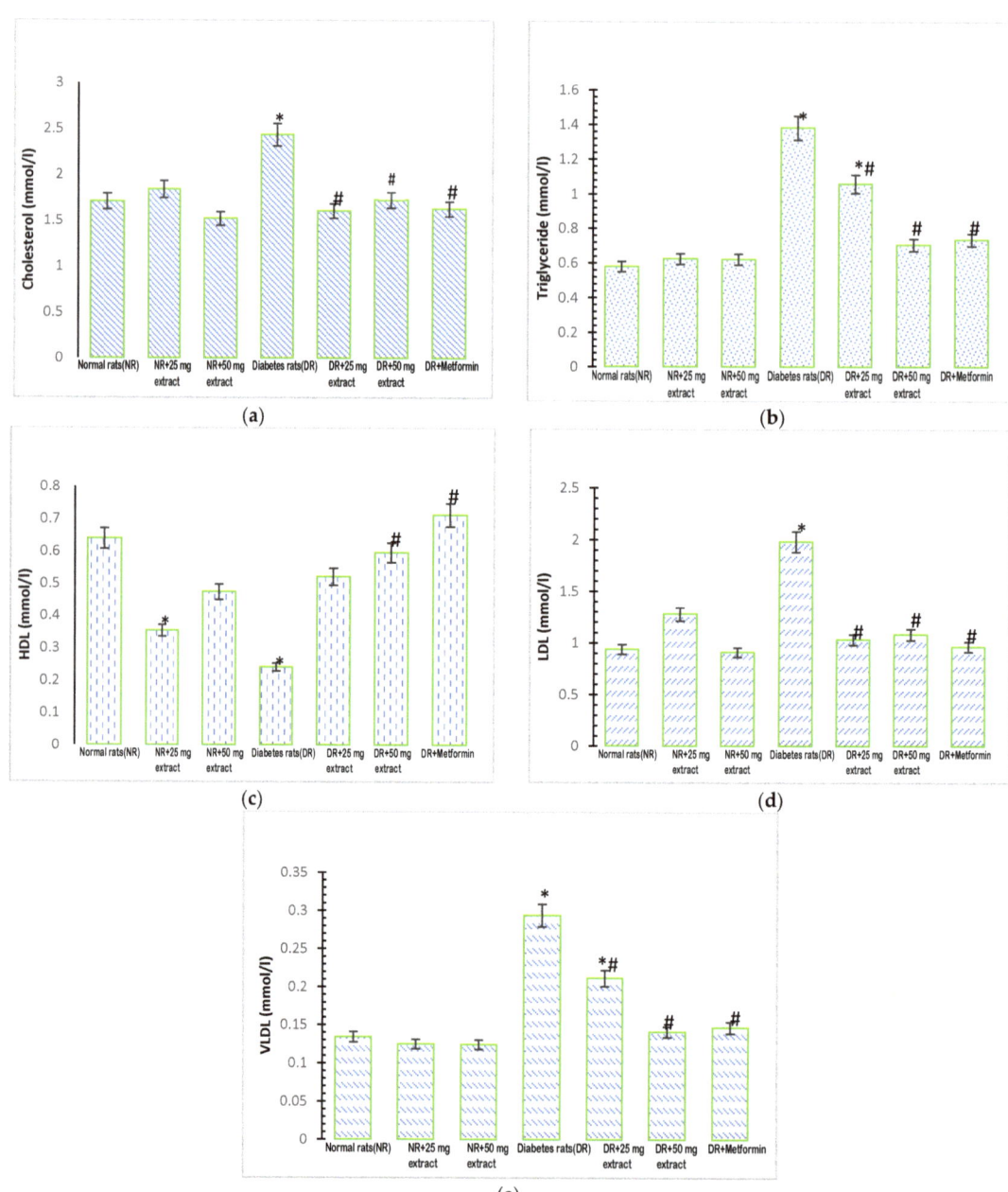

Figure 1. Lipid profile of rats treated with FFMTSE. (**a**) Concentration of cholesterol, (**b**) triglycerides, (**c**) HDL-Cholesterol, (**d**) LDL cholesterol, and (**e**) VLDL cholesterol in rats treated with FFMTSE. All results are expressed as mean ± SD. (*) indicates a significant difference compared to the normal control group at $p < 0.05$, and (#) indicates a significant difference compared to the diabetic control group at $p < 0.05$. FFMTSE- Flavonoid-rich fraction of *Monodora tenuifolia* seed extract.

The concentration of plasma triglycerides in the diabetic control group increased significantly ($p < 0.05$) compared with that in the normal control group (Figure 1b). Treatment of the diabetic rats with the extracts (25 mg/kg FFMTSE and 50 mg/kg FFMTSE) and metformin resulted in a significant decrease in plasma triglyceride concentrations compared with that in the diabetic control group.

There was a significant reduction ($p < 0.05$) in the concentration of plasma HDL-cholesterol in the diabetic control group (Figure 1c) compared with that in the normal control group. However, when the diabetic groups were treated with the plant extract (50 mg/kg FFMTSE) and metformin, there was a significant increase in HDL-cholesterol concentrations compared with that in the diabetic control group.

The concentration of plasma LDL-cholesterol in the diabetic control group increased significantly ($p < 0.05$) compared with that in the normal control group (Figure 1d). When the diabetic groups were treated with the plant extracts (25 mg/kg FFMTSE and 50 mg/kg FFMTSE) and metformin, the results showed a significant decrease in LDL-cholesterol concentrations compared with that in the diabetic control group.

The concentration of plasma VLDL was significantly increased ($p < 0.05$) in the diabetic control group (Figure 1e) when compared with that in the normal control group. Treatment with the extracts (25 mg/kg FFMTSE and 50 mg/kg FFMTSE) and metformin led to a significant reduction in VLDL concentrations in the treated diabetic groups compared with the diabetic control group. However, VLDL concentrations in the diabetic rats treated with 25 mg/kg FFMTSE were significantly higher than that in the normal rats.

3.3. Effect of FFMTSE on Kidney Biomarkers

Plasma urea concentrations showed a significant increase ($p < 0.05$) in the diabetic control group (Figure 2a), compared with that in the normal control group. The administration of 25 mg/kg FFMTSE to the diabetic rats caused a significant reduction in urea concentrations compared with that observed in the diabetic control group. However, the urea concentrations in diabetic rats treated with 50 mg/kg FFMTSE and metformin were significantly higher than that in the normal rats.

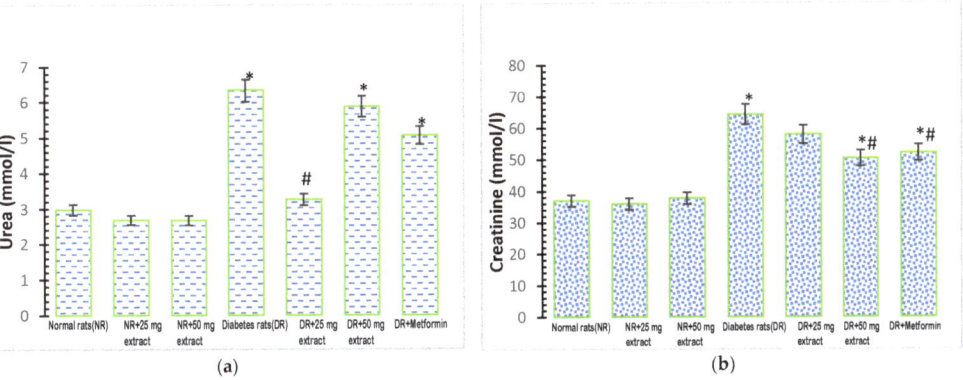

Figure 2. Kidney biomarkers in rats treated with FFMTSE. (**a**) Concentration of urea and (**b**) creatinine in rats treated with FFMTSE. All results are expressed as mean ± SD, (*) indicates a significant difference compared to the normal control group at $p < 0.05$, and (#) indicates a significant difference compared to the diabetic control group at $p < 0.05$. FFMTSE: flavonoid-rich fraction of *Monodora tenuifolia* seed extract.

Plasma creatinine concentration was significantly increased ($p < 0.05$) in the diabetic control group, compared with that in the normal control group (Figure 2b). Moreover, 50 mg/kg FFMTSE and metformin significantly decreased creatinine concentrations in diabetic rats, while those treated with 25 mg/kg FFMTSE showed no significant reduction in creatinine concentration. In addition, creatinine concentrations in diabetic rats treated with 50 mg/kg FFMTSE and metformin were significantly higher than that in the normal rats.

3.4. Effect of FFMTSE on Cardiac Biomarkers

The activity of plasma creatine kinase MB was significantly increased ($p < 0.05$) in the diabetic control group when compared with that in the normal control group (Figure 3a). In addition, the administration of *M. tenuifolia* extracts (25 mg/kg FFMTSE and 50 mg/kg FFMTSE) to the diabetic rats significantly decreased creatine kinase activity, compared with that in the diabetic control group, while creatine kinase activity in the diabetic rats treated with 25 mg/kg FFMTSE and 50 mg/kg FFMTSE as well as metformin were significantly higher than that in the normal rats.

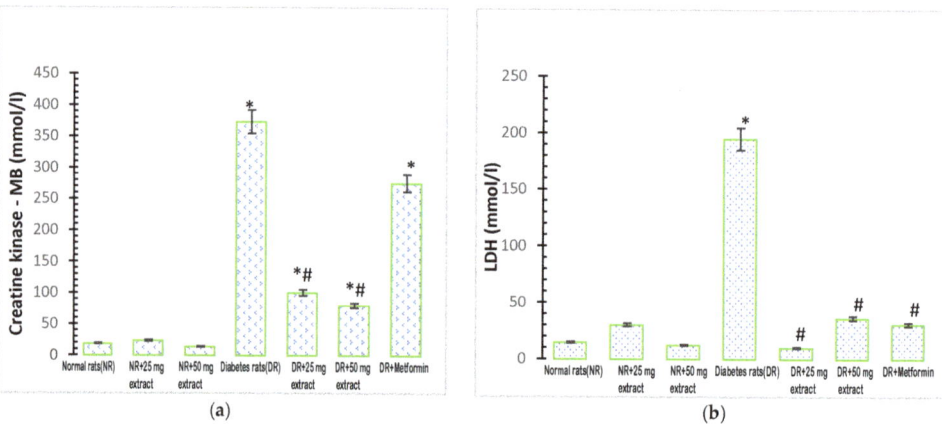

Figure 3. Cardiac biomarkers in rats treated with FFMTSE. (**a**) Activity of creatine kinase-MB (CK-MB) and (**b**) Lactate dehydrogenase (LDH) in rats treated with FFMTSE. All results are expressed as mean ± SD, (*) indicates a significant difference compared to the normal control group at $p < 0.05$, and (#) indicates a significant difference compared to the diabetic control group at $p < 0.05$. FFMTSE: flavonoid-rich fraction of *Monodora tenuifolia* seed extract.

There was a significant increase ($p < 0.05$) in the activity of plasma LDH in the diabetic control group compared with that in the normal control group (Figure 3b). However, the administration of the extracts (25 mg/kg FFMTSE and 50 mg/kg FFMTSE) to the diabetic rats significantly reduced the activity of LDH compared with that in the diabetic control group.

4. Discussion

In this study, flavonoid was found in the ethylacetate fraction of *Monodora tenuifolia* seeds, which supports the findings of Akinwunmi and Oyedapo [20] and Ekanyanwu and Njoku [16], who have previously shown that *Monodora tenuifolia* and its family species are rich in flavonoids. Diabetic patients have impaired lipid metabolism (dyslipidemia), accompanied by the risk of cardiovascular arteriosclerosis [32]. Our findings also revealed accumulated levels of lipids in diabetic rats, suggesting that impaired lipid metabolism is associated with diabetes. Type 2 diabetes occurs when body cells or organs are insensitive to the presence of insulin in circulation, and pancreatic β-cells fail to produce enough insulin to compensate for the ongoing insulin resistance. It is closely correlated with dyslipidemia, characterized by increased levels of LDL and triglycerides as well as low levels of HDL [33,34]. The clinical analysis of autopsy specimens carried out by Regan and coworkers on diabetic persons demonstrated increased deposition of cholesterol and triglycerides compared with those observed in persons without the disease [35]. In patients with type 2 diabetes, hyperinsulinemia, insulin resistance, and β-cell failure are related to diabetes dyslipidemia due to elevated plasma levels of fasting triglyceride-rich lipoproteins, small-dense LDL-particles, and low levels of high-density lipoprotein (HDL) cholesterol [36]. The present study showed increased concentrations of LDL-c, triglyceride, VLDL, and cholesterol with reduced concentrations of HDL-c in the plasma of diabetic rats. Treatment with the plant extracts at both test concentrations (25 mg/kg FFMTSE and 50 mg/kg FFMTSE) significantly reduced the concentrations of LDL-c, triglycerides, VLDL, and cholesterol. This indicates that Monodora tenufolia seeds have the potential to control lipid metabolism in diabetic conditions. When the diabetic groups were treated with 50 mg/kg FFMTSE and metformin, there was a significant increase in HDL-cholesterol concentrations compared with that in the diabetic control group; however, 25 mg/kg FFMTSE did not show any significant increase in HDL-cholesterol. The effects of the drug on the bodies of animals can be influenced by different factors, including the route of administration, drug concentration, and internal body homeostatic changes. The lower dosage of the plant extract at 25 mg/kg FFMTSE could have caused poor synthesis or metabolism of HDL in the plasma of the rats.

Diabetic nephropathy is a leading cause of chronic and end-stage renal disease, and it is relatively associated with elevated cardiovascular disease risk and mortality. Prolonged hyperglycemia and increased lipid mobilization and accumulation cause glucotoxicity and lipotoxicity, which are associated with chronic renal disease in diabetes. This present study showed significantly increased concentrations of creatinine and urea in diabetic rats, indicating serious diabetes-induced kidney damage. Increased serum levels of lipids in the kidneys of patients with diabetes and experimental animals have been reported [37,38]. The administration of plant extracts (25 mg/kg FFMTSE and 50 mg/kg FFMTSE) significantly reduced urea concentration in diabetic rats. However, only 50 mg/kg FFMTSE was able to reduce creatinine concentration in the diabetic rats, as 25 mg/kg FFMTSE showed no significant decrease in the creatinine concentration. High creatinine level in plasma is an indication of kidney malfunction; the plant extract was expected to lower creatinine levels in diabetic rats and enhance the glomerular filtration of the kidney. The non-significant effect exerted by 25 mg/kg FFMTSE could be attributed to the inability of the extract at this dose to confer any effect on glomerular filtration in the kidney. Nevertheless, at 50 mg/kg, FFMTSE significantly improved the creatinine level and enhanced glomerular filtration in the kidney.

Cardiac lipid accumulation commonly occurs in type 2 diabetes and has been suggested to play a direct causal role in the development of cardiomyopathy and heart failure in a process known as cardiac lipotoxicity [39]. Fatty acid mobilization and a significant increase in cholesterol availability in plasma are some of the characteristics of diabetes mellitus [40]. In this study, there was a significant increase in the activities of cardiac enzymes (LDH and CK-MB) in diabetic rats, which indicated structural damage, functional alteration in the heart, and the excessive release of these enzymes into the bloodstream. The present work supports the finding of Sharma et al. [41], who showed that intra-myocardial lipid overload in heart disease is greater in people with diabetes than in those without diabetes. Cardiac dysfunction induced by the excess accumulation of lipids, termed lipotoxic cardiomyopathy or fatty heart, demonstrates the importance of lipids in the development of diabetic cardiomyopathy and heart failure [42]. Cardiac dysfunction observed in individuals with diabetes is a net result of both lipid-driven cardiac dysfunction due to the effects of lipids on the cardiovascular as well as a direct pathological effect of lipids on the myocardium-promoting cardiomyopathy [43]. FFMTSE (25 and 50 mg/kg) significantly reduced the activities of cardiac enzymes (LDH and CK-MB) in diabetic rats.

5. Conclusions

Medicinal plants have been a promising source of phytochemicals that possess medicinal potential in the treatment of many diseases. This study demonstrated the capacity of FFMTSE to influence lipid metabolism through the reduction of blood concentrations of LDL-cholesterol, triglycerides, and VLDL-cholesterol and the improvement of HDL-cholesterol levels in diabetic rats. In addition, kidney parameters (creatinine and urea concentrations) and activities of cardiac enzymes improved in diabetic rats upon treatment with FFMTSE. Overall, the study showed that the flavonoid-rich fraction of *Monodora tenuifolia* seed could help to ameliorate complications arising from kidney and cardiac damage in diabetic conditions. Further investigations may be required to determine the mechanisms of the actions of the flavonoids in *Monodora tenuifolia* against kidney and cardiac dysfunctions in diabetes mellitus.

Author Contributions: S.N., A.A. and O.O. (Oluboade Oyedapo)—conceptualization; S.N.—analysis, data interpretation; S.N.—manuscript writing; A.A., O.O. (Oluboade Oyedapo), A.M., O.O. (Oluwafemi Oguntibeju) and M.N.—critical revisions and final approval of the manuscript. All authors have read and agreed to the published version of the manuscript.

Funding: This research received no external funding. APC was funded by the University of South Africa.

Institutional Review Board Statement: The animal study protocol was approved by the Ethical Review Committee of Adeleke University (AUERC) to conduct this study with the reference number AUERC/FOS/BCH/04. AUERC requires compliance with institutional guidelines and regulations and ensures that all adverse events are reported promptly to the AUERC.

Informed Consent Statement: Not applicable.

Data Availability Statement: Samples of the extract are available from the authors.

Conflicts of Interest: The authors declare no conflict of interest.

References

1. Ajuwon, O.R.; Ayeleso, A.O.; Adefolaju, G.A. The potential of South African herbal tisanes, rooibos and honeybush in the management of type 2 diabetes mellitus. *Molecules* **2018**, *23*, 3207. [CrossRef] [PubMed]
2. Gomathi, D.; Kalaiselvi, M.; Ravikumar, G.; Devaki, K.; Uma, C. Evaluation of Antioxidants in the Kidney of Streptozotocin Induced Diabetic Rats. *Indian J. Clin. Biochem.* **2014**, *29*, 221–226. [CrossRef] [PubMed]
3. Zheng, Y.; Ley, S.H.; Hu, F.B. Global aetiology and epidemiology of type 2 diabetes mellitus and its complications. *Nat. Rev. Endocrinol.* **2018**, *14*, 88–98. [CrossRef] [PubMed]
4. Shah, S.R.; Iqbal, S.M.; Alweis, R.; Roark, S. A closer look at heart failure in patients with concurrent diabetes mellitus using glucose lowering drugs. *Expert Rev. Clin. Pharmacol.* **2019**, *12*, 45–52. [CrossRef] [PubMed]
5. WHO. *Global Report on Diabetes*; World Health Organization: Geneva, Switzerland, 2016; Available online: https://apps.who.int/iris/handle/10665/204871 (accessed on 18 October 2022).
6. Hasler, C.M.; Blumberg, J.B. Symposium on Phytochemicals: Biochemistry and Physiology. *J. Nutr.* **1999**, *129*, 756–757. [CrossRef]
7. Mamta, S.; Jyoti, S.; Rajeev, N.; Dharmendra, S.; Abhishek, G. Phytochemistry of Medicinal Plants. *J. Pharmacogn. Phytochem.* **2013**, *1*, 168–182.
8. Saeed, A.; Marwat, M.S.; Shah, A.H.; Naz, R.; Zain-Ul-Abidin, S.; Akbar, S.; Khan, R.; Navid, M.T.; Saeed, A.; Bhatti, M.Z. Assessment of total phenolic and flavonoid contents of selected fruits and vegetables. *Indian J. Tradit. Knowl.* **2019**, *18*, 686–693.
9. Raina, H.; Soni, G.; Jauhari, N.; Sharma, N.; Bharadvaja, N. Phytochemical importance of medicinal plants as potential sources of anticancer agents. *Turk. J. Bot.* **2014**, *38*, 1027–1035. [CrossRef]
10. Mustafa, G.; Arif, R.; Atta, A.; Sharif, S.; Jamil, A. Bioactive Compounds from Medicinal Plants and Their Importance in Drug Discovery in Pakistan. *Matrix Sci. Pharma* **2017**, *1*, 17–26. [CrossRef]
11. Gupta, A.; Khamkar, P.R.; Chaphalkar, S. Applications and uses of active ingredients from medicinal plants. *Indian J. Nov. Drug Deliv.* **2014**, *6*, 106–111.
12. Njoku, U.O.; Akah, P.A.; Okonkwo, C.C. Antioxidant activity of seed extracts Monodora tenuifolia (Annonoaceae). *Int. J. Basic Appl. Sci.* **2012**, *12*, 80–87.
13. Nielsen, M. *Introduction to the Flowering Plants of West Africa*; University of London Press Ltd.: London, UK, 1979; p. 90.
14. Onyenibe, N.S.; Fowokemi, K.T.; Emmanuel, O.B. African Nutmeg (*Monodora Myristica*) Lowers Cholesterol and Modulates Lipid Peroxidation in Experimentally Induced Hypercholesterolemic Male Wistar Rats. *Int. J. Biomed. Sci.* **2015**, *11*, 86–92. [PubMed]
15. Ezenwali, M.O.; Njoku, O.U.; Okoli, C.O. Studies on the antidiarrhoeal properties of seed extract of *Monodora tenuifolia*. *Int. J. Appl. Res. Nat. Prod.* **2009**, *2*, 20–26.
16. Ekeanyanwu, R.C.; Njoku, O.U. Acute and subacute oral toxicity study on the flavonoid rich fraction of *Monodora tenuifolia* seed in albino rats. *Asian Pac. J. Trop. Biomed.* **2014**, *4*, 194–202. [CrossRef]
17. Irvine, F.R. *Woody Plants of Ghana with Special Reference to Their Uses*; Oxford University Press: London, UK, 1961.
18. Bele, M.Y.; Focho, D.A.; Egbe, E.A.; Chuyong, B.G. Ethnobotanical survey of the uses of Annonaceae around mount Cameroon. *Afr. J. Plant Sci.* **2011**, *5*, 237–247.

19. Akinwunmi, K.F.; Oyedapo, O.O. In vitro anti-inflammatory evaluation of African nutmeg (*Monodora* myristica) seeds. *Eur. J. Med. Plants* **2015**, *8*, 167–174. [CrossRef]
20. Akinwunmi, F.F.; Oyedapo, O.O. Evaluation of antioxidant potentials of *Monodora* myristica (Gaertn) dunel seeds. *Afr. J. Food Sci.* **2013**, *7*, 317–324.
21. Chukwuma, E.R.; Chiamaka, J.G. Ameliorative Effect of the Flavonoid Rich Fraction of *Monodora* myristica (Gaertn) Dunel Seed Extract against Carbon Tetrachloride-Induced Hepatotoxicity and Oxidative Stress in Rats. *Biochem. Pharmacol.* **2017**, *6*, 232. [CrossRef]
22. Gupta, A.; Sheth, N.R.; Pandey, S.; Yadav, J.S.; Joshi, S.V. Screening of flavonoids rich fractions of three Indian medicinal plants used for the management of liver diseases. *Rev. Bras. Farmacogn.* **2015**, *25*, 485–490. [CrossRef]
23. Bala, S.Z.; Hassan, M.; Sani, A. Effect of Flavonoid Rich Fraction of *Irvingia gabonensis* Seed Extract on Tetrachloromethane (CCl4)—Induced Liver Damage in Mice. *Int. J. Sci. Glob. Sustain.* **2021**, *7*, 102–110.
24. Kostic, D.A.; Dimitrijevic, D.S.; Mitic, S.S.; Stojanovic, G.S.; Zivanovic, A.V. Phenols from the methanolic extract of Miconia albicans (Sw.) Trian Leaves. *Molecules* **2013**, *16*, 9440–9450.
25. Hamid, H.Y.; Zuki, A.B.Z.; Yimer, N.; Haron, A.W.; Noordin, M.M.; Goh, Y.M. Effects of elevated ambient temperature on embryo implantation in rats. *Afr. J. Biotechnol.* **2012**, *11*, 6624–6632.
26. Wilson, R.D.; Islam, M.S. Fructose-fed streptozotocin-injected rat: An alternative model for type 2 diabetes. *Pharmacol. Rep.* **2012**, *64*, 129–139. [CrossRef] [PubMed]
27. Friedewald, W.T.; Levy, R.I.; Fredrickson, D.S. Estimation of the concentration of low-density lipoprotein cholesterol in plasma, without use of the preparative ultracentrifuge. *Clin. Chem.* **1972**, *18*, 499–502. [CrossRef] [PubMed]
28. Fawcett, J.K.; Scott, J.E. A Rapid and Precise Method for the Determination of Urea. *J. Clin. Pathol.* **1960**, *13*, 156–159. [CrossRef]
29. Bonsnes, R.W.; Taussky, H.H. On Colorimetric Determination of Creatinine by the Jaffe Reaction. *J. Biol. Chem.* **1945**, *158*, 581–591. [CrossRef]
30. Jansson, E.; Sylvén, C. Creatine kinase MB and citrate synthase in type I and type II muscle fibres in trained and untrained men. *Eur. J. Appl. Physiol. Occup. Physiol.* **1985**, *54*, 207–209. [CrossRef]
31. Bernstein, L.H. Automated kinetic determination of lactate dehydrogenase isoenzymes in serum. *Clin. Chem.* **1977**, *23*, 1928–1930. [CrossRef]
32. Krauss, R.M. Lipids and lipoproteins in patients with type 2 diabetes. *Diabetes Care* **2004**, *27*, 1496–1504. [CrossRef]
33. Jeppesen, J.; Hein, H.O.; Suadicani, P.; Gyntelberg, F. Relation of high TG-low HDL cholesterol and LDL cholesterol to the incidence of ischemic heart disease: An 8-year follow-up in the Copenhagen Male Study. *Arterioscler. Thromb. Vasc. Biol.* **1997**, *17*, 1114–1120. [CrossRef]
34. Bulut, T.; Demirel, F.; Metin, A. The prevalence of dyslipidemia and associated factors in children and adolescents with type 1 diabetes. *J. Pediatr. Endocrinol. Metab.* **2017**, *30*, 18. [CrossRef] [PubMed]
35. Regan, T.J.; Lyons, M.M.; Ahmed, S.S.; Levinson, G.E.; Oldewurtel, H.A.; Ahmad, M.R.; Haider, B. Evidence for cardiomyopathy in familial diabetes mellitus. *J. Clin Investig.* **1977**, *60*, 884–899. [CrossRef] [PubMed]
36. Chapman, M.J.; Ginsberg, H.N.; Amarenco, P.; Andreotti, F.; Borén, J.; Catapano, A.L.; Descamps, O.S.; Fisher, E.; Kovanen, P.T.; Kuivenhoven, J.A.; et al. Triglyceride-rich lipoproteins and high-density lipoprotein cholesterol in patients at high risk of cardiovascular disease: Evidence and guidance for management. *Eur. Heart J.* **2011**, *32*, 1345–1361. [CrossRef] [PubMed]
37. Sun, L.; Halaihel, N.; Zhang, W.; Rogers, T.; Levi, M. Role of sterol regulatory element-binding protein 1 in regulation of renal lipid metabolism and glomerulosclerosis in diabetes mellitus. *J. Biol. Chem.* **2002**, *277*, 18919–18927. [CrossRef]
38. Thongnak, L.; Pongchaidecha, A.; Lungkaphin, A. Renal Lipid Metabolism and Lipotoxity in Diabetes. *Am. J. Med. Sci.* **2020**, *359*, 84–99. [CrossRef]
39. Ritchie, R.H.; Zerenturk, E.J.; Prakoso, D.; Calkin, A.C. Lipid metabolism and its implications for type 1 diabetes-associated cardiomyopathy. *J. Mol. Endocrinol.* **2017**, *58*, 225–240. [CrossRef]
40. Mahato, R.V.; Gyawali, P.; Raut, P.P.; Regmi, P.; Khelanand, P.S.; Dipendra, R.P.; Gyawali, P. Association between glycaemic control and serum lipid profile in type 2 diabetic patients: Glycated haemoglobin as a dual biomarker. *Biomed. Res.* **2011**, *22*, 375–380.
41. Sharma, S.; Adrogue, J.V.; Golfman, L.; Uray, I.; Lemm, J.; Youker, K.; Noon, G.P.; Frazier, O.H.; Taegtmeyer, H. Intramyocardial lipid accumulation in the failing human heart resembles the lipotoxic rat heart. *FASEB J.* **2004**, *18*, 1692–1700. [CrossRef]
42. Szczepaniak, L.S.; Dobbins, R.L.; Metzger, G.J.; Sartoni-D'Ambrosia, G.; Arbique, D.; Vongpatanasin, W.; Unger, R.; Victor, R.G. Myocardial triglycerides and systolic function in humans: In vivo evaluation by localized proton spectroscopy and cardiac imaging. *Magn. Reson. Med.* **2003**, *49*, 417–423. [CrossRef]
43. Rubler, S.; Dlugash, J.; Yuceoglu, Y.Z.; Kumral, T.; Branwood, A.W.; Grishman, A. New type of cardiomyopathy associated with diabetic glomerulosclerosis. *Am. J. Cardiol.* **1972**, *30*, 595–602. [CrossRef]

Disclaimer/Publisher's Note: The statements, opinions and data contained in all publications are solely those of the individual author(s) and contributor(s) and not of MDPI and/or the editor(s). MDPI and/or the editor(s) disclaim responsibility for any injury to people or property resulting from any ideas, methods, instructions or products referred to in the content.

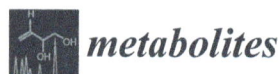

Article

Quercetin, a Plant Flavonol Attenuates Diabetic Complications, Renal Tissue Damage, Renal Oxidative Stress and Inflammation in Streptozotocin-Induced Diabetic Rats

Arshad Husain Rahmani [1,*], Mohammed A. Alsahli [1], Amjad Ali Khan [2] and Saleh A. Almatroodi [1]

[1] Department of Medical Laboratories, College of Applied Medical Sciences, Qassim University, Buraydah 52571, Saudi Arabia
[2] Department of Basic Health Science, College of Applied Medical Sciences, Qassim University, Buraydah 52571, Saudi Arabia
* Correspondence: ah.rahmani@qu.edu.sa

Abstract: Diabetes mellitus is a metabolic syndrome characterized by increased glucose levels, oxidative stress, hyperlipidemia, and frequently decreased insulin levels. The current research was carried out for eight consecutive weeks to evaluate the possible reno-protective effects of quercetin (50 mg/kg b.w.) on streptozotocin (STZ) (55 mg/kg b.w.) induced diabetes rat models. Various physiological, biochemical, and histopathological parameters were determined in control, diabetic control, and quercetin-treated diabetic rats. The current findings demonstrated that diabetes control rats showed significantly decreased body weights (198 ± 10 vs. 214 ± 13 g) and insulin levels (0.28 ± 0.04 vs. 1.15 ± 0.05 ng/mL) in comparison to normal control. Besides this, the other parameters showed increased values, such as fasting blood glucose, triglyceride (TG), and total cholesterol levels (99 ± 5 vs. 230 ± 7 mg/dL, 122.9 ± 8.7 vs. 230.7 ± 7.2 mg/dL, 97.34 ± 5.7 vs. 146.3 ± 8 mg/dL) ($p < 0.05$). In addition, the urea and creatinine levels (39.9 ± 1.8 mg/dL and 102.7 ± 7.8 µmol/L) were also high in diabetes control rats. After 8 weeks of quercetin treatment in STZ-treated animals, body weight, insulin, and fasting blood sugar levels were significantly restored ($p < 0.05$). The inflammatory markers (TNF-α, IL-6, and IL-1β) were significantly increased (52.64 ± 2, 95.64 ± 3, 23.3 ± 1.2 pg/mL) and antioxidant enzymes levels (SOD, GST, CAT, and GSH) were significantly decreased (40.3 ± 3 U/mg, 81.9 ± 10 mU/mg, 14.2 ± 2 U/mg, 19.9 ± 2 µmol/g) in diabetic rats. All the parameters in diabetic animals treated with quercetin were restored towards their normal values. Histopathological findings revealed that the quercetin-treated group showed kidney architecture maintenance, reduction of fibrosis, and decreased expression of COX-2 protein. These results determined that quercetin has reno-protective effects, and conclude that quercetin possesses a strong antidiabetic potential and might act as a therapeutic agent in the prevention or delay of diabetes-associated kidney dysfunction.

Keywords: quercetin; anti-diabetic activity; oxidative stress; reno-protective effect; anti-inflammatory activity

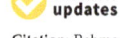

Citation: Rahmani, A.H.; Alsahli, M.A.; Khan, A.A.; Almatroodi, S.A. Quercetin, a Plant Flavonol Attenuates Diabetic Complications, Renal Tissue Damage, Renal Oxidative Stress and Inflammation in Streptozotocin-Induced Diabetic Rats. *Metabolites* 2023, 13, 130. https://doi.org/10.3390/metabo13010130

Academic Editors: Cosmin Mihai Vesa and Dana Zaha

Received: 10 December 2022
Revised: 6 January 2023
Accepted: 12 January 2023
Published: 15 January 2023

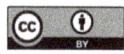

Copyright: © 2023 by the authors. Licensee MDPI, Basel, Switzerland. This article is an open access article distributed under the terms and conditions of the Creative Commons Attribution (CC BY) license (https://creativecommons.org/licenses/by/4.0/).

1. Introduction

Diabetes is one of the main public health concerns worldwide. Type 2 diabetes mellitus accounts for more than 90% of all diabetes cases and is a chronic metabolic disease of multifactorial origin [1]. Hyperglycemia is a chief contributor to the overall oxidative stress that leads to the production of reactive oxygen species (ROS) [2,3]. Furthermore, increased levels of ROS resulting from hyperglycemia disturbs the insulin signaling cascades and encourages the development of insulin resistance [4,5]. In addition, lipid abnormalities are prevalent in diabetes mellitus due to insulin resistance or metabolic disturbances that affect key enzymes and pathways of lipid metabolism [6]. Diabetic dyslipidemia is generally measured by higher serum levels of cholesterol and lower levels of HDL-cholesterol and triglyceride [7,8].

Several approaches are used for diabetes treatment: via the intake of healthy food and diet control, using insulin injections, or standard hypoglycemic chemical drugs. These factors increase pancreatic islet survival in addition to the regeneration of β-cells through islet neogenesis-related proteins [9,10]. The current modes of treatment for this disease may be effective but lead to adverse complications. It is common to anticipate the effectiveness of traditional herbal medicines in the prevention and treatment of diabetes with minimum or no side effects [11]. Consequently, for the treatment of diabetes mellitus a significant number of medicinal plants have been preferred as a natural source of drugs [12] as they are considered to be safe, less toxic, and more readily available than synthetic drugs [13].

In this regard, quercetin is a vital polyphenolic flavonoid present in vegetables and fruits and its role in promoting health has been demonstrated previously [14,15]. Quercetin consumption has been confirmed to affect energy production, mitochondrial biogenesis, electron transport chain performance, modification of reactive oxygen production, and mitochondrial defects [16,17]. Furthermore, its role as an anti-inflammatory, antioxidant, and anti-angiogenesis was proven in the previous study [18].

It was described that pre-treatment with quercetin protected hippocampal CA1 pyramidal neurons from ischemic injury [19]. Cigarette smoking damages human osteoblasts via the accumulation of ROS. Quercetin can reduce this damage by scavenging the radicals and upregulating the expression of HO-1 and SOD-1 [20]. It was reported that quercetin had a role in the restoration of antioxidant enzyme activity in kidney tissue of Diclofenac-treated rats. Furthermore, in the presence of quercetin, Diclofenac was unable to enhance the expression of pro-inflammatory cytokines, advocating that quercetin may have anti-inflammatory potential [21]. Its role in cancer has been documented through the modulation of various biological activities [22].

In the present study, the protective role of quercetin on streptozotocin (STZ)-induced renal damage in rats was examined via oxidative stress, lipid profile, and inflammation. In addition, histopathological analysis was performed to evaluate kidney tissue damage amongst treatment group animals.

2. Materials and Methods

2.1. Chemicals

Streptozotocin (STZ) (S0130), and quercetin (Q4951) were purchased from Sigma-Aldrich Inc., St. Louis, MO, USA. The kits of catalase (ab83464), superoxide dismutase (SOD) (ab65354), and glutathione S-transferases (GST) (ab65326) were purchased from Abcam, U.K. Inflammatory markers (TNF-α (ab46070), IL-1β (ab100767), and IL-6 (ab119548) ELISA based kits were also procured from Abcam, UK. Myeloperoxidase (MPO) (ab105136) and Nitric oxide assay kit (ab65328) were also procured from Abcam, UK. Trichrome Stain Kit (Connective Tissue Stain) (ab150686) and Picro Sirius red stain kit (ab150681) procured from Abcam, UK. H&E Staining Kit (Hematoxylin and Eosin) kit (ab245880), COX-2 primary antibody (ab15191), Mouse and Rabbit Specific HRP/DAB (ABC) Detection IHC kit (ab64264) was purchased from Abcam, UK. All supportive chemicals used in this study were of high purity grade.

2.2. Animal Ethics

The animal treatment procedures followed the guidelines provided by the animal care unit of CAMS, Qassim University (QU). The study was approved by the Laboratory Animal Ethics Committee (ethics committee no. 2019-2-2-I-5623) of the QU. All protocols were followed to minimize the rats' suffering.

2.3. Animals and Treatment

Adult male Wistar albino rats (180–220 g) were obtained from King Saud University, Saudi Arabia. The animals were housed in plastic cages at the central animal facility unit of the College of Applied Medical Science (CAMS), Qassim University. All rats had free access to rat chow and tap water throughout the study. All animals were handled/treated in accordance with the guidelines of the Committee for the Control and Supervision of Experiments on Animals, CAMS, Saudi Arabia. The animals were grouped as 8 animals/group and were treated as described below.

The animals were rested for 7 days to reduce any transportation stress. Streptozotocin was freshly prepared in 0.05 M sodium citrate buffer (pH 4.5). The diabetes was induced by injecting intraperitoneally STZ (55 mg/kg b.w.) [23] solution in all animals except the normal control. Quercetin (50 mg/kg b.w.) was prepared in 1% dimethyl sulfoxide (DMSO) solution and was given orally by gavage to the treatment animals. Vehicle and quercetin treatments were given twice weekly after one week of diabetes induction [24], and were continued for eight consecutive weeks. The positive control rats were also given glibenclamide (5mg/kg b.w.) twice weekly. The STZ-induced rats were considered to have hyperglycemia when their fasting blood glucose levels were more than 200 mg/dL.

2.4. Animal Groups and Treatment Plan

Group Name	Short Name	Treatment Plan
Normal control	C	Rats with free access to rat pellets and orally given saline as a placebo
Negative control	NC	STZ-induced diabetic rats at 55 mg/kg b.w. [23] and orally given saline.
Positive control	PC	STZ-induced diabetic rats and oral gavage treatment with glibenclamide (5 mg/kg b.w.) [25] as a standard drug.
Quercetin Treatment	QT	STZ-induced diabetic rats and oral gavage treatment with quercetin (50 mg/kg b.w.)

2.5. Measurement of Body Weight

In all four groups, the body weights of the rats were measured weekly to check for changes in their overall weight, and the results were analyzed accordingly.

2.6. Fasting Blood Glucose and Insulin Level Measurement

The fasting blood glucose (FBG) was checked weekly in all experimental rats after overnight fasting, throughout the treatment plan. Blood samples were obtained from the tail vein, and FBG was measured through a standard glucometer. The level of insulin was checked at the end of the experimental design.

2.7. Measurement of Lipid Profile

After overnight fasting was completed, blood samples were obtained from each rat. The serum was isolated using centrifugation at $400 \times g$ for 10–12 min. The total cholesterol (TC), high-density lipoprotein cholesterol (HDL-C), and triglycerides (TG) were measured accordingly.

2.8. Oral Glucose Tolerance Test (OGTT)

After continuous treatment for 8 weeks, the OGTT was performed. For OGTT, fasting rats were orally given glucose at a dose of 2 g/kg b.w. Blood samples were obtained from the tail vein at different intervals such as 0, 30, 60, 90, and 120 min after administration. The blood glucose level was measured and the results were analyzed.

2.9. Measurement of Kidney Function Parameters

The kidney function parameters were determined by the estimation of urea and creatinine levels in serum samples from all the experimental animals and the results were interpreted accordingly.

2.10. Measurement of TNF-α, IL-6 and IL-1β Pro-Inflammatory Parameters

Enzyme-Linked Immunosorbent Assay (ELISA) is an in vitro enzyme-linked immunosorbent test for the quantitative evaluation of different inflammatory markers. The experiment was accomplished as per the manufacturer's instructions for the evaluation of TNF-α, IL-6, and IL-1β levels, and the absorbance was measured at 450 nm.

2.11. Measurement of Lipid Peroxidation

Malondialdehyde (MDA) was assessed via thiobarbituric acid (TBA) reactive substance at high temperature, forming a colored complex according to manufacturer guidelines. The absorbance of the resultant product was measured at 532 nm.

2.12. Determination of SOD, GST, CAT and GSH Levels

Kidney tissue was taken from all groups of rats and kept in a phosphate buffer saline solution. Furthermore, the tissue samples were homogenized as well as centrifuged at $1100\times g$ for 15 min. Blood samples were obtained and the serum was isolated by centrifugation at $400\times g$ for 12 min. The antioxidant enzymes were measured as per the kit guidelines.

2.13. Histopathological Examination

For microscopic evaluation, kidney tissue samples were fixed in a 10% formalin. Tissues were processed using an automated tissue processor. Paraffin was used to embed the tissue, and paraffin-embedded blocks were made for sectioning. The tissue samples were sectioned at 5 µm using a rotatory microtome. Haematoxylin/eosin (H&E) staining was performed to stain the sections. Two independent pathologists evaluated the slides in a blinded manner. H&E staining images were analyzed under a light microscope (Nikon Corporation, Tokyo, Japan) and the results were interpreted accordingly.

2.14. Masson's Trichrome Staining

The collagen fiber deposition was evaluated using Masson's trichrome staining kit. Briefly, kidney sections were deparaffinized using xylene and properly hydrated in distilled water. Bouin's fluid was preheated in a water bath to almost 60 °C in a fume hood and slides were placed in preheated Bouin's fluid for one hour followed by a 10 min cooling period. Sections were cleared in distilled water. Equal parts of Weigert's (A) and Weigert's (B) solutions were mixed properly and slides were stained with working Weigert's Iron Haematoxylin for 5–6 min. Slides were rinsed in running tap water for 2 min. Biebrich Scarlet/Acid Fuchsin solution was applied to each slide for 15 min. All slides were properly rinsed in distilled water. Phosphomolybdic/Phosphotungstic acid solution was used to differentiate. Aniline blue solution was applied to slides for 5–10 min and rinsed in distilled water. Acetic Acid Solution (1%) was applied to slides for 3–5 min and dehydrated rapidly in 95% alcohol, followed by changes of absolute alcohol. All slides were cleared using xylene and mounted using mounting media. The resultant formation of blue stains from the collagen deposition was examined. Two independent pathologists evaluated the slides in a blinded manner. Masson's trichrome staining images were analyzed under a light microscope and the results were interpreted accordingly.

2.15. Picro Sirius Red Staining

The fiber deposition was evaluated using the Picro sirius red staining kit of Abcam, UK. Sections were deparaffinized and hydrated with distilled water. Adequate Picro sirius red solution was applied to fully cover the tissue sections and incubated for one hour. Slides were rinsed for 2 changes of acetic acid solution. Slides were rinsed in alcohol and dehydrated in absolute alcohol. Slides were cleared, mounted, and examined accordingly.

2.16. Expressional Evaluation of COX-2 Protein through Immunohistochemical Staining

Briefly, formalin-fixed paraffin-embedded tissue sections were deparaffinized using xylene, rehydrated, and washed in phosphate-buffered saline (pH 7.0), and the remaining protocols were followed as per the method described earlier [26,27]. The COX-2 protein of Abcam, Cambridge, U.K. was used as primary antibodies and incubated for 1 h at 4 °C, followed by incubation with the secondary antibody for 60 min, then streptavidin–biotin enzyme complex for 1 h. Diaminobenzidine (DAB) (Abcam, Cambridge, UK, ab 64259) chromogen was then applied accordingly, and hematoxylin was used as a counterstain. Finally, the results were analyzed under a light microscope.

2.17. Statistical Analysis

The values are described as the means ± standard deviation. For assessments in multiple groups, one-way analysis of variance (ANOVA) was performed accordingly. The $p < 0.05$ was considered statistically significant.

3. Results

3.1. Quercetin Effects on Body Weight

The effect of orally given quercetin on the body weight of rats was examined. Diabetic control rats showed a reduction in body weight as compared to non-diabetic rats (Table 1). At the end of 8 weeks of continuous treatment, the body weight of the rats in the normal control, diabetic control plus quercetin, and diabetic control plus glibenclamide increased significantly.

Table 1. Body weight of different animal groups measured at start and end of the treatment plan. The animals were divided equally among different groups (n = 8 per group). The data is represented as mean ± standard error of the mean (SEM). * $p < 0.05$ (significant difference of final body weight between NC vs. C), # $p < 0.05$ (significant difference of final boy wight between NC vs. QT).

Animal Groups	Body Weight (0 Days) (g)	Body Weight (After 8 Weeks) (g)
Control (C)	216 ± 12	295 ± 10
Negative Control (NC)	214 ± 13	198 ± 10 *
Positive Control (PC)	213 ± 11	272 ± 12
Quercetin Treatment (QT)	219 ± 12	263 ± 14 #

3.2. Effect of Quercetin on Glucose and Insulin Levels

The glucose and insulin levels were measured in all experimental groups. The diabetic control rats revealed high FBG levels (230 ± 7.2 mg/dL) and low insulin levels (0.28 ± 0.04 ng/mL) as compared with normal control rats (Figure 1, Supplementary File S1). Moreover, the diabetic control animals treated with quercetin showed decreased FBG levels (151 ± 6.8 mg/dL) and increased insulin levels (0.75 ± 0.06 ng/mL). However, based on these findings, it was revealed that quercetin plays a vital role in the inhibition of kidney pathogenesis through the regulation of glucose and insulin levels.

3.3. Effect of Quercetin on Oral Glucose Tolerance Tests

The effect of quercetin on diabetic rats was measured through oral glucose tolerance tests. Glucose solution (2 g/kg b.w.) was administrated by oral gavage feeding. After oral glucose intake, compared with normal control rats, diabetic rats exhibited higher blood glucose levels. Quercetin supplementation was established to improve glucose tolerance (Figure 2).

3.4. Effect of Quercetin on Lipid Profile

The serum levels of triglycerides (TG), total cholesterol (TC), and high-density lipoprotein cholesterol (HDL-C) were measured in experimental animals in each group. STZ treatment showed a significant increase of TC (146.37 ± 8.7 mg/dL), TG (230.7 ± 7.2 mg/dL), and a reduction in HDL-C levels (45.6 ± 7.2) as compared to the normal control rats ($p < 0.05$, Figure 3, Supplementary File S1). Moreover, a significant reduction in TC (123.23 ± 4.7 mg/dL), TG (193.23 ± 9.4 mg/dL), and elevation of HDL-C (52.9 ± 9.4 mg/dL) was observed in diabetic rats treated with quercetin ($p < 0.05$).

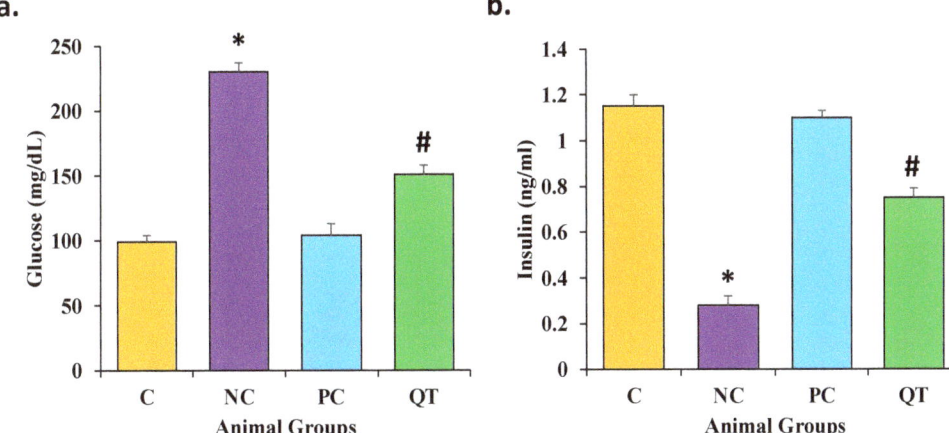

Figure 1. The concentration of (**a**) glucose and (**b**) insulin in serum in various animal groups after 8 weeks of continuous treatment. The animals were proportionally divided into each group (n = 8 animals per group). The data is described as mean ± SEM. * $p < 0.05$ (significant difference of b.w. (final) between NC vs. C), # $p < 0.05$ (significant difference of b.w. (final) between negative control (NC) vs. Quercetin Treatment (QT)).

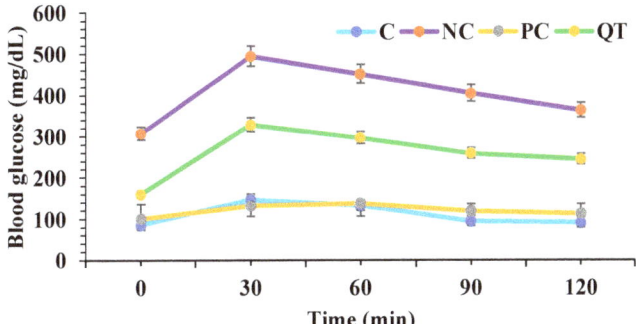

Figure 2. Effect of quercetin (50 mg/kg b.w.) on oral glucose tolerance test. Data are described as mean ± SEM ($n = 8$).

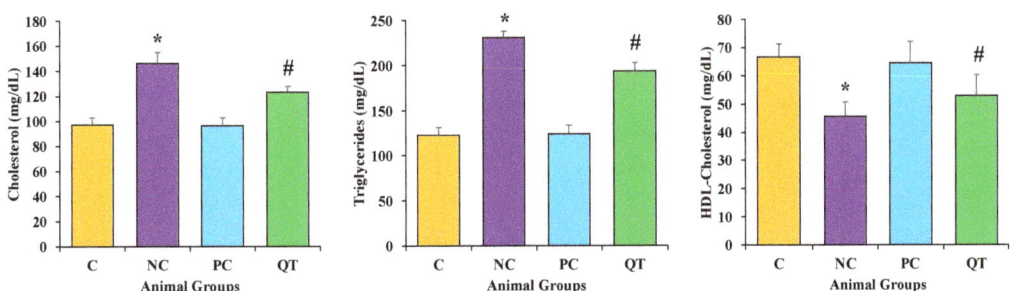

Figure 3. The measurement of lipid profile in different animal groups. The animals were proportionally divided into each group (n = 8 rats/group). The data is described as mean ± SEM. * $p < 0.05$ (significant difference of b.w. (final) between NC vs. C), # $p < 0.05$ (significant difference of b.w. (final) between negative control (NC) vs. quercetin Treatment (QT)).

3.5. Effect of Quercetin on Kidney Function Profile

The serum levels of urea and creatinine were measured in experimental animals in each group. STZ treatment showed significant increases in these parameters (urea as 39.9 ± 1.8 mg/dL; creatinine as 102.7 ± 7.8 µmol/L) as compared to the normal control rats ($p < 0.05$) (Figure 4). However, a significant reduction in urea (18.6 ± 2.6 mg/dL) and creatinine levels (81.5 ± 6.9 µmol/L) were observed among the diabetic animals treated with quercetin ($p < 0.05$).

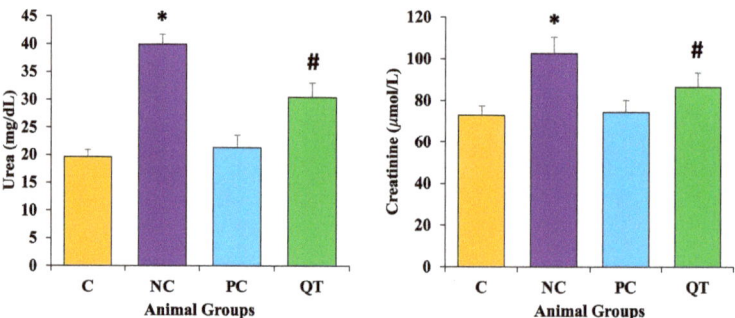

Figure 4. The level of urea and creatinine in different animal groups. The animals were proportionally divided into each group (n = 8 rats/group). The data is described as mean ± SEM. * $p < 0.05$ (significant difference of b.w. (final) between NC vs. C), # $p < 0.05$ (significant difference of b.w. (final) between negative control (NC) vs. quercetin Treatment (QT)).

3.6. Effect of Quercetin on Oxidative Stress

Antioxidants enzyme (CAT, SOD, GST) and GSH levels were measured to evaluate the antioxidant potential of quercetin. The results revealed that diabetic rats showed a decrease in these enzyme levels (CAT as 14.2 ± 2.2 U/mg protein, SOD as 40.3 ± 3.2 U/mg protein, GST as 81.9 ± 10.1 mU/mg protein). However, in diabetic rats treated with quercetin at doses of 50 mg/kg b.w., it showed a prominent protective effect in kidney function. The results revealed significantly increased levels of these parameters (CAT as 20.6 ± 1.1 U/mg protein, SOD as 51.8 ± 9.2 U/mg protein, and GST as 125.4 ± 8.2 mU/mg protein) after the quercetin treatment for eight consecutive weeks (Figure 5, Supplementary File S1).

3.7. Effect of Quercetin Extract on Lipid Peroxidation

Malondialdehyde (MDA) and nitric oxide (NO) content were measured to examine the protective role of quercetin on oxidative stress. Results revealed that diabetic rats showed enhanced levels of both MDA (149.3 ± 3.2 nmol/g) and NO (32.4 ± 2.4 µmol/L) content as compared to the control rats. However, the diabetic rats treated with quercetin showed a prominent reduction of these parameters (MDA as 123.3 ± 7.2 nmol/g and NO as 22.3 ± 1.9 µmol/L) (Figure 6).

3.8. Effect of Quercetin on Inflammatory Markers Level

The levels of InterlukinL-6, TNF-α, and IL-1β levels were raised significantly in diabetic control rats (IL-6 as 95.64 ± 3.2 pg/mL, IL-1β as 23.30 ± 1.2 pg/mL, and TNF-α as 52.64 ± 2.2 pg/mL) when compared to the control group ($p < 0.05$). The treatment of diabetic rats with quercetin significantly decreased the level of these pro-inflammatory markers (IL-6 as, 70.29 ± 9.3 pg/mL, IL-1β as 21.10 ± 1.4 pg/mL, and TNF-α as 42.29 ± 1.3 pg/mL) towards the normal levels ($p < 0.05$) (Figure 7).

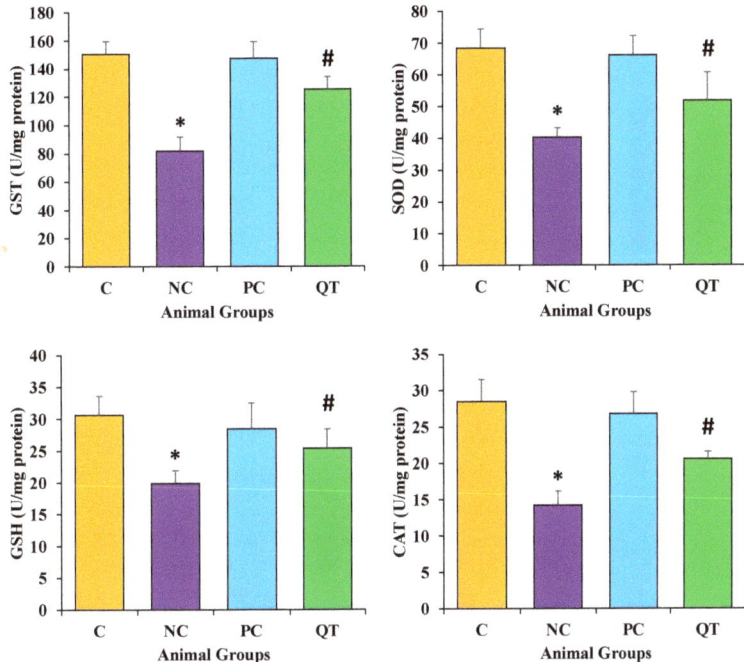

Figure 5. The antioxidant enzymes and antioxidant profile among different animal groups. The animals were equally divided (n = 8 animals/group). * $p < 0.05$ (significant difference of b.w. (final) between NC vs. C), # $p < 0.05$ (significant difference of b.w. (final) between negative control (NC) vs. Quercetin Treatment (QT)).

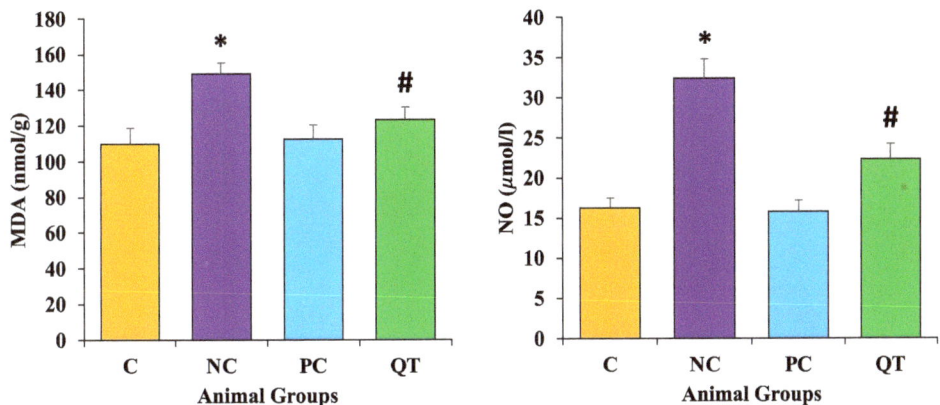

Figure 6. The malondialdehyde and nitric oxide levels in different animal groups. The animals were equally divided (n = 8 animals/group). * The data is described as mean ± SEM. * $p < 0.05$ (significant difference of b.w. (final) between NC vs. C), # $p < 0.05$ (significant difference of b.w. (final) between negative control (NC) vs. Quercetin Treatment (QT)).

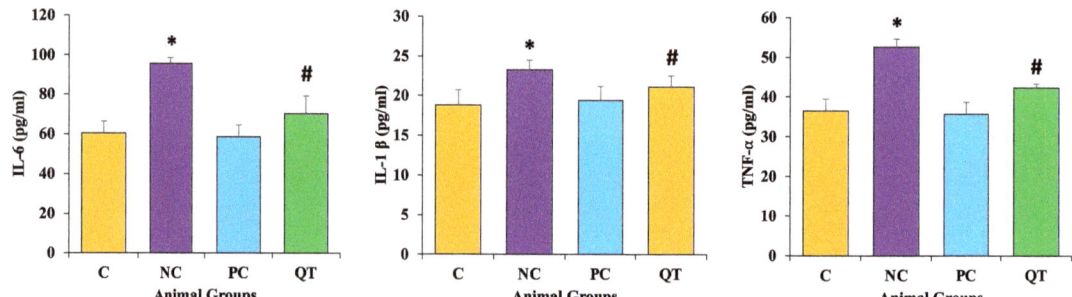

Figure 7. The level of different inflammatory markers in various animal groups. The animals were proportionally divided into each group (n = 8 rats/group). The data is described as mean ± SEM. * $p < 0.05$ (significant difference of b.w. (final) between NC vs. C), # $p < 0.05$ (significant difference of b.w. (final) between negative control (NC) vs. quercetin Treatment (QT)).

3.9. Effect of Quercetin on Kidney Histology

To evaluate the effect of quercetin on renal structural changes in all experimental animals, renal morphology was examined through Haematoxylin and Eosin staining. Histological study of normal control groups showed normal renal architecture as normal glomerulus, proximal and distal tubules with normal epithelium. The histopathological sections of kidneys in diabetic rats showed distorted glomerular morphology, congestion, and infiltration of lymphocytes, demonstrating kidney injury. On the other hand, pathological changes of the kidney tissues in diabetic groups that received quercetin showed less damage as less congestion and fewer inflammatory cells were observed as compared to the diabetes control group (Figure 8).

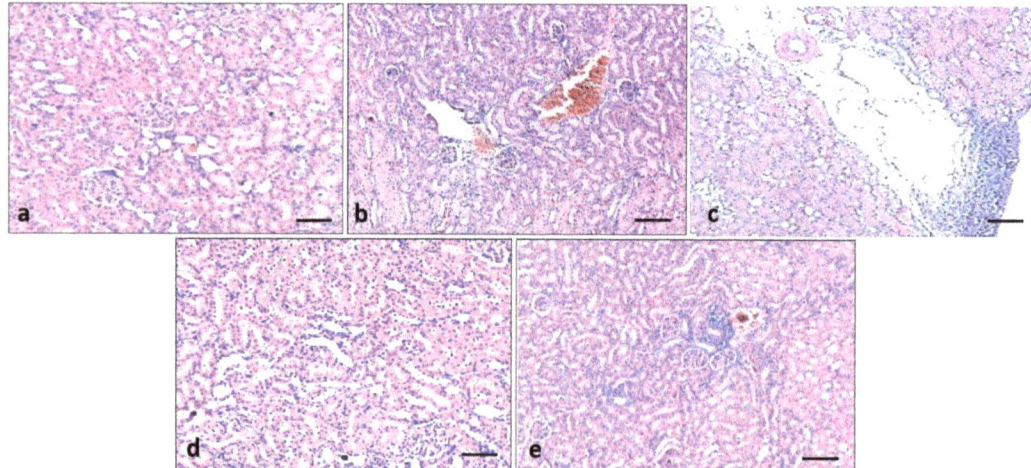

Figure 8. Effect of quercetin extract in kidney tissue architecture. Light photomicrographs of kidney sections from the control group: normal architecture was noticed (**a**), streptozotocin (STZ) group (Negative control): showed infiltration of lymphocytes, and congestion (**b,c**), STZ + glibenclamide (Positive control) showed normal kidney architecture (**d**), STZ + quercetin (50 mg/kg b.w.) displayed mild inflammation and congestion (**e**).

3.10. Effect of Quercetin on Renal Fibrosis

Collagen fiber was examined using Masson's trichrome staining to detect the effects of quercetin on renal fibrosis and changes in collagen fiber in the control and experimental groups. Furthermore, this staining established that collagen fiber (blue staining) was significantly high in diabetic rats. Quercetin treatment (50 mg/kg) reduced the collagen deposition in the renal tissue of diabetic rats when compared to the STZ-induced diabetes group (Figure 9).

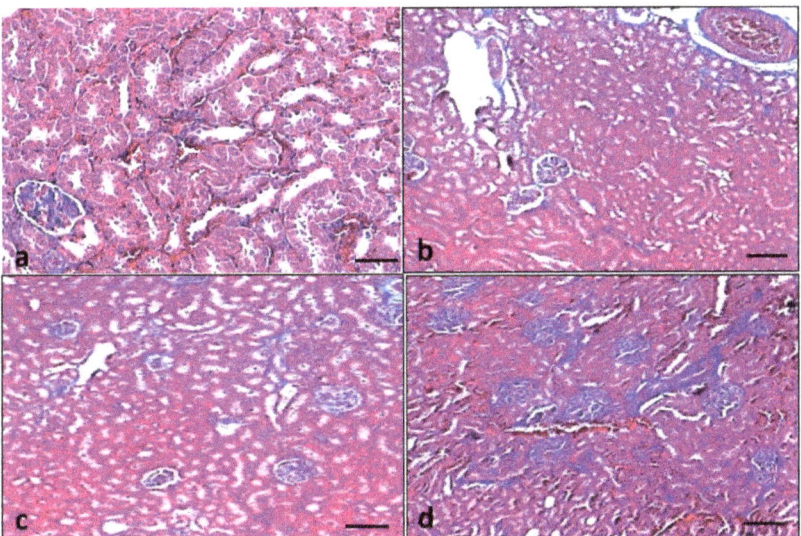

Figure 9. Quercetin decreases collagen fiber in the kidney tissues. Light photomicrographs of kidney sections from the control group: collagen fiber not seen (**a**), streptozotocin (STZ) group (Negative control): high deposition of collagen fiber noticed (**b**), STZ + glibenclamide (Positive control) collagen fiber was significantly less (**c**), STZ + quercetin (50 mg/kg b.w.): showed less collagen fiber (**d**).

3.11. Effect of Quercetin on Renal Fibrosis of STZ-Induced Diabetic Rats

Picro sirius staining was performed on all experimental groups to evaluate the reno-protective effect of quercetin. Picro sirius staining demonstrated that fibrosis (red staining) was significantly high in the disease control group (diabetic rats). Quercetin treatment (50 mg/kg) plays a reno-protective role through the reduction of fibrosis in the renal tissue of diabetic rats when compared to the STZ-induced diabetes group (Figure 10).

3.12. Effect of Quercetin on COX-2 Protein Expression of STZ-Induced Diabetic Rats

Immunohistochemistry staining was performed on all experimental groups to evaluate the COX-2 protein expression. The expression of COX-2 was high in the diseases control group (diabetic rats). Quercetin treatment (50 mg/kg) plays a reno-protective role through the decrease of COX-2 protein expression in the renal tissue of diabetic rats when compared to the STZ-induced diabetes group (Figure 11).

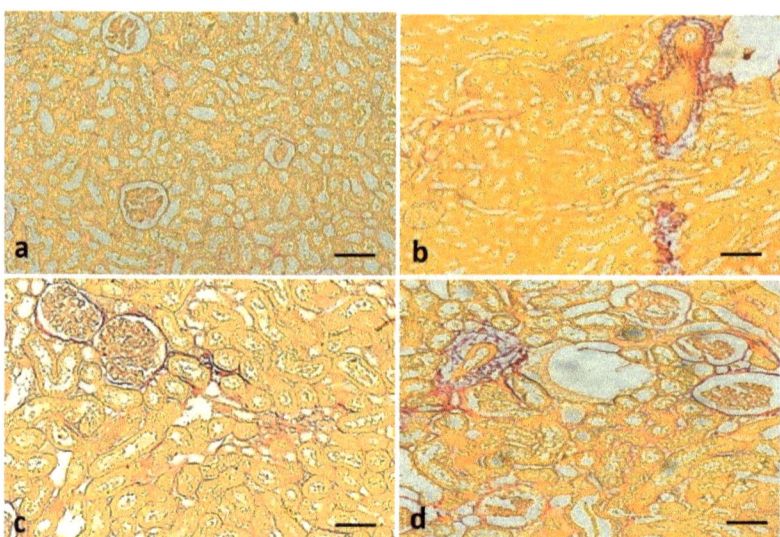

Figure 10. Quercetin decreases fiber in renal tissue. Kidney sections from the control group: did not show fibrosis (**a**), streptozotocin (STZ) group (Negative control): deposition of fiber (red color) was significantly high (**b**), STZ + glibenclamide (Positive control) showed almost no fibrosis (**c**), STZ + quercetin (50 mg/kg b.w.): showed less fiber as compared to streptozotocin (STZ) group (Negative control) (**d**).

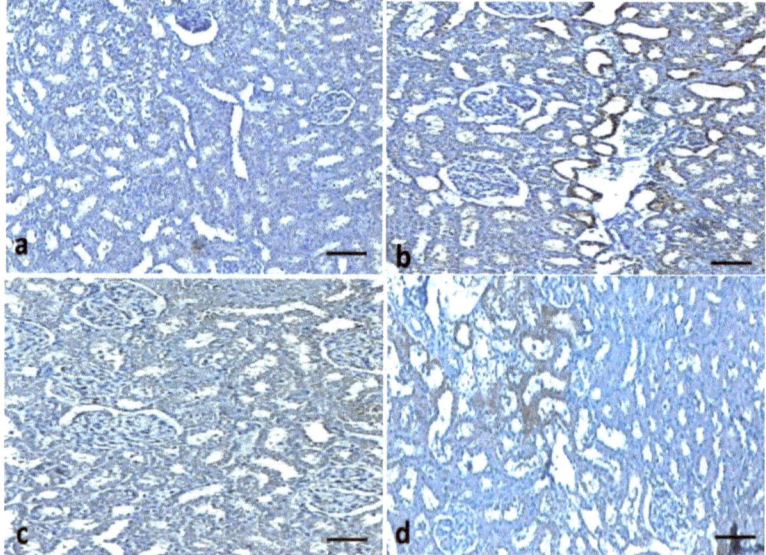

Figure 11. Quercetin decreases COX-2 protein in the renal tissues. Kidney sections from the control group: did not show any expression (**a**), streptozotocin (STZ) group (Negative control): expression of COX-2 protein was high (**b**), STZ + glibenclamide (Positive control) fiber showed almost no expression (**c**), STZ + quercetin (50 mg/kg b.w.): showed less expression as compared to the streptozotocin (STZ) group (Negative control) (**d**).

4. Discussion

Diabetes is a metabolic disorder and is characterized by chronic hyperglycemia with altered metabolism of carbohydrates, proteins, and fats resulting from altered insulin secretion, action, or both [28]. Hyperglycemia is one of the main contributors to the production of ROS and oxidative stress [2,3]. In addition, increased levels of ROS also disturb the cascade of insulin-signaling, inspiring the development of insulin resistance [3,4]. Therefore, the recognized altered state is associated with ROS over-production which causes a state of oxidative stress that is involved in the pathogenesis as well the progression of diabetes and diabetes-linked complications [29].

Natural compounds, as whole or specific active compounds of medicinal plants, play an important role in the inhibition of pathogenesis including diabetes [30–33]. To know whether quercetin has a role in the management of diabetes mellitus, it was examined by checking its role as an anti-hyperglycemic, oxidative stress, anti-inflammatory activity, and in kidney tissue architecture at a dose of 50 mg/kg b.w. in rats. STZ-induced diabetic rats treated with quercetin (50 mg/kg b.w.) showed a significant increase in body weight. All animals in the diabetic control group showed a decrease in body weight when compared to the normal control and STZ-induced diabetic rats treated with quercetin. Our results are consistent with those of earlier studies and it was reported that STZ-induced diabetes is characterized by a major loss in body weight resulting from increased muscle destruction or degradation of structural proteins [34]. Moreover, the treatment with quercetin in STZ-induced diabetic rats prevented the changes in body weight and blood glucose [35]. In addition, quercetin improved the decrease in body weight gain, and it possibly prevented reductions in body weight gain and polyuria [36]. This result is justified by previous findings as better glycemic control, with a reduction of the lipolytic response, and the consequential normalization of triglyceridemia [37,38].

After the oral administration of quercetin, the STZ-induced diabetic rats showed a significant decrease in blood glucose levels and increased insulin levels. These results are in accordance with earlier findings of antidiabetic studies that reported elevated serum blood glucose levels and insulin levels in diabetic rats were significantly improved by quercetin, resveratrol, and combined treatments [39].

It is well recognized that uncontrolled type 2 diabetes mellitus leads to increased triglycerides, *LDL* and VLDL-C, and decreased HDL-C, which promotes coronary artery diseases [40,41]. Furthermore, it has been shown that insulin deficiency in diabetes mellitus leads to a variety of derangements in metabolic and regulatory processes, which in turn lead to the accumulation of lipids like triglycerides and TC in diabetic patients [42]. In the current study, STZ treatment showed a significant increase in total cholesterol, triglycerides, and a reduction in HDL-C levels as compared to the normal control rats. Moreover, a significant reduction in TC, TG, and an elevation of HDL-C was noticed in diabetic rats treated with quercetin. Earlier findings were in agreement with the current findings and the study revealed that administration of quercetin showed significant improvements in the profiles of high-density lipoprotein, triglycerides, and total cholesterol in STZ-induced diabetic rats [43].

Streptozotocin causes major oxidative stress in diabetic animals and possibly causes the peroxidation of polyunsaturated fatty acids, important for the formation of MDA. which is a by-product of lipid peroxidation [44]. Oxidative stress plays a major role in the disturbance of cellular functions in the kidney and causes vascular permeability enhancement and tissue damage [45]. This suggestion is evidenced by the previous results [38,46] which show indications of renal oxidative stress in diabetic rats [47–50].

Measurements of MDA as a final product of the lipid peroxidation reveal the degree of oxidative stress [51]. STZ injections were administered to illustrate the cellular oxidative damage as it produces ROS and decreases the antioxidant potential in the pancreas, which is known to deteriorate this organ [52]. Antioxidants play a significant role in the reduction of MDA levels. In the current study, it is reported that diabetic rats showed a decrease in antioxidant enzymes (CAT, SOD, and GST) and GSH levels. However, in diabetic rats, quercetin treatments at doses of 50 mg/kg b.w. produced a prominent protective effect. The results revealed significantly increased levels of MDA and NO in the kidneys of diabetic rats. On the other hand, treating diabetic rats with 50 mg/kg b.w. quercetin for 8 weeks considerably improved the oxidative status through significant decreases in levels of MDA and NO, and increases in antioxidant enzyme levels. In this context, the previous study was in accord with the current findings as after 8 weeks of continuous treatment, diabetic rats displayed renal dysfunction, as confirmed by decreased urea clearance and creatinine, and proteinuria nearby with a noticeable increase in oxidative stress, as determined by lipid peroxidation. Whereas treatment with quercetin significantly reduced oxidative stress and renal dysfunction in diabetic rats [53].

STZ treatment showed a significant increase in urea and creatinine levels as compared to the normal control. However, an important reduction in urea and creatinine levels were detected among the diabetic animals treated with quercetin. The previous findings were in accordance with the current findings as quercetin treatment decreased proteinuria and high plasma levels of uric acid, urea, and creatinine [37].

Quercetin has a proven role in the inhibition of pathogenesis, including kidney damage through the maintenance of kidney architecture. The histopathological sections of kidney in diabetic rats showed congestion, fibrosis and infiltration of lymphocytes, and deposition of collagen fiber demonstrating kidney injury. Whereas pathological changes of the kidney tissue in the diabetic groups that received quercetin showed less injury and reduced fibrosis as compared to the diabetes control group. The renoprotective effect of quercetin has been proven in other studies as diabetic rats showed changes such as brush border loss and peritubular infiltration, epithelial desquamation, swelling, and intracytoplasmic vacuolization. Moreover, sclerotic changes and basement membrane thickening were seen in the glomerulus, whereas, quercetin significantly reduced such histopathological changes [48]. Other study findings were consistent with the current study's results and it was reported that STZ-induced rats showed inflammatory cell infiltration in the renal tubular and glomerulus. These kidney pathological alterations in this model were improved by treatment with quercetin [47].

Oxidative stress can cause inflammation through numerous mechanisms [54] and inflammation played an important role in the pathogenesis of diabetes [55,56]. STZ treatment showed significant enhancement of inflammatory marker levels and COX-2 protein expression as compared to the normal control. However, a decrease in inflammatory markers was observed among the diabetic animals treated with quercetin. In other novel research work, it was reported that quercetin treatment for diabetic rats led to significant decreases in oxidative stress, inflammation, and apoptosis levels [57]

In the current study, STZ-induced diabetic rats showed significant fibrosis in the kidney tissue, which was reduced by quercetin. The results established that quercetin could improve kidney injury through the maintenance of kidney architecture and reduction of fibrosis. These results are consistent with the previous reports as quercetin and crocin inhibit renal fibrosis as confirmed by Masson trichrome staining [58]. Another study reported similar findings based on *Myrciaria cauliflora* extract as increased collagen deposition was also observed in the STZ group when compared to the control group. Furthermore, the collagen deposition was inhibited by *Myrciaria cauliflora* extract in a dose-dependent manner [59].

5. Conclusions

The current findings reveal the anti-diabetic, antihyperlipidemic, anti-inflammatory, and reno-protective effects of quercetin against STZ-induced diabetes. Quercetin enhanced antioxidant enzyme levels and maintained kidney architecture. This study determines that the effects of quercetin have the potential for use in the management of diabetes mellitus, however, comprehensive, detailed biochemical and molecular studies should be performed to identify the exact mechanisms of quercetin's renoprotective effects.

Supplementary Materials: The following supporting information can be downloaded at: https://www.mdpi.com/article/10.3390/metabo13010130/s1, Supplementary File S1: supplementary data.

Author Contributions: Conceptualization, A.H.R., A.A.K., M.A.A. and S.A.A.; methodology, A.H.R. and A.A.K.; investigation, A.H.R., M.A.A., A.A.K. and S.A.A.; writing—original draft preparation, A.H.R. and A.A.K.; writing—review and editing, M.A.A., A.A.K., S.A.A. and A.H.R.; supervision, S.A.A. and M.A.A. All authors have read and agreed to the published version of the manuscript.

Funding: Deputyship for Research & Innovation, Ministry of Education, Saudi Arabia, project number (QU-IF-02-01-28388).

Institutional Review Board Statement: The animals were maintained at animal facility of the College of Applied Medical Sciences (CAMS) followed by the standards of the Qassim University on Animal Care. The animal experiments were carried out as per the guidelines of CAMS, Qassim University.

Informed Consent Statement: Not applicable.

Data Availability Statement: The data used to support the findings of this study are included within the article.

Acknowledgments: The authors extend their appreciation to the Deputyship for Research & Innovation, Ministry of Education, Saudi Arabia for funding this research work through the project number (QU-IF-02-01-28388). The authors also thank to Qassim University for technical support.

Conflicts of Interest: The authors declare no conflict of interest.

References

1. International Diabetes Federation. *IDF Diabetes Atlas*, 8th ed.; International Diabetes Federation: Brussels, Belgium, 2017.
2. Nowotny, K.; Jung, T.; Hohn, A.; Weber, D.; Grune, T. Advanced glycation end products and oxidative stress in type 2 diabetes mellitus. *Biomolecules* **2015**, *5*, 194–222. [CrossRef]
3. Abdali, D.; Samson, S.E.; Grover, A.K. How effective are antioxidant supplements in obesity and diabetes? *Med. Princ. Pract.* **2015**, *24*, 201–215. [CrossRef] [PubMed]
4. Gurzov, E.N.; Tran, M.; Fernandez-Rojo, M.A.; Merry, T.L.; Zhang, X.; Xu, Y.; Fukushima, A.; Waters, M.J.; Watt, M.J.; Andrikopoulos, S.; et al. Hepatic oxidative stress promotes insulin-STAT-5 signaling and obesity by inactivating protein tyrosine phosphatase N_2. *Cell Metab.* **2014**, *20*, 85–102. [CrossRef]
5. Wang, X.; Zhang, W.; Chen, H.; Liao, N.; Wang, Z.; Zhang, X.; Hai, C. High selenium impairs hepatic insulin sensitivity through opposite regulation of ROS. *Toxicol. Lett.* **2014**, *224*, 16–23. [CrossRef]
6. Taskinen, M.R. Diabetic dyslipidemia. *Atheroscler. Suppl.* **2002**, *3*, 47–51. [CrossRef] [PubMed]
7. Bandeira, F.; Gharib, H.; Golbert, A.; Griz, L.; Faria, M. An overview on management of diabetic dyslipidemia. *J. Diabetes Endocrinol.* **2014**, *4*, 27–36.
8. Wu, L.; Parhofer, K.G. Diabetic dyslipidemia. *Metab. Clin. Exp.* **2014**, *63*, 1469–1479. [CrossRef] [PubMed]
9. Krentz, A.J. Comparative safety of newer oral antidiabetic drugs. *Expert Opin. Drug Saf.* **2006**, *5*, 827–834. [CrossRef] [PubMed]
10. Rafaeloff, R.; Pittenger, G.L.; Barlow, S.W.; Qin, X.F.; Yan, B.; Rosenberg, L.; Duguid, W.P.; Vinik, A.I. Cloning and sequencing of the pancreatic islet neogenesis associated protein (INGAP) gene and its expression in islet neogenesis in hamsters. *J. Clin. Investig.* **1997**, *99*, 2100–2109. [CrossRef] [PubMed]
11. Yin, J.; Zhang, H.; Ye, J. Traditional Chinese medicine in treatment of metabolic syndrome. *Endocr. Metab. Immune Disord. Drug Targets* **2008**, *8*, 99–111. [CrossRef]
12. Dhasarathan, P.; Theriappan, P. Evaluation of anti-diabetic activity of *Strychonous potatorum* in alloxan induced diabetic rats. *J. Med. Sci.* **2011**, *2*, 670–674.
13. Ramesh, B.; Pugalendi, K.V. Anti-hyperglycemic effect of Umbelliferone in Streptozotocin diabetic rats. *J. Med. Plants.* **2006**, *9*, 562–566.
14. Anand David, A.V.; Arulmoli, R.; Parasuraman, S. Overviews of Biological Importance of Quercetin: A Bioactive Flavonoid. *Pharmacogn. Rev.* **2016**, *10*, 84–89. [PubMed]
15. Dabeek, W.M.; Marra, M.V. Dietary quercetin and kaempferol: Bioavailability and potential cardiovascular-related bioactivity in humans. *Nutrients* **2019**, *11*, 2288. [CrossRef] [PubMed]
16. Davis, J.M.; Murphy, A.; Carmichael, M.D.; Davis, B. Quercetin increases brain and muscle mitochondrial biogenesis and exercise tolerance. *Am. J. Physiol. Regul. Integr. Comp. Physiol.* **2009**, *296*, R1071–R1077. [CrossRef] [PubMed]
17. Saeedi-Boroujeni, A.; Mahmoudian-Sani, M.-R. Anti-inflammatory potential of Quercetin in COVID-19 treatment. *J. Inflamm.* **2021**, *18*, 3.
18. Alzohairy, M.A.; Khan, A.A.; Ansari, M.A.; Babiker, A.Y.; Alsahli, M.A.; Almatroodi, S.A.; Rahmani, A.H. Protective Effect of Quercetin, a Flavonol against Benzo(a)pyrene-Induced Lung Injury via Inflammation, Oxidative Stress, Angiogenesis and Cyclooxygenase-2 Signalling Molecule. *Appl. Sci.* **2021**, *11*, 8675. [CrossRef]

19. Chen, B.H.; Park, J.H.; Ahn, J.H.; Cho, J.H.; Kim, I.H.; Lee, J.C.; Won, M.H.; Lee, C.H.; Hwang, I.K.; Kim, J.D.; et al. Pretreated quercetin protects gerbil hippocampal CA1 pyramidal neurons from transient cerebral ischemic injury by increasing the expression of antioxidant enzymes. *Neural Regen Res.* **2017**, *12*, 220–227.
20. Braun, K.F.; Ehnert, S.; Freude, T.; Egaña, J.T.; Schenck, T.L.; Buchholz, A.; Schmitt, A.; Siebenlist, S.; Schyschka, L.; Neumaier, M.; et al. Quercetin protects primary human osteoblasts exposed to cigarette smoke through activation of the antioxidative enzymes HO-1 and SOD-1. *Sci. World J.* **2011**, *11*, 2348–2357. [CrossRef]
21. Izak-Shirian, F.; Najafi-Asl, M.; Azami, B.; Heidarian, E.; Najafi, M.; Khaledi, M.; Nouri, A. Quercetin exerts an ameliorative effect in the rat model of diclofenac-induced renal injury through mitigation of inflammatory response and modulation of oxidative stress. *Eur. J. Inflamm.* **2022**, *20*, 1721727X221086530. [CrossRef]
22. Almatroodi, S.A.; Alsahli, M.A.; Almatroudi, A.; Verma, A.K.; Aloliqi, A.; Allemailem, K.S.; Khan, A.A.; Rahmani, A.H. Potential therapeutic targets of quercetin, a plant flavonol, and its role in the therapy of various types of cancer through the modulation of various cell signaling pathways. *Molecules* **2021**, *26*, 1315.
23. Strugała, P.; Dzydzan, O.; Brodyak, I.; Kucharska, A.Z.; Kuropka, P.; Liuta, M.; Kaleta-Kuratewicz, K.; Przewodowska, A.; Michałowska, D.; Gabrielska, J.; et al. Antidiabetic and Antioxidative Potential of the Blue Congo Variety of Purple Potato Extract in Streptozotocin-Induced Diabetic Rats. *Molecules* **2019**, *24*, 3126. [CrossRef]
24. Ola, M.S.; Ahmed, M.M.; Shams, S.; Al-Rejaie, S.S. Neuroprotective effects of quercetin in diabetic rat retina. *Saudi J. Biol. Sci.* **2017**, *24*, 1186–1194. [CrossRef]
25. Nazir, N.; Zahoor, M.; Nisar, M.; Khan, I.; Ullah, R.; Alotaibi, A. Antioxidants Isolated from *Elaeagnus umbellata* (Thunb.) Protect against Bacterial Infections and Diabetes in Streptozotocin-Induced Diabetic Rat Model. *Molecules* **2021**, *26*, 4464. [CrossRef] [PubMed]
26. Husain, N.E.; Babiker, A.Y.; Albutti, A.S.; Alsahli, M.A.; Aly, S.M.; Rahmani, A.H. Clinicopathological Significance of Vimentin and Cytokeratin Protein in the Genesis of Squamous Cell Carcinoma of Cervix. *Obstet. Gynecol. Int.* **2016**, *2016*, 8790120.
27. Babiker, A.Y.; Almatroudi, A.; Allemailem, K.S.; Husain, N.E.O.; Alsammani, M.A.; Alsahli, M.A.; Rahmani, A.H. Clinicopathologic Aspects of Squamous Cell Carcinoma of the Uterine Cervix: Role of PTEN, BCL2 and P53. *Applied Sciences* **2018**, *8*, 2124. [CrossRef]
28. Khan, N.; Sultana, S. Abrogation of potassium bromate-induced renal oxidative stress and subsequent cell proliferation response by soy isoflavones in Wistar rats. *Toxicology* **2004**, *201*, 173–184. [CrossRef] [PubMed]
29. Bigagli, E.; Lodovici, M. Circulating oxidative stress biomarkers in clinical studies on type 2 diabetes and its complications. *Oxid. Med. Cell. Longev.* **2019**, *2019*, 5953685. [PubMed]
30. Rahmani, A.H.; Aldebasi, Y.H.; Srikar, S.; Khan, A.A.; Aly, S.M. *Aloe vera*: Potential candidate in health management via modulation of biological activities. *Pharmacogn. Rev.* **2015**, *9*, 120–126. [CrossRef] [PubMed]
31. Rahmani, A.H. Cassia fistula Linn: Potential candidate in the health management. *Pharmacogn. Res.* **2015**, *7*, 217–224. [CrossRef]
32. Rahmani, A.H.; Aly, S.M.; Ali, H.; Babiker, A.Y.; Srikar, S.; Khan, A.A. Therapeutic effects of date fruits (*Phoenix dactylifera*) in the prevention of diseases via modulation of anti-inflammatory, anti-oxidant and anti-tumour activity. *Int. J. Clin. Exp. Med.* **2014**, *7*, 483–491.
33. Almatroodi, S.A.; Almatroudi, A.; Alsahli, M.A.; Rahmani, A.H. Grapes and their Bioactive Compounds: Role in Health Management Through Modulating Various Biological Phcogj.com Activities. *Pharmacogn. J.* **2020**, *12*, 1455–1462. [CrossRef]
34. Priscilla, D.H.; Jayakumar, M.; Thirumurgan, K. Flavanone naringenin: An effective antihyperglycemic and antihyperlipidemic nutraceutical agent on high fat diet fed streptozotocin induced type 2 diabetic rats. *J. Func. Foods* **2015**, *14*, 363–373.
35. Bhutada, P.; Mundhada, Y.; Bansod, K.; Bhutada, C.; Tawari, S.; Dixit, P.; Mundhada, D. Ameliorative effect of quercetin on memory dysfunction in streptozotocin-induced diabetic rats. *Neurobiol. Learn Mem.* **2010**, *94*, 293–302. [CrossRef]
36. Gomes, I.B.S.; Porto, M.L.; Santos, M.C.L.F.S.; Campagnaro, B.P.; Gava, A.L.; Meyrelles, S.S.; Pereira, T.M.C.; Vasquez, E.C. The protective effects of oral low-dose quercetin on diabetic nephropathy in hypercholesterolemic mice. *Front. Physiol.* **2015**, *6*, 247. [CrossRef] [PubMed]
37. Gomes, I.; Porto, M.L.; Santos, M.C.L.; Campagnaro, B.P.; Pereira, T.; Meyrelles, S.S.; Vasquez, E.C. Renoprotective, anti-oxidative and anti-apoptotic effects of oral low-dose quercetin in the C57BL/6J model of diabetic nephropathy. *Lipids Health Dis.* **2014**, *13*, 184. [CrossRef] [PubMed]
38. Ozcelik, D.; Tuncdemir, M.; Ozturk, M.; Uzun, H. Evaluation of trace elements and oxidative stress levels in the liver and kidney of streptozotocin-induced experimental diabetic rat model. *Gen. Physiol. Biophys.* **2011**, *30*, 356–363. [CrossRef] [PubMed]
39. Yang, D.K.; Kang, H.S. Anti-Diabetic Effect of Cotreatment with Quercetin and Resveratrol in Streptozotocin-Induced Diabetic Rats. *Biomol. Ther.* **2018**, *26*, 130–138. [CrossRef] [PubMed]
40. Arvind, K.; Pradeep, R.; Deepa, R.; Mohan, V. Diabetes and coronary artery diseases. *Indian J. Med. Res.* **2002**, *116*, 163–176.
41. Palumbo, P.J. Metformin: Effect on cardiovascular risk factor in patients with non-insulin dependent diabetes mellitus. *J. Diabetes Its Complicat.* **1998**, *12*, 110–119. [CrossRef]
42. Goldberg, R.B. Lipid disorders in diabetes. *Diabetes Care* **1981**, *4*, 561–572. [CrossRef] [PubMed]
43. Srinivasan, P.; Vijayakumar, S.; Kothandaraman, S.; Palani, M. Anti-diabetic activity of quercetin extracted from Phyllanthus emblica L. fruit: In silico and in vivo approaches. *J. Pharm. Anal.* **2018**, *8*, 109–118. [CrossRef] [PubMed]
44. Ma, Q.; Guo, Y.; Sun, L.; Zhuang, Y. Anti-Diabetic Effects of Phenolic Extract from Rambutan Peels (*Nephelium lappaceum*) in High-Fat Diet and Streptozotocin-Induced Diabetic Mice. *Nutrients* **2017**, *9*, 801. [CrossRef]

45. Brown, W.V. Microvascular complications of diabetes mellitus: Renal protection accompanies cardiovascular protection. *Am. J. Cardiol.* **2008**, *102*, 10L–13L. [CrossRef] [PubMed]
46. Oršolić, N.; Gajski, G.; Garaj-Vrhovac, V.; Dikić, D.; Prskalo, Z.Š.; Sirovina, D. DNA-protective effects of quercetin or naringenin in alloxan-induced diabetic mice. *Eur. J. Pharmacol.* **2011**, *656*, 110–118. [CrossRef]
47. Wang, C.; Pan, Y.; Zhang, Q.Y.; Wang, F.M.; Kong, L.D. Quercetin and allopurinol ameliorate kidney injury in STZ-treated rats with regulation of renal NLRP3 inflammasome activation and lipid accumulation. *PLoS ONE* **2012**, *7*, e38285. [CrossRef]
48. Elbe, H.; Vardi, N.; Esrefoglu, M.; Ates, B.; Yologlu, S.; Taskapan, C. Amelioration of streptozotocin-induced diabetic nephropathy by melatonin, quercetin, and resveratrol in rats. *Hum. Exp. Toxicol.* 2014; *epub ahead of priint*.
49. Chen, P.; Chen, J.; Zheng, Q.; Chen, W.; Wang, Y.; Xu, X. Pioglitazone, extract of compound Danshen dripping pill, and quercetin ameliorate diabetic nephropathy in diabetic rats. *J. Endocrinol. Invest.* **2013**, *36*, 422–427.
50. Lai, P.B.; Zhang, L.; Yang, L.Y. Quercetin ameliorates diabetic nephropathy by reducing the expressions of transforming growth factor-β1 and connective tissue growth factor in streptozotocin-induced diabetic rats. *Ren. Fail.* **2012**, *34*, 83–87. [CrossRef]
51. Oh, P.S.; Lee, S.J.; Lim, K.T. Hypolipidemic and antioxydative effects of the plant glycoprotein (36 kDa) from *Rhus verniciflua* stokes fruit in triton Wr-1339 induced hyperlipidemic mice. *Biosci. Biotechnol. Biochem.* **2006**, *70*, 447–456. [CrossRef]
52. Coskun, O.; Kanter, M.; Korkmaz, A.; Oter, S. Quercetin, a flavonoid antioxidant, prevents and protects streptozotocin-induced oxidative stress and beta-cell damage in rat pancreas. *Pharmacol. Res.* **2005**, *51*, 117–123. [CrossRef]
53. Anjaneyulu, M.; Chopra, K. Quercetin, an anti-oxidant bioflavonoid, attenuates diabetic nephropathy in rats. *Clin. Exp. Pharmacol. Physiol.* **2004**, *31*, 244–248. [CrossRef] [PubMed]
54. Lai, L.L.; Lu, H.Q.; Li, W.N.; Huang, H.P.; Zhou, H.Y.; Leng, E.N.; Zhang, Y.Y. Protective effects of quercetin and crocin in the kidneys and liver of obese Sprague-Dawley rats with Type 2 diabetes: Effects of quercetin and crocin on T2DM rats. *Hum. Exp. Toxicol.* **2021**, *40*, 661–672. [CrossRef] [PubMed]
55. Hsu, J.D.; Wu, C.C.; Hung, C.N.; Wang, C.J.; Huang, H.P. Myrciaria cauliflora extract improves diabetic nephropathy via suppression of oxidative stress and inflammation in streptozotocin-nicotinamide mice. *J. Food Drug Anal.* **2016**, *24*, 730–737. [CrossRef]
56. Wada, J.; Makino, H. Inflammation and the pathogenesis of diabetic nephropathy. *Clin. Sci.* **2013**, *124*, 139–152. [CrossRef] [PubMed]
57. Roslan, J.; Giribabu, N.; Karim, K.; Salleh, N. Quercetin ameliorates oxidative stress, inflammation and apoptosis in the heart of streptozotocin-nicotinamide-induced adult male diabetic rats. *Biomed. Pharmacother.* **2017**, *86*, 570–582. [CrossRef] [PubMed]
58. Lim, A.K.; Tesch, G.H. Inflammation in diabetic nephropathy. *Mediat. Inflamm.* **2012**, *2012*, 146154. [CrossRef]
59. Wu, C.C.; Hung, C.N.; Shin, Y.C.; Wang, C.J.; Huang, H.P. Myrciaria cauliflora extracts attenuate diabetic nephropathy involving the Ras signaling pathway in streptozotocin/nicotinamide mice on a high fat diet. *J. Food Drug analysis* **2016**, *24*, 136–146. [CrossRef]

Disclaimer/Publisher's Note: The statements, opinions and data contained in all publications are solely those of the individual author(s) and contributor(s) and not of MDPI and/or the editor(s). MDPI and/or the editor(s) disclaim responsibility for any injury to people or property resulting from any ideas, methods, instructions or products referred to in the content.

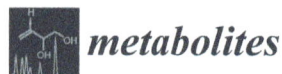

Review

Recent Updates on Source, Biosynthesis, and Therapeutic Potential of Natural Flavonoid Luteolin: A Review

Nandakumar Muruganathan [1,†], Anand Raj Dhanapal [2,3,†], Venkidasamy Baskar [4,†], Pandiyan Muthuramalingam [5], Dhivya Selvaraj [6], Husne Aara [2], Mohamed Zubair Shiek Abdullah [2] and Iyyakkannu Sivanesan [7,*]

1. Department of Plant Pathology and Microbiology, The Robert H. Smith Faculty of Agriculture, Food and Environment, The Hebrew University of Jerusalem, Rehovot 76100, Israel
2. Department of Biotechnology, Karpagam Academy of Higher Education, Coimbatore 641021, Tamil Nadu, India
3. Centre for Plant Tissue Culture & Central Instrumentation Laboratory, Karpagam Academy of Higher Education, Coimbatore 641021, Tamil Nadu, India
4. Department of Oral & Maxillofacial Surgery, Saveetha Dental College and Hospitals, Saveetha Institute of Medical and Technical Sciences (SIMATS), Saveetha University, Chennai 600077, Tamil Nadu, India
5. Division of Horticultural Science, College of Agriculture and Life Sciences, Gyeongsang National University, Jinju 52725, Republic of Korea
6. Department of Computer Science and Engineering CSE-AI, Amrita School of Engineering, Chennai 601103, Tamil Nadu, India
7. Department of Bioresources and Food Science, Institute of Natural Science and Agriculture, Konkuk University, 1 Hwayang-dong, Gwangjin-gu, Seoul 05029, Republic of Korea
* Correspondence: siva74@konkuk.ac.kr; Tel.: +82-2-450-0576
† These authors contributed equally to this work.

Abstract: Nature gives immense resources that are beneficial to humankind. The natural compounds present in plants provide primary nutritional values to our diet. Apart from food, plants also provide chemical compounds with therapeutic values. The importance of these plant secondary metabolites is increasing due to more studies revealing their beneficial properties in treating and managing various diseases and their symptoms. Among them, flavonoids are crucial secondary metabolite compounds present in most plants. Of the reported 8000 flavonoid compounds, luteolin is an essential dietary compound. This review discusses the source of the essential flavonoid luteolin in various plants and its biosynthesis. Furthermore, the potential health benefits of luteolins such as anti-cancer, anti-microbial, anti-inflammatory, antioxidant, and anti-diabetic effects and their mechanisms are discussed in detail. The activity of luteolin and its derivatives are diverse, as they help to prevent and control many diseases and their life-threatening effects. This review will enhance the knowledge and recent findings regarding luteolin and its therapeutic effects, which are certainly useful in potentially utilizing this natural metabolite.

Keywords: anti-inflammatory; anti-cancer; anti-diabetic; luteolin; secondary metabolite; flavonoid

1. Introduction

Plants have a vast majority of chemical compounds which are used daily. Due to knowledge of plant-based therapeutic benefits, bioactive compounds have been explored in past decades to treat various human diseases in addition to being utilized in their prevention [1]. The uses of these chemical compounds in dietary and therapeutic applications significantly impact well-being, as most of these compounds have beneficial activities for healthy living. Among the phytochemical compounds, flavonoids are the major group due to their beneficial properties. The flavonoids are polyphenols having a C6-C3-C6 diphenylpropane structure and two benzene rings. As of today, more than 8000 flavonoid compounds have been identified and differentiated based on their heterocyclic C-ring structure into 10 groups, among which flavones, flavanones, chalcones, flavanols, isoflavones, and anthocyanins have pharmacological benefits [2,3]. In plants, their role is involved in protecting the plant cells against ultraviolet radiation and biotic stresses. They act as anti-microbial compounds, give color to the flowers, and thus help pollination [4,5].

The flavonoid compounds structural activities depend on their hydroxyl groups. Among the flavonoids, luteolin (3',4',5,7-tetrahydroxy flavone) is an important dietary compound present in different plant species [6]. Most of the bioactivity of luteolin (LUT) is due to a hydroxyl moiety present in the position of 3', 4', 5, and 7 carbon (Figure 1). Luteolin is a widely present flavonoid compound, as its major source is fruits, vegetables, and other edible parts of plants. Research studies in the past decades explored the biological significance of the LUT compounds, revealing their antioxidant, anti-cancer, anti-inflammatory, and neuroprotective nature [7,8]. As these compounds therapeutic effects are increasing, this review will enlighten more on LUT for a deeper understanding in addition to highlighting current research.

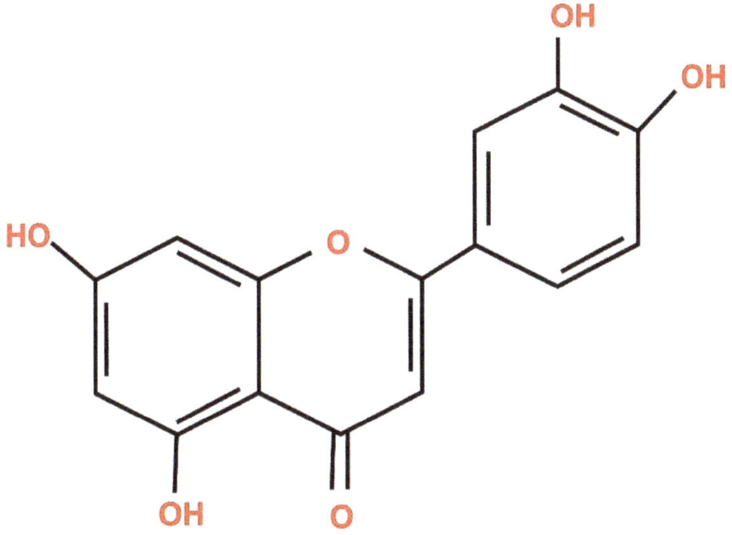

Figure 1. Diagrammatic representation of luteolin compound.

2. Source of Luteolin

Luteolin's therapeutic benefits have led the scientific community to explore its potential more. The search in the NCBI PubMed database retrieved more than five thousand articles showing its potential nature. The plant kingdom is the major source of this compound, and it is present as LUT or as luteolin glycosides. Its wide distribution among plants is well documented, as more than 300 plant species were reported to possess LUT or its derivates [9]. Its presence is even documented in the 36- and 25-million-year-old fossils of *Celtis* and *Ulmus* species, respectively [10]. The presence of LUT was identified among monocotyledons and dicotyledons. Among the plant kingdom, in the families of Asteraceae, Lamiaceae, Poaceae, Leguminosae, and Scrophulariaceae species, the LUT and its glycosides were identified in 66, 38, 13, 10, and 10 species, respectively (Figure 2).

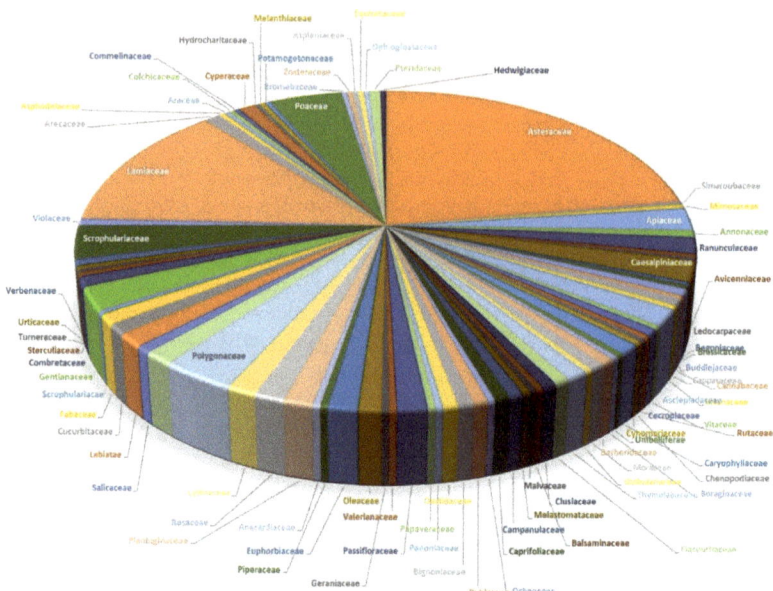

Figure 2. Distribution of luteolin compounds in the plant kingdom. The presence of luteolin in various plant families is represented in the pie chart based on the number of species in each family.

3. Luteolin Biosynthesis

Plants have an array of metabolic compounds for their basic functions and their response to various stimuli. Phenyl propanoids are compounds involved in plant development, cellular metabolism, and biotic and abiotic stimuli, and are obtained from the phenylalanine molecule [11]. The phenylpropanoid pathway starts after the shikimate pathway that has been studied for decades [12]. The LUT molecule is the product of the phenylpropanoid and flavonoid pathways, as it branches from the major secondary metabolite pathway, the phenylpropanoid pathway, where all the secondary metabolic compounds are synthesized.

The flavonoid biosynthesis starts with phenylalanine ammonia lyase converting phenylalanine (Phe) amino acid into trans-cinnamic acid, followed by trans-coumaric acid using enzyme trans-cinnamate 4-hydroxylase (C4H), p-coumaroyl CoA by enzyme coumarate 4-ligase (4CL) [11,13], which is then converted into naringenin chalcone (NC) by the enzyme chalcone synthase, a type III polyketide synthase family enzyme [14]. NC is transformed into naringenin, an important compound acting as a key step in the luteolin biosynthesis by the enzyme chalcone isomerase (CHI) [15]. Further, naringenin is converted into eriodictyol by the enzyme flavonoid 3′-hydroxylase (F3′H), as this enzyme introduces a hydroxyl group at the 3′ position in the beta ring [16]. In addition, flavone synthase (FNS) belongs to the cytochrome P450 superfamily, which produces LUT from the substrate naringenin and eriodictyol [17,18] (Figure 3).

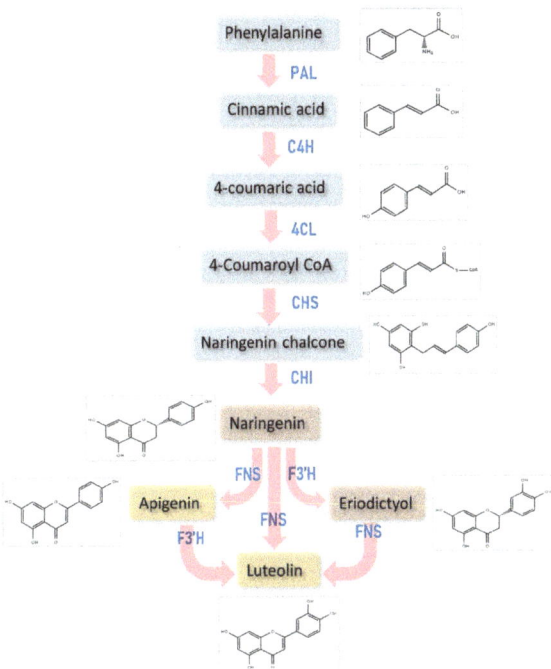

Figure 3. Diagrammatic representation of the biosynthesis of luteolin. PAL—phenylalanine ammonia lyase; C4H—cinnamate 4-hydroxylase; 4-CL—coumarate 4-ligase; CHS—chalcone synthase; F3′H—flavonoid 3′-hydroxylase; CHI—chalcone isomerase; FNS—flavone synthase.

4. Physiochemical Properties of Luteolin

The luteolin molecule in plants is widely distributed as the aglycone molecule without a sugar moiety and as a glycoside molecule with a sugar moiety bound to it. Its molecular formula is $C_{15}H_{10}O_6$ with an MW of 286.24 [19]. Luteolin has weak aqueous soluble properties [20]. Most of the LUT molecule occurs as O-glycosides, having aglycone attached with sugar moieties by one or more hydroxyl (OH) group. The OH groups are positioned at the 5, 7, 3′, and 4′ position. Among the sugar moieties, glucose is the major sugar molecule attached to luteolin. Other than that, rhamnose, rutinose, arabinose, xylose, and glucuronic acid are other sugar derivatives attached to luteolin [9,21].

5. Chemopreventive Functions of Luteolin

Luteolin is one of the natural secondary metabolites derived from plants shown to possess various chemopreventive activities such as antioxidant, anti-cancer, anti-microbial, anti-diabetic, anti-inflammatory, and neuroprotective functions.

5.1. Antioxidant Properties of Luteolin

Oxidative stress plays a major role in various cellular metabolisms and also during the pathogenesis of neurodegenerative disorders, cancer, diabetes, cardiovascular diseases, rheumatoid arthritis, aging, and hypertension [22]. Oxidative stress occurs due to the production of reactive oxygen species (ROS) formed during the oxidative phosphorylation of oxygen to produce energy by synthesizing ATP. There are different ROS molecules present, such as hydroxyl radical (OH), hydrogen peroxide (H_2O_2), peroxynitrate ($ONOO^-$), and superoxide anion (O_2^-). The balanced production of antioxidant molecules maintains balanced cellular homeostasis, whereas an imbalanced mechanism of overproduction of ROS leads to oxidative stress. Thus, the antioxidative molecules help protect from developing oxidative stress in various diseases.

Flavonoids have antioxidant properties that have been widely reported in several research findings [23,24]. The LUT molecule among the flavonoids has antioxidant activity, as it possesses anti-scavenging activity due to its glycosidic group, which helps in removing reactive nitrogen species and oxygen species [25–29]. LUT's antioxidant activity is linked to the C-glycosylation effect at various positions, which causes the intensity and changes in its scavenging properties [30]. The luteolin (50 mg/kg orally) pretreatment gives protection against renal failure through the detoxification mechanism by antioxidant activity and anti-inflammatory and anti-apoptotic mechanisms in Wister rats [31]. In addition, LUT helps in reducing the effect of mucosal damage due to intestinal mucositis caused during cancer treatment [32]. The hepatoxicity induced by carbon tetra chloride (CCl_4) in the rat model was reduced by LUT's antioxidant property by increasing the activity of various antioxidant enzymes [33].

Furthermore, the LUT antioxidant activity was proved to induce apoptosis via increasing antioxidant activity [34]. LUT from *Reseda odorata* L. reduces severe acute pancreatitis (SAP) by activating hemeoxygenase-1 (HO^{-1})-based anti-inflammatory and antioxidant activity via suppressing nuclear factor-κB (NF-κB) [35]. LUT also acts as a chemoprotective molecule during doxorubicin treatment which causes hepatorenal injuries, as it helps in the therapeutic efficiency of the drug by removing its toxic effect due to its antioxidant nature [36]. Thus, the effective role of the LUT molecule and its glycosides mediates a crucial action in various metabolic processes and acts as a protective molecule by reducing the ROS species through its antioxidant activity.

5.2. Anti-Cancer Activity

Cancer is the deadliest disease affecting human beings, as the global death ratio is ever increasing due to its uncurable nature. As it alone causes around 10 million deaths, which implies that one in every six people dies from it [37]. The most common cancers are lung, breast, colon, prostate, stomach, liver, ovary, thyroid, and rectum. The cause of the higher emergence of cancers is due to lifestyle changes such increased tobacco and alcohol consumption, enhanced body weight index, lack of physical exercise, and lower dietary food intake. Adjoining diseases such as human papillomavirus (HPV) cause nearly 30% of death due to cancer [38–40]. The luteolin molecule has anti-cancer and anti-inflammatory properties [41] (Figure 4 and Table 1). An in silico analysis of the LUT molecule from *Tridax procumbens* showed it to have high active probability and less cardio-toxicity, making it an ideal drug candidate targeting the mini chromosome maintenance (MCM7) protein which causes dysregulation of DNA and leads to various types of cancer [42].

The LUT molecule has anti-cancer properties attributed to its antioxidant and free radical quenching activity [41]. Its effective inhibitor activity against cancer cell proliferation studied both in vivo at a dosage of 3 to 50 μM and in vitro at a dosage of 5 to 10 mg/kg proved its efficiency [43]. Its ability to penetrate the skin gives the advantage of treating skin cancer. Studies involving human carcinoma cells have shown its activity against stomach cancer at an IC50 value of 7.1 μg/mL. Against lung cancer, its effective activity was seen at an IC50 value of 11.7 μg/mL, and an IC50 value of 19.5 μg/mL was found to be effective against bladder cancer [44]. Blood cancer leukemia is another major cancer affecting humans, as it produces abnormal white blood cells, causing many deaths. The LUT compound also showed an inhibitory effect on the human leukemic cell lines CEM-C1 and CEM-C7 [45,46].

In addition, its growth inhibitory effects are evidenced in a study against HL-60, the human promyelocytic leukemia cells. LUT from the fruit of *Vitex rotundifolia* has a growth inhibitory concentration of 15 μM at 96 h [47,48]. Also, when STZ-induced diabetic rat models administered with luteolin it improves cognitive function, as it reduces in the diabetic condition. The improvement in expression of growth-associated protein-43 (GAP-43) and synaptophysin (SYN) in the hippocampus after LUT treatment was also found [49].

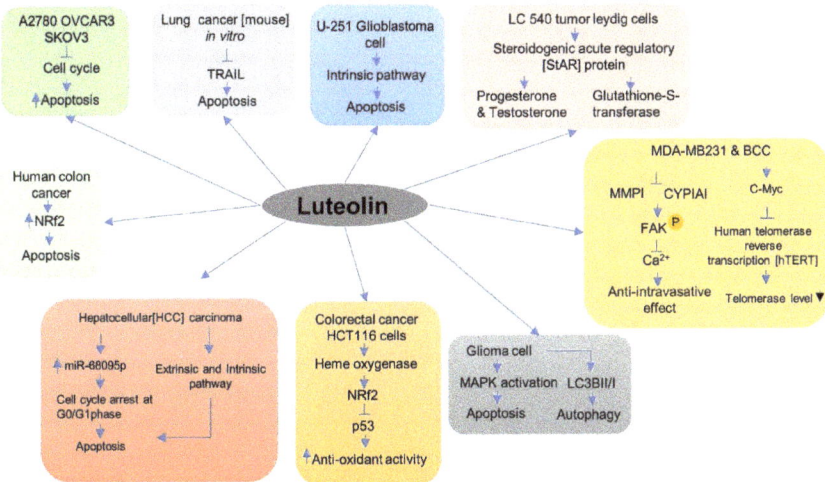

Figure 4. The anti-cancer effect of luteolin compounds against different cancer cells was sketched. The anti-cancer activity of the compound and its mechanism for preventing cancer cells involving different mechanisms.

Table 1. The mechanistic action of luteolin and its types against various types of cancer cells.

Compound	Cancer Cell	Mechanism	Reference
Luteolin	Colorectal cancer HCT116 cells	It increases the transcriptional activity of antioxidative response element in HCT116 cells.	[50]
Luteolin-7-O-glucoside and luteolin	MCF-7 cell in breast cancer	Anti-cancer activities against MC77 cells with selective index 8.0.	[51]
Apigenin and luteolin	MDA-MB231 breast cancer cells (BCC) immortalized lymph endothelial cell (LEC) monolayer	It suppresses pro intravasation trigger factors in MDA-MB 231 BCC, specifically MMP1 expression and CYP1A1 activity.	[52]
Luteolin	A2780, OVCAR3, and SKOV3	By inducing apoptosis, arrested cell cycle thus inhibits cell invasion in ovarian cancer cells.	[53]
Luteolin	Myeloid leukemia cells	It triggers leukemia cells apoptosis through modulating the differential expression of PTTG1.	[54]
Luteolin	Lung cancer (mouse) in vitro	It enhances inhibition of tumor growth, thus decreases tumor weight and increases tumor cell apoptosis in vitro.	[33]
Luteolin	Tumor cells	It reduces the tumorigenic potential and inhibits the migration of U-251 glioblastoma cells. It enhances apoptosis by an intrinsic pathway.	[55]
Nano Luteolin	Lung cancer (H292 cell) and head and neck cancer (SSCH and TU212) cell line	Nanoluteolin inhibits the effect of tumor growth of SCCHN.	[56]
Luteolin	Hepatocellular (HCC) carcinoma	It represses the growth of HCC by stimulating apoptosis and cell cycle arrest at G0/G1phase in Huh7 cells at the G2/M phase; miR-68095p mediates the growth-repressive activity of luteolin in HCC.	[57]

Table 1. Cont.

Compound	Cancer Cell	Mechanism	Reference
Luteolin	Colon cancer cells	It induces apoptosis in doxorubicin-sensitive LoVo colon cancer cells and drug-resistant LoVo/Dx cell lines. Their cytotoxic activity in LoVo/Dx cell line was considerably lower than LoVo cell line.	[58]
Luetolin-7-O-glucoside	Nasopharyngeal carcinoma (NPC-039 NPC-BM)	It reduces the proliferation of NPC cell line by inducing S and G2/M cell cycle arrest by chromatin condensation at apoptosis through AKT signaling pathway.	[59]
Luteolin	4TI breast cancer cell	It increases the apoptosis in 4TI BCC.	[60]
Luteolin	Breast cancer cell MDA-MB231	It reduces telomerase levels in a concentration-based fashion. It inhibits phosphorylation of the NF-κB inhibitor and its target gene c-Myc to repress human telomerase reverse transcription (hTERT) expression that codes the catalytic subunit of telomerase.	[61]
Luteolin	Tamoxifen resistant ER (TRER) + VE Breast cancer cells	The synergistic application of luteolin and P13K, AKT, or mTOR inhibitors synergistically enhances apoptosis in TRER+VE cells. Ras gene (K-Ras, H-Ras, and N-Ras) inducer of P13K was transcriptionally suppressed by stimulation of tumor suppressor mixed-PI3K lineage leukemia 3 (MLL3) expression.	[62]
Luteolin	Hepatocellular cancer Hep 3B cells	It induced autophagy in p53 null Hep3B cells.	[63]
Luteolin	Human colon cancer	It inhibits the expression of DNA methyltransferase, a transcription repressor that enhanced the expression of the activity of ten-eleven translocation (TET) DNA methylase a transcription activator. It also increases the interaction between Nrf2 and p53, which increases the expression of antioxidative enzymes and apoptosis-related protein.	[34]
Luteolin	Glioma cell	It inhibits glioma cell proliferation in a time- and concentration-based fashion by glioma cell apoptosis via MAPK induction (JNK, ERK, and P38) and autophagy	[64]
Luteolin	LC 540 tumor Leydig cells	It activates steroidogenic acute regulatory (StAR) protein expression and increases progesterone and testosterone production. It also controls the expression of genes that participate in stress responses such as glutathione-S-transferases Gsta1 and Gstt2 and the unfolded protein response.	[65]
Luteolin	Amelanotic melanoma C32 (CRL-1585) cells	Luteolin and its derivatives demonstrate significant cytotoxic and pro-apoptotic potential.	[66]
Luteolin-7-O-glucoside	Oral squamous cell carcinoma	It reduces the oral cancer cell migration and invasion, causing a decrement in cancer metastasis by decreasing p38 phosphorylation by reducing matrix metalloproteinase (MMP)-2 expression. It exerts an anti-migratory effect by inhibiting P38-induced enhanced expression of MMP-2 and also by the extracellular signal regulatory kinase pathway.	[67]

5.3. Anti-Diabetic Activity

Diabetes is a significant health concern worldwide. Its prevalence is felt in every developed and developing country. Nearly 451 million people are affected by it, according to the 2017 International Diabetic Federation (IDF) report, which projects a further increase to 693 million by 2045. It also has severe socio-economic effects. Diabetes among the younger population is increasing, which alarms society. Diabetes is among the top diseases that affect the world population's health and lead to various life-threatening illnesses [68]. LUT, a secondary plant metabolite, has anti-diabetic properties, as established in multiple studies. On administration, it lowers the seizure threshold due to its antiepileptic activity.

In addition, its neuroprotective property helps reduce the kainic-acid-induced neuronal cell death in the hippocampal CA3 region. When used as pretreatment, it protects the morphological appearance of the nerve cells' nucleus, mitochondria, and endoplasmic reticulum, while restoring the ultrastructure of the nerve cells [69]. Diabetes affects the heart muscles and causes myocardial I/R or damage due to oxidative stress. Upon treatment with LUT, oxidative stress and damage to the heart are reduced by the redirection in the oxidation reaction via activating the sestrin 2-Nrf2-based feedback loop [70].

Long-term diabetes impacts the cerebral cortex neurons; the administration of luteolin significantly reduces diabetic conditions, including lipid peroxidation, as it increases in diabetic rat brains and also reduces GS4, superoxide dismutase, and catalase activity, which markedly decrease in the cerebral cortex and hippocampus of rats upon administering luteolin. This implies that luteolin's antioxidant action helps improve CA1 neurons by reducing neuronal apoptosis, as ChE activity results from diabetes, leading to progressive cognitive impairment and neurological dysfunction. In treating diabetic rats with LUT, the ChE activity is inhibited, thus improving the condition [71].

An in silico molecular docking study showed that LUT binds to alpha-amylase and dipeptidyl peptidase IV (DPP IV) efficiently. Thus, it prevents glucose optimization and then binding to glutamine-fructose-6-phosphate amido transferase (GFAT1), and Forkhead box protein O1 (FOX01), suggesting that it may help to avoid hyperglycemia. This shows that LUT is a potent inhibitor of type 2 diabetes mellitus [72]. During kidney hemorrhage, LUT significantly decreases MDA levels and increases SOD activity. It also restores the enhanced level of serum lipids in diabetes mellitus, as the increased level leads to diabetic nephropathy. Its antioxidant properties help to decrease oxidative stress by stabilizing the membrane lipids and thus reducing oxidative damage. Luteolin's renoprotective effects relate to enhancing HO-1 expression and inducing antioxidants in diabetic nephropathy. Luteolin prevents the morphological damage of the kidney caused by diabetes mellitus [21]. However, intense research is warranted to examine the mechanism of luteolin's renoprotective effects.

In another study, compared to untreated cells, LUT significantly increased PI3K and IRS1/2 expression in a dose-dependent manner. These findings demonstrate that in the adipocytes IRSI 1/2 and PI3K pathway-dependent insulin sensitivity was seen. The fact that LUT prevented p65 from moving from the cytosol to the nucleus suggests that it reduces adipocyte inflammation by preventing NK-κB cell activation [73].

Luteolin is a non-competitive inhibitor of alpha-glucosidase, as it binds to enzymes, whether at low or high concentrations. It suggests that LUT has the strongest affinity for alpha-glucosidase enzymes and BACE1 [74]. Luteolin acts as a potent, highly effective, non-competitive reversible inhibitor of alpha-glucosidase [75]. Due to its low IC50, LUT exhibits the strongest dipeptidyl peptidase IV (DPP IV) inhibitory activity. A kinetic study revealed that LUT inhibits DPP IV in a non-competitive manner and binds to the S3 and S2 proteins. The side chain of amino acid residues may change in DPP IV confirmation due to S2 and S3 binding. The IC of DPP IV is required to inhibit 50% of enzyme activity [76].

5.4. Anti-Inflammatory Activities

Inflammation is a response to stimuli induced by immune cells and non-immune cells in our body by involving various biochemical pathways and different molecules. It is a natural process of how the body responds to a stimulus with the help of immune cells such as natural killer cells, macrophages, and their molecular pathways. However, the inflammation response is needed to reduce the impact of the stimuli, further affecting the normal cells, but prolonged inflammation affects normal functioning as it leads to chronic conditions, so it needs to be prevented. For managing it, anti-inflammatory molecules are administered to protect cells from adverse effects [77]. Luteolin has anti-inflammatory properties, which are shown in Figure 5. Luteolin decreases the oxLDL-activated inflammation by inhibiting a signal transducer and activator of transcription 3 (STAT3) in vitro. One study showed its interaction with STAT3 primarily through hydrogen bonds [78]. Luteolin administration alleviates lung injury by attenuating caspase-2-based pyroptosis in the lung tissue of cecal ligation and puncture (CLP). Also in the induced ALI mouse model, it regulates the mechanism related to the frequency of regulated T cells (Treg) and the Treg-derived IL-10 [79].

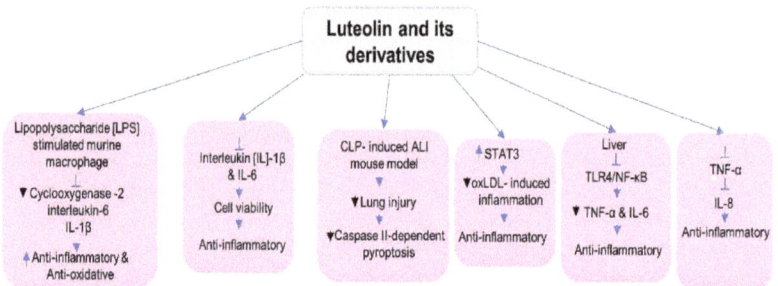

Figure 5. The figure representing the anti-inflammatory mechanism of luteolin in various cells.

Luteolin-7-O-glucuronide [L7Gn] revealed anti-inflammatory and antioxidative properties in lipopolysaccharide (LPS)-stimulated murine macrophages, as the mRNA expression of inflammatory mediators including cyclooxygenase-2 (COX-2), interleukin-6, and IL-1B was inhibited by luteolin-7-O-glucuronide treatment [80]. The co-system of LUT and quercetin was analyzed as the combination of repressed TNF-α production and IL-8 mRNA expression, thus indicating anti-inflammatory and anti-allergic activities [81]. Also in another study, Luteolin-7-O-glucoside (LUT-7G) prevents damage to cardiovascular tissues by lowering the generation of ROS is established by the inhibition of STAT3 and the downregulation of target genes involved in inflammation [82]. Luteolin could inhibit the TLR4/NF-κB pathway, thus reducing the inflammatory factor TNF-α and IL-6 in plasma, liver, and ileum to reduce liver inflammation [83].

Matrix metalloproteinase 9 (MMP-9) plays a critical role in the inflammatory response. One study established that LUT decreases MMP-9 expression to treat ischemic stroke, colon cancer, and diabetes. CASP3 is the main terminal-cleaving enzyme, and the activation of CASP3 causes apoptosis and inflammation, but LUT can increase CASP3 expression to induce apoptosis in the HaCat cells and cancer cells [84]. Luteolin significantly improved the caerulein plus LPS induced in severe acute pancreatitis (SAP) mice. Increased HO-1 levels decreased NF-κB activity and increased anti-inflammatory activity [35]. Further, LUT is reported to process anti-inflammatory activity with the mechanism of having COX-2, interleukin, and TNF as molecular targets. Luteolin-7-0-β-D-glucuronide inhibited the NO and pro-inflammatory cytokine production [85]. The research shows that TNF-α induced a considerable reduction in HNPC (human nucleus pulposus cell) viability and an increase in inflammatory factor levels. In contrast, application with LUT shows enhanced cell viability and reduced intracellular interleukin (IL)-1β and IL-6 expression levels [86].

Luteolin also reversed TNF-α-induced senescence and suppressed TNF-α, causing inflammatory injury. In addition, luteolin-3'-O-phosphate (LTP) shows better anti-inflammatory activity by inhibiting the mitogen-activated protein kinase and NF-κB more effectively than luteolin. Also, at the concentration of 10 μM, LTP showed higher anti-inflammatory activity in comparison to luteolin [87]. In a previous study, it was found that LUT caused in vitro activation of NF-κB and AP-1. However, LUT exhibited a more potent anti-inflammatory activity than luteolin-7-O-glucoside in GalN/LPS-intoxicated

ICR mice [88]. The STAT3 pathway is the potential target of LUT, which reduces renal fibrosis and delays the progress of diabetic nephropathy [89].

5.5. Protection against Alzheimer's Disease

Alzheimer's disease is a prime cause of memory loss among the world's population. The main characteristic of the disease is the accumulation of β amyloid peptides in the brain's extracellular matrix [90]. A treatment to prevent the condition has not been established. Still, research is ongoing around the globe to find the cure for Alzheimer's disease. In this view, the secondary metabolite LUT has some potential to reduce the condition. LUT effectively reduces Alzheimer's disease symptoms and the formation of Aβ42 aggregation in transgenic drosophila due to the (direct) interaction of ROS with the gene expression of an antioxidant enzyme involved in free radical scavenging. This is shown via a reduction in AchE activity in a concentration-mediated manner, which results in the slowing down of the inception of Alzheimer's disease-like symptoms [91]. Luteolin improves brain histomorphology and decreases protein plaques in 3XTg-Alzheimer's disease mice, as it inhibits neuro-inflammatory aggravation by repressing ER stress, which causes learning and memory impairment in mice [92].

Further, it significantly reduced the expression of Bax and caspase-3 and induced the expression of Bcl2. A high amount of LUT may have potential toxicity, inhibiting Aβ25-35 and inducing cell apoptosis. It also activates the ER/ERK/MAPK signaling pathway to protect Bcl2 cells against Aβ25-35 and induce apoptosis via specifically acting on ERβ [93]. Luteolin may decrease brain insulin resistance. The present studies found that the LUT treatment potentiated insulin signaling in the hippocampus and increased glucose metabolism by increasing hepatic insulin sensitivity and the tight regulation of β-cell function [94].

5.6. Luteolin in Parkinson's Disease (PD) Treatment

Luteolin produced during counteraction in the in vitro effect on oxidation is associated with the abnormal enhancement of endogenous free radical suppression of the mitochondrial viability of mitochondria membrane potential and a decrease in the glutathione content. The catalyzing activity indicates that the multilayer modulatory pathway plays a role in luteolin neuroprotection activity. The protection is a result of possible balancing in the pro-oxidation or antioxidation ratio. Further, the neuroprotective mechanism helps to restore the depressed endogenous enzymatic and non-enzymatic antioxidative defense system known as ROS scavenging activity [95]. Luteolin-7-O-glucoside helps to protect against dopaminergic neuro injury in the SH-SY5Y human dopaminergic neuronal cell line, where it increased the cell viability of a 1-methyl-4-phenylpyridinium iodide (MPP+)-treated SH-SY5Y cell line by suppressing apoptosis, as was visible by decreased nuclear condensation.

Furthermore, it increases the Bcl2/Bax ratio by reducing caspase-3, and also prevents the depletion of TH+ve neurons in the substantia nigra (SN) and neuro fibers in the striatum, thus improving mice behavior in the pole trait and traction test and implicating its potential in applied PD therapy [96]. The cell viability is lost due to 6-OHDA-induced apoptosis in PC12 cells, during which the Bax/Bcl2 ratio is enhanced along with p53 expression. The 6-OHDA induces BIM and TRB3 mRNA expression, affecting cellular viability. Treating with the LUT inhibits 6-OHDA-induced apoptosis and blocks BIM and TRB3 mRNA expression, thus increasing cell viability loss. This indicates neuroprotective activity [97,98]. Further, the luteolin administration reduces the H_2O_2-induced cell apoptosis through the Bcl2 pathway, thus improving neuronal synaptic plasticity.

The superoxide dismutase activity is enhanced due to LUT, which helps to decompose OH-mediated lipid peroxidation. Luteolin suppresses the higher expression of Cyclin-dependent kinase-5 (Cdk5) and p35 due to oxidation stress. Thus it proves its effectiveness in influencing the extracellular signal-regulated kinase 1/2 (Erk1/2)- and dynamin-related protein 1 (Drp 1)-dependent survival pathways [99] (Figure 6).

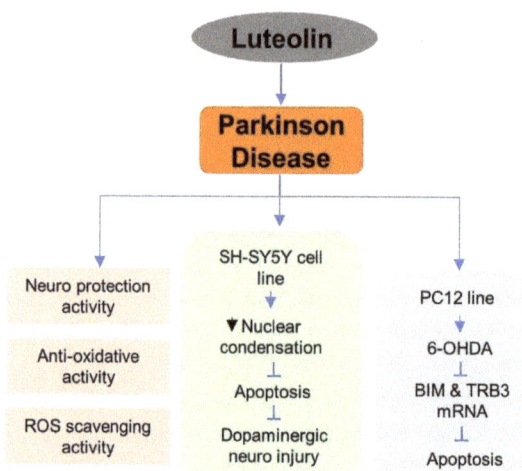

Figure 6. Protective role of luteolin in Parkinson's treatment.

5.7. Luteolin in Cardiac Health

The luteolin compound in various plant sources has many beneficial properties in favor of a healthy and disease-preventive lifestyle for humans. It possesses the property of managing heart ailments such as myocardial infarction. Cardiovascular diseases (CVDs) can result from various factors such as unhealthy lifestyle, unbalanced diet, and sedentary lifestyle. They can be prevented by eating healthy food and having an active lifestyle. The luteolin molecule helps to reduce the risk of myocardial infarction, as its inclusion in food may help in reducing CVD. In a study involving myocardial ischemia/reperfusion (I/R) (MIRM) rats, the luteolin compound treatment reduced the damage to the heart valves by reducing the Src homology 2 domain-containing protein tyrosine phosphatase 1 (SHP-1) regulation and upregulating the STAT3 pathway, resulting in decreased inflammatory response [100].

The reduced damage to heart muscles is due to the luteolin treatment, as it reduces the cytokine level in the serum of the treated animal models. In addition, luteolin helps in balancing the Siti1/NLRP3/NF-κB pathway, as it was affected in the MIRM rats [101]. The administration of luteolin to MIRM rats also proved to increase the sarcoplasmic/endoplasmic reticulum Ca^{2+}-ATPase (SERCA) protein level by SUMOylation, and the expression of the SERCA was modulated by the Sp1 transcription factor, which has positive regulation over the *SERCA* gene. This process helped recover the heart tissue injury caused by myocardial infarction compared to the control [102,103].

The anti-apoptosis property is important in preventing heart tissue damage. In one study, administering luteolin reduced apoptosis in the simulated ischemia/reperfusion (sI/R) model by upregulating the AKT signaling [104]. Cardiac wellness is improved by luteolin, as it helps in preventing cardiac abnormalities such as contractile dysfunction and Ca^{2+} transport, which reduce in the failing cardiomyocytes and are prevented by upregulating the *SERCA2a* gene [105]. The importance of the SERCA proteins in cardiac health is evident. Luteolin helps to upregulate its expression by activating the p38 MAPK pathway in the sI/R rat models and in the cardiomyocytes [106]. The cardiac protective effect of the luteolin molecule is proved in animal models and cell lines, implying its possible effectiveness in humans. Its intake as a dietary compound could play a possible preventive role against life-threatening heart disease.

5.8. Luteolin in Obesity Treatment

Another lifestyle disorder is obesity, which is the high accumulation of fats. It leads to many non-communicable disorders such as cardiac arrest and diabetes, musculoskeletal disorders such osteoarthritis, and cancers such as colon, ovarian, breast, liver, prostate, kidney, and gallbladder [107]. Luteolin, through dietary supplements, has proved to manage obesity. A study on rat models showed that luteolin supplementation decreased adipokine/cytokine dysregulation and macrophage infiltration by modifying the Toll-like receptor (TLR) signaling pathway [108]. In another study, the luteolin compound helped in overcoming diet-induced obesity and also increased the metabolomic rates by activating the AMPK/PGC1α pathway [109]. The luteolin compound helps fight obesity by acting against adipocyte differentiation by regulating the TF peroxisome proliferator-activated receptor γ (PPARγ) [110].

The obesity studies involving C57BL/6N mice showed that artichoke leaves (AR), having luteolin, helped in reducing the obesity-related complications in mice when given along with a high-fat diet [111]. The obesity adipocyte inflammation observed on administering luteolin reduces inflammation by reducing the proinflammatory mediators in macrophages such as tumor necrosis factor-α (TNFα), monocyte chemoattractant protein (MCP-1), and NO, while co-cultivating with 3T3-L1 adipocytes and RAW264 macrophages. This is evidenced by the activity of luteolin in reducing the inflammation in the adipose tissue [112]. In another study involving diet-induced obesity mice, luteolin was involved in the regulation of cholesterol efflux genes such as liver X receptor α (*LXR-α*), scavenger receptor class B member 1 (*SRB1*), and ATP-binding cassette transporter G1 (*ABCG1*). It showed that luteolin reduces cholesterol by regulating the various genes involved in the cholesterol efflux pathway [113]. Thus, the luteolin compound helps in managing obesity by acting on various cellular mechanisms and helps manage and control obesity in model animals, which could be translated into treating humans.

6. Cytotoxic Studies

The phytocompounds used in managing or treating a particular disease or its related symptoms must be in a precise dose, so that other cellular functions are not affected by the compound administration. Thus, toxicity studies help provide crucial information for the compounds used in the study. The LUT compound toxicity was studied by treating human retinal microvascular endothelial cells (HRMECs) against the anti-angiogenic effect. The treatment with 10 µM of LUT had no toxic effect but increasing the concentration up to 100 µM affected the cells [114,115]. In another study, LUT treated with human lymphoblastoid TK6 cells showed cytotoxic activity at 24 h with a minimal lethal dose concentration of 2.5 µM. In addition, DNA damage was observed at the concentrations of 5 and 10 µM, measured by the alkaline comet assay and the γH2A.X protein level [116].

In a study involving *Verbena officinalis*, a traditional medicinal herb containing luteolin 3′-methyl ether 7-glucuronosyl-(1-2)-glucuronide, resulted in prenatal toxicity when administered in high doses during the gestation period in female Sprague Dawley rats [117]. In another study, 100 µg/ml of LUT caused DNA damage in Vero cells and lymphocytes [118]. The toxicity studies emphasize the safe usage of LUT in therapeutic treatments, as the higher dosage may cause side effects. Therefore, intense studies exploring the toxicity of the luteolin phytocompound will give more insight into the effective concentration of its doses for disease treatments.

7. Clinical Trials

Clinical studies for the compound LUT have been carried out with various objectives. According to the clinical trials website, 18 entries were found to be involved in using the LUT compound. Among them, three studies are in starting phase, seven studies have been completed, and two were terminated. A clinical study to treat the olfactory dysfunction of Severe Acute Respiratory Syndrome Coronavirus 2 (SARS-CoV-2)-affected persons showed that the administration of palmitoylethanolamide (PEA) and luteolin helped in the recovery of olfactory functions [119]. In another randomized clinical trial in hepatocellular carcinoma (HCC) patients, a standard transcatheter arterial chemoembolization (TACE) therapy was synergized with a traditional Chinese medicine Fuzheng Jiedu Xiaoji formulation (FZJDXJ) that constitutes several phytocompounds, including luteolin. The results showed that the synergistic application of LUT resulted in the prolongation of one-year overall survival (OS) and progression-free survival (PFS) cases in the trials, as the anti-cancer activity was proven in animal models by their role in influencing the AKT/CyclinD1/p21/p27 pathway [120].

Another clinical study involved LUT treatment of delirium, a condition of cognition and awareness disorder. Post-operative delirium conditions were prevented when subjects were administrated with 700 mg of co-ultra-micronized palmitoylethanolamide (PEA) + 70 mg luteolin [121]. The product Altilix® contains LUT as one of the components used to treat cardiovascular and liver function in metabolic syndrome. The results of one study showed that intake of Altilix® supplementation helps to improve liver and cardiovascular functions [122]. In another study, LUT enhanced exercise performance by increasing oxygen extraction in muscle and brain oxygenation in low and high doses [123]. The efficiency of LUT in treating autism spectrum disorders (ASD) was studied in a control clinical study in which results showed adaptive functioning improvement among the subjects. This proves the effectiveness of the LUT compound in treating complex disorders such as autism [124]. The clinical trials using LUT compounds prove its effectiveness in managing and treating several diseases and health issues. Future studies will further explore the therapeutic benefits of luteolin against several diseases.

8. Conclusions

The plant-derived phytocompound LUT is present in most plants on earth. Plants containing the LUT compound have been used in various traditional medicines. The advent of modern analytical techniques highlighted the occurrence of LUT in plants as an important secondary metabolite in different cellular responses. Meanwhile, LUT is currently being explored for its beneficial activity in treating various human ailments. It has been made clear that the plant-obtained compound is a potential candidate in the treatment of various diseases, as it possesses the properties of anti-cancer, anti-inflammatory, anti-diabetic, and antioxidative effects. These beneficial activities of LUT have been proven and validated in multiple studies.

From a future perspective, the synergistic application of LUT with other natural or synthetic drugs in chemopreventive studies could be carried out, as this approach will be more effective in controlling and managing diseases. In addition, the bioavailability of LUT can be enhanced by nanoformulation using nanotechnology, which will increase its efficacy in administration to humans and also caters to specific and efficient disease management. To make this possible, comprehensive studies should be carried out to unravel the role of LUT in treating several other diseases at a molecular level and explore the exact mechanism behind its beneficial activity. This paves the way for different strategies to employ in studies aimed at improving the well-being of humankind.

Author Contributions: Conceptualization, N.M., A.R.D., V.B. and I.S.; writing—original draft preparation, N.M., A.R.D. and V.B.; writing—review and editing, N.M., A.R.D., V.B., P.M., D.S., H.A., M.Z.S.A. and I.S.; funding acquisition, I.S. All authors have read and agreed to the published version of the manuscript.

Funding: This research received no external funding.

Institutional Review Board Statement: Not applicable.

Informed Consent Statement: Not applicable.

Data Availability Statement: Not applicable.

Acknowledgments: This article was supported by the KU Research Professor Program of Konkuk University.

Conflicts of Interest: The authors declare no conflict of interest.

References

1. Imran, M.; Rauf, A.; Abu-Izneid, T.; Nadeem, M.; Shariati, M.A.; Khan, I.A.; Imran, A.; Orhan, I.E.; Rizwan, M.; Atif, M.; et al. Luteolin, a Flavonoid, as an Anticancer Agent: A Review. *Biomed. Pharmacother.* **2019**, *112*, 108612. [CrossRef] [PubMed]
2. Bravo, L. Polyphenols: Chemistry, Dietary Sources, Metabolism, and Nutritional Significance. *Nutr. Rev.* **2009**, *56*, 317–333. [CrossRef] [PubMed]
3. Nabavi, S.F.; Braidy, N.; Gortzi, O.; Sobarzo-Sanchez, E.; Daglia, M.; Skalicka-Woźniak, K.; Nabavi, S.M. Luteolin as an Anti-Inflammatory and Neuroprotective Agent: A Brief Review. *Brain Res. Bull.* **2015**, *119*, 1–11. [CrossRef] [PubMed]
4. Harborne, J.B.; Williams, C.A. Advances in Flavonoid Research since 1992. *Phytochemistry* **2000**, *55*, 481–504. [CrossRef]
5. Hartmann, T. Diversity and Variability of Plant Secondary Metabolism: A Mechanistic View. *Entomol. Exp. Appl.* **1996**, *80*, 177–188. [CrossRef]
6. Ross, J.A.; Kasum, C.M. Dietary Flavonoids: Bioavailability, Metabolic Effects, and Safety. *Annu. Rev. Nutr.* **2002**, *22*, 19–34. [CrossRef]
7. Ou, H.-C.; Pandey, S.; Hung, M.-Y.; Huang, S.-H.; Hsu, P.-T.; Day, C.-H.; Pai, P.; Viswanadha, V.P.; Kuo, W.-W.; Huang, C.-Y. Luteolin: A Natural Flavonoid Enhances the Survival of HUVECs against Oxidative Stress by Modulating AMPK/PKC Pathway. *Am. J. Chin. Med.* **2019**, *47*, 541–557. [CrossRef]
8. Cook, M.T. Mechanism of Metastasis Suppression by Luteolin in Breast Cancer. *Breast Cancer Targets Ther.* **2018**, *10*, 89–100. [CrossRef]
9. Lopez-Lazaro, M. Distribution and Biological Activities of the Flavonoid Luteolin. *Mini-Rev. Med. Chem.* **2009**, *9*, 31–59. [CrossRef]
10. Giannasi, D.E.; Niklas, K.J. Flavonoid and Other Chemical Constituents of Fossil Miocene Celtis and Ulmus (Succor Creek Flora). *Science* **1977**, *197*, 765–767. [CrossRef]
11. Vogt, T. Phenylpropanoid Biosynthesis. *Mol. Plant* **2010**, *3*, 2–20. [CrossRef] [PubMed]
12. Herrmann, K.M.; Weaver, L.M. The Shikimate Pathway. *Annu. Rev. Plant Physiol. Plant Mol. Biol.* **1999**, *50*, 473–503. [CrossRef] [PubMed]
13. Ferrer, J.-L.; Austin, M.B.; Stewart, C.; Noel, J.P. Structure and Function of Enzymes Involved in the Biosynthesis of Phenylpropanoids. *Plant Physiol. Biochem.* **2008**, *46*, 356–370. [CrossRef] [PubMed]
14. Noel, J.P.; Ferrer, J.-L.; Jez, J.M.; Bowman, M.E.; Dixon, R.A. Structure of Chalcone Synthase and the Molecular Basis of Plant Polyketide Biosynthesis. *Nat. Struct. Biol.* **1999**, *6*, 775–784. [CrossRef] [PubMed]
15. Noel, J.P.; Jez, J.M.; Bowman, M.E.; Dixon, R.A. Structure and Mechanism of the Evolutionarily Unique Plant Enzyme Chalcone Isomerase. *Nat. Struct. Biol.* **2000**, *7*, 786–791. [CrossRef] [PubMed]
16. CROFT, K.D. The Chemistry and Biological Effects of Flavonoids and Phenolic Acidsa. *Ann. N. Y. Acad. Sci.* **1998**, *854*, 435–442. [CrossRef] [PubMed]
17. Martens, S.; Mithöfer, A. Flavones and Flavone Synthases. *Phytochemistry* **2005**, *66*, 2399–2407. [CrossRef] [PubMed]
18. Nabavi, S.M.; Šamec, D.; Tomczyk, M.; Milella, L.; Russo, D.; Habtemariam, S.; Suntar, I.; Rastrelli, L.; Daglia, M.; Xiao, J.; et al. Flavonoid Biosynthetic Pathways in Plants: Versatile Targets for Metabolic Engineering. *Biotechnol. Adv.* **2020**, *38*, 107316. [CrossRef] [PubMed]
19. Yang, K.; Song, Y.; Ge, L.; Su, J.; Wen, Y.; Long, Y. Measurement and Correlation of the Solubilities of Luteolin and Rutin in Five Imidazole-Based Ionic Liquids. *Fluid Phase Equilibria* **2013**, *344*, 27–31. [CrossRef]
20. Shakeel, F.; Haq, N.; Alshehri, S.; Ibrahim, M.A.; Elzayat, E.M.; Altamimi, M.A.; Mohsin, K.; Alanazi, F.K.; Alsarra, I.A. Solubility, Thermodynamic Properties and Solute-Solvent Molecular Interactions of Luteolin in Various Pure Solvents. *J. Mol. Liq.* **2018**, *255*, 43–50. [CrossRef]
21. Wang, Z.; Zeng, M.; Wang, Z.; Qin, F.; Chen, J.; He, Z. Dietary Luteolin: A Narrative Review Focusing on Its Pharmacokinetic Properties and Effects on Glycolipid Metabolism. *J. Agric. Food Chem.* **2021**, *69*, 1441–1454. [CrossRef] [PubMed]
22. Valko, M.; Leibfritz, D.; Moncol, J.; Cronin, M.T.D.; Mazur, M.; Telser, J. Free Radicals and Antioxidants in Normal Physiological Functions and Human Disease. *Int. J. Biochem. Cell Biol.* **2007**, *39*, 44–84. [CrossRef] [PubMed]
23. Rice-Evans, C. Flavonoid Antioxidants. *Curr. Med. Chem.* **2001**, *8*, 797–807. [CrossRef]
24. Pietta, P.-G. Flavonoids as Antioxidants. *J. Nat. Prod.* **2000**, *63*, 1035–1042. [CrossRef] [PubMed]
25. Choi, C.-W.; Jung, H.A.; Kang, S.S.; Choi, J.S. Antioxidant Constituents and a New Triterpenoid Glycoside From Flos Lonicerae. *Arch. Pharmacal Res.* **2007**, *30*, 1–7. [CrossRef] [PubMed]
26. Wu, M.-J.; Huang, C.-L.; Lian, T.-W.; Kou, M.-C.; Wang, L. Antioxidant Activity Of Glossogyne Tenuifolia. *J. Agric. Food Chem.* **2005**, *53*, 6305–6312. [CrossRef]
27. Cai, Q.; Rahn, R.O.; Zhang, R. Dietary Flavonoids, Quercetin, Luteolin and Genistein, Reduce Oxidative DNA Damage and Lipid Peroxidation and Quench Free Radicals. *Cancer Lett.* **1997**, *119*, 99–107. [CrossRef]
28. Horváthová, K.; Chalupa, I.; Šebová, L.; Tóthová, D.; Vachálková, A. Protective Effect of Quercetin and Luteolin in Human Melanoma HMB-2 Cells. *Mutat. Res. Genet. Toxicol. Environ. Mutagen.* **2005**, *565*, 105–112. [CrossRef]
29. Cheng, I.F.; Breen, K. On the Ability of Four Flavonoids, Baicilein, Luteolin, Naringenin, and Quercetin, to Suppress the Fenton Reaction of the Iron-ATP Complex. *BioMetals* **2000**, *13*, 77–83. [CrossRef]
30. Choi, J.S.; Islam, M.N.; Ali, M.Y.; Kim, Y.M.; Park, H.J.; Sohn, H.S.; Jung, H.A. The Effects of C-Glycosylation of Luteolin on Its Antioxidant, Anti-Alzheimer's Disease, Anti-Diabetic, and Anti-Inflammatory Activities. *Arch. Pharmacal Res.* **2014**, *37*, 1354–1363. [CrossRef]

31. Albarakati, A.J.A.; Baty, R.S.; Aljoudi, A.M.; Habotta, O.A.; Elmahallawy, E.K.; Kassab, R.B.; Abdel Moneim, A.E. Luteolin Protects against Lead Acetate-Induced Nephrotoxicity through Antioxidant, Anti-Inflammatory, Anti-Apoptotic, and Nrf2/HO-1 Signaling Pathways. *Mol. Biol. Rep.* **2020**, *47*, 2591–2603. [CrossRef]
32. Boeing, T.; Souza, P.; Speca, S.; Somensi, L.B.; Mariano, L.N.B.; Cury, B.J.; Ferreira dos Anjos, M.; Quintão, N.L.M.; Dubuqoy, L.; Desreumax, P.; et al. Luteolin Prevents Irinotecan-Induced Intestinal Mucositis in Mice through Antioxidant and Anti-Inflammatory Properties. *Br. J. Pharmacol.* **2020**, *177*, 2393–2408. [CrossRef] [PubMed]
33. Yan, Y.; Jun, C.; Lu, Y.; Jiangmei, S. Combination of Metformin and Luteolin Synergistically Protects Carbon Tetrachloride-Induced Hepatotoxicity: Mechanism Involves Antioxidant, Anti-Apoptotic, Antiapoptotic, and Nrf2/HO-1 Signaling Pathway. *BioFactors* **2019**, *45*, 598–606. [CrossRef] [PubMed]
34. Kang, K.A.; Piao, M.J.; Hyun, Y.J.; Zhen, A.X.; Cho, S.J.; Ahn, M.J.; Yi, J.M.; Hyun, J.W. Luteolin Promotes Apoptotic Cell Death via Upregulation of Nrf2 Expression by DNA Demethylase and the Interaction of Nrf2 with P53 in Human Colon Cancer Cells. *Exp. Mol. Med.* **2019**, *51*, 1–14. [CrossRef]
35. Xiong, J.; Wang, K.; Yuan, C.; Xing, R.; Ni, J.; Hu, G.; Chen, F.; Wang, X. Luteolin Protects Mice from Severe Acute Pancreatitis by Exerting HO-1-Mediated Anti-Inflammatory and Antioxidant Effects. *Int. J. Mol. Med.* **2016**, *39*, 113–125. [CrossRef] [PubMed]
36. Owumi, S.; Lewu, D.; Arunsi, U.; Oyelere, A. Luteolin Attenuates Doxorubicin-Induced Derangements of Liver and Kidney by Reducing Oxidative and Inflammatory Stress to Suppress apoptosis. *Hum. Exp. Toxicol.* **2021**, *40*, 1656–1672. [CrossRef] [PubMed]
37. World Health Organization Cancer. Available online: https://www.who.int/news-room/fact-sheets/detail/cancer (accessed on 6 October 2022).
38. de Martel, C.; Georges, D.; Bray, F.; Ferlay, J.; Clifford, G.M. Global Burden of Cancer Attributable to Infections in 2018: A Worldwide Incidence Analysis. *Lancet Glob. Health* **2020**, *8*, e180–e190. [CrossRef]
39. Sung, H.; Ferlay, J.; Siegel, R.L.; Laversanne, M.; Soerjomataram, I.; Jemal, A.; Bray, F. Global Cancer Statistics 2020: GLOBOCAN Estimates of Incidence and Mortality Worldwide for 36 Cancers in 185 Countries. *CA Cancer J. Clin.* **2021**, *71*, 209–249. [CrossRef]
40. Ferlay, J.; Colombet, M.; Soerjomataram, I.; Parkin, D.M.; Piñeros, M.; Znaor, A.; Bray, F. Cancer Statistics for the Year 2020: An Overview. *Int. J. Cancer* **2021**, *149*, 778–789. [CrossRef]
41. Ganai, S.A.; Sheikh, F.A.; Baba, Z.A.; Mir, M.A.; Mantoo, M.A.; Yatoo, M.A. Anticancer Activity of the Plant Flavonoid Luteolin against Preclinical Models of Various Cancers and Insights on Different Signalling Mechanisms Modulated. *Phytother. Res.* **2021**, *35*, 3509–3532. [CrossRef]
42. Lakhera, S.; Rana, M.; Devlal, K.; Celik, I.; Yadav, R. A Comprehensive Exploration of Pharmacological Properties, Bioactivities and Inhibitory Potentiality of Luteolin from Tridax Procumbens as Anticancer Drug by In-Silico Approach. *Struct. Chem.* **2022**, *33*, 703–719. [CrossRef] [PubMed]
43. Kawaii, S.; Tomono, Y.; Katase, E.; Ogawa, K.; Yano, M. Antiproliferative Activity of Flavonoids on Several Cancer Cell Lines. *Biosci. Biotechnol. Biochem.* **1999**, *63*, 896–899. [CrossRef] [PubMed]
44. Cherng, J.-M.; Shieh, D.-E.; Chiang, W.; Chang, M.-Y.; Chiang, L.-C. Chemopreventive Effects of Minor Dietary Constituents in Common Foods on Human Cancer Cells. *Biosci. Biotechnol. Biochem.* **2007**, *71*, 1500–1504. [CrossRef] [PubMed]
45. Post, J.F.M.; Varma, R.S. Growth Inhibitory Effects of Bioflavonoids and Related Compounds on Human Leukemic CEM-C1 and CEM-C7 Cells. *Cancer Lett.* **1992**, *67*, 207–213. [CrossRef]
46. Seelinger, G.; Merfort, I.; Wölfle, U.; Schempp, C. Anti-Carcinogenic Effects of the Flavonoid Luteolin. *Molecules* **2008**, *13*, 2628–2651. [CrossRef]
47. Ko, W.G.; Kang, T.H.; Lee, S.J.; Kim, Y.C.; Lee, B.H. Effects of Luteolin on the Inhibition of Proliferation and Induction of Apoptosis in Human Myeloid Leukaemia Cells. *Phytother. Res.* **2002**, *16*, 295–298. [CrossRef]
48. Lin, Y.; Shi, R.; Wang, X.; Shen, H.-M. Luteolin, a Flavonoid with Potential for Cancer Prevention and Therapy. *Curr. Cancer Drug Targets* **2008**, *8*, 634–646. [CrossRef]
49. Gu, J.; Cheng, X.; Luo, X.; Yang, X.; Pang, Y.; Zhang, X.; Zhang, Y.; Liu, Y. Luteolin Ameliorates Cognitive Impairments by Suppressing the Expression of Inflammatory Cytokines and Enhancing Synapse-Associated Proteins GAP-43 and SYN Levels in Streptozotocin-Induced Diabetic Rats. *Neurochem. Res.* **2018**, *43*, 1905–1913. [CrossRef]
50. Jang, C.H.; Moon, N.; Oh, J.; Kim, J.-S. Luteolin Shifts Oxaliplatin-Induced Cell Cycle Arrest at G0/G1 to Apoptosis in HCT116 Human Colorectal Carcinoma Cells. *Nutrients* **2019**, *11*, 770. [CrossRef]
51. Goodarzi, S.; Tabatabaei, M.J.; Jafari, M.; Shemirani, F.; Tavakoli, S.; Mofasseri, M.; Tofighi, Z. Cuminum cyminum Fruits as Source of Luteolin-7-O-Glucoside, Potent Cytotoxic Flavonoid against Breast Cancer Cell Lines. *Nat. Prod. Res.* **2018**, *34*, 1602–1606. [CrossRef]
52. Hong, J.; Fristiohady, A.; Nguyen, C.H.; Milovanovic, D.; Huttary, N.; Krieger, S.; Hong, J.; Geleff, S.; Birner, P.; Jäger, W.; et al. Apigenin and Luteolin Attenuate the Breaching of MDA-MB231 Breast Cancer Spheroids through the Lymph Endothelial Barrier in Vitro. *Front. Pharmacol.* **2018**, *9*, 220. [CrossRef] [PubMed]
53. Tavsan, Z.; Kayali, H.A. Flavonoids Showed Anticancer Effects on the Ovarian Cancer Cells: Involvement of Reactive Oxygen Species, Apoptosis, Cell Cycle and Invasion. *Biomed. Pharmacother.* **2019**, *116*, 109004. [CrossRef] [PubMed]
54. Chen, P.-Y.; Tien, H.-J.; Chen, S.-F.; Horng, C.-T.; Tang, H.-L.; Jung, H.-L.; Wu, M.-J.; Yen, J.-H. Response of Myeloid Leukemia Cells to Luteolin Is Modulated by Differentially Expressed Pituitary Tumor-Transforming Gene 1 (PTTG1) Oncoprotein. *Int. J. Mol. Sci.* **2018**, *19*, 1173. [CrossRef] [PubMed]

55. Franco, Y.E.; de Lima, C.A.; Rosa, M.N.; Viviane, S.; Reis, R.M.; Priolli, D.G.; Carvalho, P.O.; do Nascimento, J.R.; da Rocha, C.Q.; Longato, G.B. Investigation of U-251 Cell Death Triggered by Flavonoid Luteolin: Towards a Better Understanding on Its Anticancer Property against Glioblastomas. *Nat. Prod. Res.* **2020**, *35*, 4807–4813. [CrossRef] [PubMed]
56. Majumdar, D.; Jung, K.-H.; Zhang, H.; Nannapaneni, S.; Wang, X.; Amin, A.R.M.R.; Chen, Z.; Chen, Z.G.; Shin, D.M. Luteolin Nanoparticle in Chemoprevention: In Vitro and In Vivo Anticancer Activity. *Cancer Prev. Res.* **2014**, *7*, 65–73. [CrossRef] [PubMed]
57. Yang, P.-W.; Lu, Z.-Y.; Pan, Q.; Chen, T.-T.; Feng, X.-J.; Wang, S.-M.; Pan, Y.-C.; Zhu, M.-H.; Zhang, S.-H. MicroRNA-6809-5p Mediates Luteolin-Induced Anticancer Effects against Hepatoma by Targeting Flotillin 1. *Phytomedicine* **2019**, *57*, 18–29. [CrossRef] [PubMed]
58. Palko-Labuz, A.; Sroda-Pomianek, K.; Uryga, A.; Kostrzewa-Suslow, E.; Michalak, K. Anticancer Activity of Baicalein and Luteolin Studied in Colorectal Adenocarcinoma LoVo Cells and in Drug-Resistant LoVo/Dx Cells. *Biomed. Pharmacother.* **2017**, *88*, 232–241. [CrossRef] [PubMed]
59. Ho, H.; Chen, P.; Lo, Y.; Lin, C.; Chuang, Y.; Hsieh, M.; Chen, M. Luteolin-7-O-Glucoside Inhibits Cell Proliferation and Modulates apoptosis through the AKT Signaling Pathway in Human Nasopharyngeal Carcinoma. *Environ. Toxicol.* **2021**, *36*, 2013–2024. [CrossRef]
60. Poppy, H.; Harahap, U.; Sitorus, P.; Satria, D. The Anticancer Activities of *Vernonia Amygdalina* Delile. Leaves on 4T1 Breast Cancer Cells through Phosphoinositide 3-Kinase (PI3K) Pathway. *Heliyon* **2020**, *6*, e04449. [CrossRef]
61. Huang, L.; Jin, K.; Lan, H. Luteolin Inhibits Cell Cycle Progression and Induces Apoptosis of Breast Cancer Cells through Downregulation of Human Telomerase Reverse Transcriptase. *Oncol. Lett.* **2019**, *17*, 3842–3850. [CrossRef]
62. Wu, H.-T.; Liu, Y.-E.; Hsu, K.-W.; Wang, Y.-F.; Chan, Y.-C.; Chen, Y.; Chen, D.-R. MLL3 Induced by Luteolin Causes Apoptosis in Tamoxifen-Resistant Breast Cancer Cells through H3K4 Monomethylation and Suppression of the PI3K/AKT/MTOR Pathway. *Am. J. Chin. Med.* **2020**, *48*, 1221–1241. [CrossRef]
63. Lee, Y.; Kwon, Y.H. Regulation of Apoptosis and Autophagy by Luteolin in Human Hepatocellular Cancer Hep3B Cells. *Biochem. Biophys. Res. Commun.* **2019**, *517*, 617–622. [CrossRef]
64. You, Y.; Wang, R.; Shao, N.; Zhi, F.; Yang, Y.P. Luteolin Suppresses Tumor Proliferation through Inducing Apoptosis and Autophagy via MAPK Activation in Glioma. *Onco Targets Ther.* **2019**, *12*, 2383–2396. [CrossRef]
65. Couture, R.; Mora, N.; Bittar, A.; Najih, M.; Touaibia, M.; Martin, L.J. Luteolin Modulates Gene Expression Related to Steroidogenesis, Apoptosis, and Stress Response in Rat LC540 Tumor Leydig Cells. *Cell Biol. Toxicol.* **2019**, *36*, 31–49. [CrossRef]
66. Juszczak, A.M.; Czarnomysy, R.; Strawa, J.W.; Zovko Končić, M.; Bielawski, K.; Tomczyk, M. In Vitro Anticancer Potential of Jasione Montana and Its Main Components against Human Amelanotic Melanoma Cells. *Int. J. Mol. Sci.* **2021**, *22*, 3345. [CrossRef]
67. Velmurugan, B.K.; Lin, J.-T.; Mahalakshmi, B.; Chuang, Y.-C.; Lin, C.-C.; Lo, Y.-S.; Hsieh, M.-J.; Chen, M.-K. Luteolin-7-o-Glucoside Inhibits Oral Cancer Cell Migration and Invasion by Regulating Matrix Metalloproteinase-2 Expression and Extracellular Signal-Regulated Kinase Pathway. *Biomolecules* **2020**, *10*, 502. [CrossRef]
68. Lin, X.; Xu, Y.; Pan, X.; Xu, J.; Ding, Y.; Sun, X.; Song, X.; Ren, Y.; Shan, P.-F. Global, Regional, and National Burden and Trend of Diabetes in 195 Countries and Territories: An Analysis from 1990 to 2025. *Sci. Rep.* **2020**, *10*, 14790. [CrossRef]
69. Lin, T.Y.; Lu, C.W.; Wang, S.J. Luteolin Protects the Hippocampus against Neuron Impairments Induced by Kainic Acid in Rats. *Neurotoxicology* **2016**, *55*, 48–57. [CrossRef]
70. Zhou, X.-R.; Ru, X.-C.; Xiao, C.; Pan, J.; Lou, Y.-Y.; Tang, L.-H.; Yang, J.-T.; Qian, L.-B. Sestrin2 Is Involved in the Nrf2-Regulated Antioxidative Signaling Pathway in Luteolin-Induced Prevention of the Diabetic Rat Heart from Ischemia/Reperfusion Injury. *Food Funct.* **2021**, *12*, 3562–3571. [CrossRef]
71. Liu, Y.; Tian, X.; Gou, L.; Sun, L.; Ling, X.; Yin, X. Luteolin Attenuates Diabetes-Associated Cognitive Decline in Rats. *Brain Res. Bull.* **2013**, *94*, 23–29. [CrossRef]
72. Davella, R.; Mamidala, E. Luteolin: A Potential Multiple Targeted Drug Effectively Inhibits Diabetes Mellitus Protein Targets. *J. Pharm. Res. Int.* **2021**, *33*, 161–171. [CrossRef]
73. Kim, D.-K.; Nepali, S.; Son, J.-S.; Poudel, B.; Lee, J.-H.; Lee, Y.-M. Luteolin Is a Bioflavonoid That Attenuates Adipocyte-Derived Inflammatory Responses via Suppression of Nuclear Factor-KB/Mitogen-Activated Protein Kinases Pathway. *Pharmacogn. Mag.* **2015**, *11*, 627. [CrossRef]
74. Wagle, A.; Seong, S.H.; Shrestha, S.; Jung, H.A.; Choi, J.S. Korean Thistle (Cirsium Japonicum Var. Maackii (Maxim.) Matsum.): A Potential Dietary Supplement against Diabetes and Alzheimer's Disease. *Molecules* **2019**, *24*, 649. [CrossRef]
75. Djeujo, F.M.; Ragazzi, E.; Urettini, M.; Sauro, B.; Cichero, E.; Tonelli, M.; Froldi, G. Magnolol and Luteolin Inhibition of α-Glucosidase Activity: Kinetics and Type of Interaction Detected by in Vitro and in Silico Studies. *Pharmaceuticals* **2022**, *15*, 205. [CrossRef] [PubMed]
76. Fan, J.; Johnson, M.H.; Lila, M.A.; Yousef, G.; Gonzalez, E. Berry and Citrus Phenolic Compounds Inhibit Dipeptidyl Peptidase IV: Implications in Diabetes Management. *Evid. Based Complement. Altern. Med.* **2013**, *2013*, 479505. [CrossRef]
77. Aziz, N.; Kim, M.-Y.; Cho, J.Y. Anti-Inflammatory Effects of Luteolin: A Review of in Vitro, in Vivo, and in Silico Studies. *J. Ethnopharmacol.* **2018**, *225*, 342–358. [CrossRef]
78. Ding, X.; Zheng, L.; Yang, B.; Wang, X.; Ying, Y. Luteolin Attenuates Atherosclerosis via Modulating Signal Transducer and Activator of Transcription 3-Mediated Inflammatory Response. *Drug Des. Dev. Ther.* **2019**, *13*, 3899–3911. [CrossRef]
79. Zhang, Z.; Zhang, D.; Xie, K.; Wang, C.; Xu, F. Luteolin Activates Tregs to Promote IL-10 Expression and Alleviating Caspase-11-Dependent Pyroptosis in Sepsis-Induced Lung Injury. *Int. Immunopharmacol.* **2021**, *99*, 107914. [CrossRef]

80. Cho, Y.-C.; Park, J.; Cho, S. Anti-Inflammatory and Anti-Oxidative Effects of Luteolin-7-O-Glucuronide in LPS-Stimulated Murine Macrophages through TAK1 Inhibition and Nrf2 Activation. *Int. J. Mol. Sci.* **2020**, *21*, 2007. [CrossRef]
81. Mizuno, M.; Yamashita, S.; Hashimoto, T. Enhancement of Anti-Inflammatory and Anti-Allergic Activities with Combination of Luteolin and Quercetin in *in Vitro* Co-Culture System. *Food Sci. Technol. Res.* **2017**, *23*, 811–818. [CrossRef]
82. Stefano, D.; Caporali, S.; Daniele, D.; Rovella, V.; Cardillo, C.; Schinzari, F.; Minieri, M.; Pieri, M.; Candi, E.; Bernardini, S.; et al. Anti-Inflammatory and Proliferative Properties of Luteolin-7-O-Glucoside. *Int. J. Mol. Sci.* **2021**, *22*, 1321. [CrossRef] [PubMed]
83. Sun, W.-L.; Yang, J.-W.; Dou, H.-Y.; Li, G.-Q.; Li, X.-Y.; Shen, L.; Ji, H.-F. Anti-Inflammatory Effect of Luteolin Is Related to the Changes in the Gut Microbiota and Contributes to Preventing the Progression from Simple Steatosis to Nonalcoholic Steatohepatitis. *Bioorganic Chem.* **2021**, *112*, 104966. [CrossRef] [PubMed]
84. Pandey, S.; Rana, M. Anti-Inflammatory Activity and Isolation of Luteolin from Plagiochasma Appendiculatum Methanol Extract. *Asian Pac. J. Health Sci.* **2022**, *9*, 76–79. [CrossRef]
85. Ma, Q.; Jiang, J.-G.; Zhang, X.-M.; Zhu, W. Identification of Luteolin 7-O-β-D-Glucuronide from Cirsium Japonicum and Its Anti-Inflammatory Mechanism. *J. Funct. Foods* **2018**, *46*, 521–528. [CrossRef]
86. Xie, T.; Yuan, J.; Mei, L.; Li, P.; Pan, R. Luteolin Suppresses TNF-α-Induced Inflammatory Injury and Senescence of Nucleus Pulposus Cells via the Sirt6/NF-KB Pathway. *Exp. Ther. Med.* **2022**, *24*, 469. [CrossRef]
87. Kim, J.-H.; Park, T.-J.; Park, J.-S.; Kim, M.-S.; Chi, W.-J.; Kim, S.-Y. Luteolin-3′-O-Phosphate Inhibits Lipopolysaccharide-Induced Inflammatory Responses by Regulating NF-KB/MAPK Cascade Signaling in RAW 264.7 Cells. *Molecules* **2021**, *26*, 7393. [CrossRef]
88. Park, C.M.; Song, Y.-S. Luteolin and Luteolin-7-O-Glucoside Protect against Acute Liver Injury through Regulation of Inflammatory Mediators and Antioxidative Enzymes in GalN/LPS-Induced Hepatic ICR Mice. *Nutr. Res. Pract.* **2019**, *13*, 473. [CrossRef]
89. Zhang, M.; He, L.; Liu, J.; Zhou, L. Luteolin Attenuates Diabetic Nephropathy through Suppressing Inflammatory Response and Oxidative Stress by Inhibiting STAT3 Pathway. *Exp. Clin. Endocrinol. Diabetes* **2020**, *129*, 729–739. [CrossRef]
90. Uwishema, O.; Mahmoud, A.; Sun, J.; Correia, I.F.S.; Bejjani, N.; Alwan, M.; Nicholas, A.; Oluyemisi, A.; Dost, B. Is Alzheimer's Disease an Infectious Neurological Disease? A Review of the Literature. *Brain Behav.* **2022**, *12*, e2728. [CrossRef]
91. Ali, F.; Jyoti, S.; Naz, F.; Ashafaq, M.; Shahid, M.; Siddique, Y.H. Therapeutic Potential of Luteolin in Transgenic Drosophila Model of Alzheimer's Disease. *Neurosci. Lett.* **2019**, *692*, 90–99. [CrossRef]
92. Kou, J.; Shi, J.; He, Y.; Hao, J.; Zhang, H.; Luo, D.; Song, J.; Yan, Y.; Xie, X.; Du, G.; et al. Luteolin Alleviates Cognitive Impairment in Alzheimer's Disease Mouse Model via Inhibiting Endoplasmic Reticulum Stress-Dependent Neuroinflammation. *Acta Pharmacol.* **2021**, *43*, 840–849. [CrossRef] [PubMed]
93. Wang, H.-R.; Pei, S.-Y.; Fan, D.-X.; Liu, Y.-H.; Pan, X.-F.; Song, F.-X.; Deng, S.-H.; Qiu, H.-B.; Zhang, N. Luteolin Protects Pheochromocytoma (PC-12) Cells against Aβ25-35-Induced Cell Apoptosis through the ER/ERK/MAPK Signalling Pathway. *Evid. Based Complement. Altern. Med.* **2020**, *2020*, 2861978. [CrossRef] [PubMed]
94. Park, S.; Kim, D.S.; Kang, S.; Kim, H.J. The Combination of Luteolin and L-Theanine Improved Alzheimer Disease–like Symptoms by Potentiating Hippocampal Insulin Signaling and Decreasing Neuroinflammation and Norepinephrine Degradation in Amyloid-β–Infused Rats. *Nutr. Res.* **2018**, *60*, 116–131. [CrossRef]
95. Zhao, G.; Yao-Yue, C.; Qin, G.-W.; Guo, L.-H. Luteolin from Purple Perilla Mitigates ROS Insult Particularly in Primary Neurons. *Neurobiol. Aging* **2012**, *33*, 176–186. [CrossRef]
96. Qin, L.; Chen, Z.; Yang, L.; Shi, H.; Wu, H.; Zhang, B.; Zhang, W.; Xu, Q.; Huang, F.; Wu, X. Luteolin-7-O-Glucoside Protects Dopaminergic Neurons by Activating Estrogen-Receptor-Mediated Signaling Pathway in MPTP-Induced Mice. *Toxicology* **2019**, *426*, 152256. [CrossRef] [PubMed]
97. Hu, L.-W.; Yen, J.-H.; Shen, Y.-T.; Wu, K.-Y.; Wu, M.-J. Luteolin Modulates 6-Hydroxydopamine-Induced Transcriptional Changes of Stress Response Pathways in PC12 Cells. *PLoS ONE* **2014**, *9*, e97880. [CrossRef]
98. Guo, D.-J.; Li, F.; Yu, P.H.-F.; Chan, S.-W. Neuroprotective Effects of Luteolin against Apoptosis Induced by 6-Hydroxydopamine on Rat Pheochromocytoma PC12 Cells. *Pharm. Biol.* **2012**, *51*, 190–196. [CrossRef]
99. Reudhabibadh, R.; Binlateh, T.; Chonpathompikunlert, P.; Nonpanya, N.; Prommeenate, P.; Chanvorachote, P.; Hutamekalin, P. Suppressing Cdk5 Activity by Luteolin Inhibits MPP+-Induced Apoptotic of Neuroblastoma through Erk/Drp1 and Fak/Akt/GSK3β Pathways. *Molecules* **2021**, *26*, 1307. [CrossRef]
100. Liu, D.; Luo, H.; Qiao, C. SHP-1/STAT3 Interaction Is Related to Luteolin-Induced Myocardial Ischemia Protection. *Inflammation* **2021**, *45*, 88–99. [CrossRef]
101. Zhao, L.; Zhou, Z.; Zhu, C.; Fu, Z.; Yu, D. Luteolin Alleviates Myocardial Ischemia Reperfusion Injury in Rats via Siti1/NLRP3/NF-KB Pathway. *Int. Immunopharmacol.* **2020**, *85*, 106680. [CrossRef]
102. Du, Y.; Liu, P.; Xu, T.; Pan, D.; Zhu, H.; Zhai, N.; Zhang, Y.; Li, D. Luteolin Modulates SERCA2a Leading to Attenuation of Myocardial Ischemia/ Reperfusion Injury via Sumoylation at Lysine 585 in Mice. *Cell. Physiol. Biochem.* **2018**, *45*, 883–898. [CrossRef]
103. Hu, Y.; Zhang, C.; Zhu, H.; Wang, S.; Zhou, Y.; Zhao, J.; Xia, Y.; Li, D. Luteolin Modulates SERCA2a via Sp1 Upregulation to Attenuate Myocardial Ischemia/Reperfusion Injury in Mice. *Sci. Rep.* **2020**, *10*, 15407. [CrossRef] [PubMed]
104. Hu, W.; Xu, T.; Wu, P.; Pan, D.; Chen, J.; Chen, J.; Zhang, B.; Zhu, H.; Li, D. Luteolin Improves Cardiac Dysfunction in Heart Failure Rats by Regulating Sarcoplasmic Reticulum Ca2+-ATPase 2a. *Sci. Rep.* **2017**, *7*, 41017. [CrossRef]

105. Fang, F.; Li, D.; Pan, H.; Chen, D.; Qi, L.; Zhang, R.; Sun, H. Luteolin Inhibits Apoptosis and Improves Cardiomyocyte Contractile Function through the PI3K/Akt Pathway in Simulated Ischemia/Reperfusion. *Pharmacology* **2011**, *88*, 149–158. [CrossRef] [PubMed]
106. Zhu, S.; Xu, T.; Luo, Y.; Zhang, Y.; Xuan, H.; Ma, Y.; Pan, D.; Li, D.; Zhu, H. Luteolin Enhances Sarcoplasmic Reticulum Ca2+-ATPase Activity through P38 MAPK Signaling Thus Improving Rat Cardiac Function after Ischemia/Reperfusion. *Cell. Physiol. Biochem.* **2017**, *41*, 999–1010. [CrossRef] [PubMed]
107. World Health Organization Obesity and Overweight. Available online: https://www.who.int/news-room/fact-sheets/detail/obesity-and-overweight (accessed on 6 October 2022).
108. Kwon, E.-Y.; Choi, M.-S. Luteolin Targets the Toll-like Receptor Signaling Pathway in Prevention of Hepatic and Adipocyte Fibrosis and Insulin Resistance in Diet-Induced Obese Mice. *Nutrients* **2018**, *10*, 1415. [CrossRef]
109. Zhang, X.; Zhang, Q.-X.; Wang, X.; Zhang, L.; Qu, W.; Bao, B.; Liu, C.-A.; Liu, J. Dietary Luteolin Activates Browning and Thermogenesis in Mice through an AMPK/PGC1α Pathway-Mediated Mechanism. *Int. J. Obes.* **2016**, *40*, 1841–1849. [CrossRef]
110. Park, H.-S.; Kim, S.-H.; Kim, Y.S.; Ryu, S.Y.; Hwang, J.-T.; Yang, H.J.; Kim, G.-H.; Kwon, D.Y.; Kim, M.-S. Luteolin Inhibits Adipogenic Differentiation by Regulating PPARγ Activation. *BioFactors* **2009**, *35*, 373–379. [CrossRef]
111. Kwon, E.-Y.; Kim, S.; Choi, M.-S. Luteolin-Enriched Artichoke Leaf Extract Alleviates the Metabolic Syndrome in Mice with High-Fat Diet-Induced Obesity. *Nutrients* **2018**, *10*, 979. [CrossRef]
112. Ando, C.; Takahashi, N.; Hirai, S.; Nishimura, K.; Lin, S.; Uemura, T.; Goto, T.; Yu, R.; Nakagami, J.; Murakami, S.; et al. Luteolin, a Food-Derived Flavonoid, Suppresses Adipocyte-Dependent Activation of Macrophages by Inhibiting JNK Activation. *FEBS Lett.* **2009**, *583*, 3649–3654. [CrossRef]
113. Park, H.; Lee, K.; Kim, S.; Hong, M.J.; Jeong, N.; Kim, M. Luteolin Improves Hypercholesterolemia and Glucose Intolerance through LXRα-Dependent Pathway in Diet-Induced Obese Mice. *J. Food Biochem.* **2020**, *44*, e13358. [CrossRef] [PubMed]
114. Caporali, S.; De Stefano, A.; Calabrese, C.; Giovannelli, A.; Pieri, M.; Savini, I.; Tesauro, M.; Bernardini, S.; Minieri, M.; Terrinoni, A. Anti-Inflammatory and Active Biological Properties of the Plant-Derived Bioactive Compounds Luteolin and Luteolin 7-Glucoside. *Nutrients* **2022**, *14*, 1155. [CrossRef] [PubMed]
115. Park, S.W.; Cho, C.S.; Jun, H.O.; Ryu, N.H.; Kim, J.H.; Yu, Y.S.; Kim, J.S.; Kim, J.H. Anti-Angiogenic Effect of Luteolin on Retinal Neovascularization via Blockade of Reactive Oxygen Species Production. *Investig. Ophthalmol. Vis. Sci.* **2012**, *53*, 7718–7726. [CrossRef] [PubMed]
116. Li, X.; He, X.; Chen, S.; Le, Y.; Bryant, M.S.; Guo, L.; Witt, K.L.; Mei, N. The Genotoxicity Potential of Luteolin Is Enhanced by CYP1A1 and CYP1A2 in Human Lymphoblastoid TK6 Cells. *Toxicol. Lett.* **2021**, *344*, 58–68. [CrossRef] [PubMed]
117. Fateh, A.H.; Mohamed, Z.; Chik, Z.; Alsalahi, A.; Md Zin, S.R.; Alshawsh, M.A. Prenatal Developmental Toxicity Evaluation of Verbena Officinalis during Gestation Period in Female Sprague-Dawley Rats. *Chem. Biol. Interact.* **2019**, *304*, 28–42. [CrossRef]
118. Cariddi, L.N.; Sabini, M.C.; Escobar, F.M.; Montironi, I.; Mañas, F.; Iglesias, D.; Comini, L.R.; Sabini, L.I.; Dalcero, A.M. Polyphenols as Possible Bioprotectors against Cytotoxicity and DNA Damage Induced by Ochratoxin A. *Environ. Toxicol. Pharmacol.* **2015**, *39*, 1008–1018. [CrossRef]
119. D'Ascanio, L.; Vitelli, F.; Cingolani, C.; Maranzano, M.; Brenner, M.J.; Di Stadio, A. Randomized clinical trial "olfactory dysfunction after COVID-19: Olfactory rehabilitation therapy vs. intervention treatment with Palmitoylethanolamide and Luteolin": Preliminary results. *Eur. Rev. Med. Pharmacol. Sci.* **2021**, *25*, 4156–4162. [CrossRef] [PubMed]
120. Yang, X.; Feng, Y.; Liu, Y.; Ye, X.; Ji, X.; Sun, L.; Gao, F.; Zhang, Q.; Li, Y.; Zhu, B.; et al. FuzhengJieduXiaoji Formulation Inhibits Hepatocellular Carcinoma Progression in Patients by Targeting the AKT/CyclinD1/P21/P27 Pathway. *Phytomedicine* **2021**, *87*, 153575. [CrossRef]
121. Lunardelli, M.L.; Crupi, R.; Siracusa, R.; Cocuzza, G.; Cordaro, M.; Martini, E.; Impellizzeri, D.; Di Paola, R.; Cuzzocrea, S. Co-UltraPEALut: Role in Preclinical and Clinical Delirium Manifestations. *CNS Neurol. Disord. Drug Targets* **2019**, *18*, 530–554. [CrossRef]
122. Castellino, G.; Nikolic, D.; Magán-Fernández, A.; Malfa, G.A.; Chianetta, R.; Patti, A.M.; Amato, A.; Montalto, G.; Toth, P.P.; Banach, M.; et al. Altilix® Supplement Containing Chlorogenic Acid and Luteolin Improved Hepatic and Cardiometabolic Parameters in Subjects with Metabolic Syndrome: A 6 Month Randomized, Double-Blind, Placebo-Controlled Study. *Nutrients* **2019**, *11*, 2580. [CrossRef]
123. Gelabert-Rebato, M.; Wiebe, J.C.; Martin-Rincon, M.; Galvan-Alvarez, V.; Curtelin, D.; Perez-Valera, M.; Juan Habib, J.; Pérez-López, A.; Vega, T.; Morales-Alamo, D.; et al. Enhancement of Exercise Performance by 48 Hours, and 15-Day Supplementation with Mangiferin and Luteolin in Men. *Nutrients* **2019**, *11*, 344. [CrossRef] [PubMed]
124. Taliou, A.; Zintzaras, E.; Lykouras, L.; Francis, K. An Open-Label Pilot Study of a Formulation Containing the Anti-Inflammatory Flavonoid Luteolin and Its Effects on Behavior in Children with Autism Spectrum Disorders. *Clin. Ther.* **2013**, *35*, 592–602. [CrossRef] [PubMed]

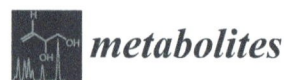 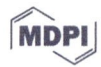

Article

The Combined Intervention of Aqua Exercise and Burdock Extract Synergistically Improved Arterial Stiffness: A Randomized, Double-Blind, Controlled Trial

Min-Seong Ha [1,*,†], Jae-Hoon Lee [2], Woo-Min Jeong [3], Hyun Ryun Kim [4] and Woo Hyeon Son [5,*,†]

1. Department of Sports Culture, College of the Arts, Dongguk University-Seoul, 30 Pildong-ro 1-gil, Jung-gu, Seoul 04620, Korea
2. Department of Sports Science, University of Seoul, 163 Seoulsiripdae-ro, Dongdaemun-gu, Seoul 02504, Korea
3. Wellcare Korea Co. Ltd., 26 Wadong-ro, Danwon-gu, Ansan-si 15265, Korea
4. Department of Physical Education, Woosuk University, 443 Samnye-ro, Samnye-eup, Wanju-gun 55338, Korea
5. Institute of Convergence Bio-Health, Dong-A University, 26 Daesingongwon-ro, Seo-gu, Busan 49201, Korea
* Correspondence: haminseong@dgu.ac.kr (M.-S.H.); physical365@gmail.com (W.H.S.); Tel.: +82-2-2290-1926 (M.-S.H.); +82-10-2886-6819 (W.H.S.)
† These authors contributed equally to this work.

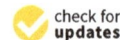

Citation: Ha, M.-S.; Lee, J.-H.; Jeong, W.-M.; Kim, H.R.; Son, W.H. The Combined Intervention of Aqua Exercise and Burdock Extract Synergistically Improved Arterial Stiffness: A Randomized, Double-Blind, Controlled Trial. Metabolites 2022, 12, 970. https://doi.org/10.3390/metabo12100970

Academic Editors: Petr G. Lokhov and Silvia Ravera

Received: 14 July 2022
Accepted: 11 October 2022
Published: 13 October 2022

Publisher's Note: MDPI stays neutral with regard to jurisdictional claims in published maps and institutional affiliations.

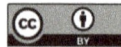

Copyright: © 2022 by the authors. Licensee MDPI, Basel, Switzerland. This article is an open access article distributed under the terms and conditions of the Creative Commons Attribution (CC BY) license (https://creativecommons.org/licenses/by/4.0/).

Abstract: Metabolic syndrome (MS), characterized by the presence of risk factors for various metabolic disorders, including impaired glucose tolerance, dyslipidemia, hypertension, and insulin resistance, has a high incidence in the Asian population. Among the various approaches used for improving MS, the combination of exercise and nutrition is of increasing importance. In this randomized controlled trial, we evaluated the effects of combined aqua exercise and burdock extract intake on blood pressure, insulin resistance, arterial stiffness, and vascular regulation factors in older women with MS. A total of 42 participants were randomly assigned into one of four groups (control, exercise, burdock, and exercise + burdock) and underwent a 16-week double-blinded intervention. Blood pressure, insulin resistance, arterial stiffness, and vascular regulation factors were evaluated before and after the intervention. The 16-week intervention of aqua exercise decreased the levels of insulin, glucose, homeostasis model assessment of insulin resistance, and thromboxane A2, but increased the levels of the quantitative insulin sensitivity check index and prostaglandin I2. The combined burdock extract intake and aqua exercise intervention had an additional effect, improving the augmentation index, augmentation index at 75 beats per min, and pulse wave velocity. In conclusion, aqua exercise could improve insulin resistance and vascular regulation factors in older women with MS. Furthermore, combined treatment with burdock extract intake could improve arterial stiffness via a synergistic effect.

Keywords: aqua exercise; burdock extract; metabolic syndrome; cardiovascular disease; vascular endothelial function

1. Introduction

Metabolic syndrome (MS) is characterized by the presence of risk factors for various metabolic disorders, including impaired glucose tolerance, dyslipidemia, hypertension, and insulin resistance [1]. According to the criteria of the National Cholesterol Education Program—Adult Treatment Panel III, MS is defined based on the presence of three or more of the following five risk indicators: abdominal obesity, hyperglycemia, hypertension, reduced levels of high-density lipoprotein (HDL) cholesterol, and increased levels of triglycerides (TG) [2]. Compared with that in Caucasians and African-Americans, the incidence of MS is high among Asians [3].

With insulin resistance and atherosclerosis as key factors, MS accelerates the increase in the risk of cardiovascular disease (CVD) [4]. Moreover, complications often arise in relation to diabetes and reduced vascular function [4]. In this regard, the incidence of

CVD is correlated with the incidence of insulin resistance or hyperinsulinemia through sympathetic activation and parasympathetic inhibition [5].

Furthermore, individuals with MS have impaired endothelial function [6]. Indeed, the incidence of atherosclerosis is increased by MS, which was shown to reduce the ability of vascular endothelial cells to regulate the secretion of various compounds that promote healthy blood flow, including vasodilators—nitric oxide (NO) and prostacyclin (prostaglandin I2; PGI2)—and vasoconstrictors—endothelin-1, angiotensin II, and thromboxane A2 (TXA2) [7–11].

According to the obesity, hypertension, and dyslipidemia criteria, MS results from increased arterial stiffness due to carotid artery hypertrophy and increased central arterial pressure. Accordingly, individuals with MS have increased pulse wave velocity (PWV) [12,13]. In addition, CVD-related mortality is three-fold higher among individuals with MS than among healthy individuals [14,15]. Furthermore, CVD and MS risks are higher in women than in men [3,16], and older women are more susceptible to MS due to an increase in adipose tissue and insulin resistance caused by hormonal imbalances after menopause [17]. Thus, it is essential to reduce the risk of CVD in this population through effective interventions that will achieve improvement in insulin resistance and vascular function.

Exercise is a non-invasive method for increasing the resistance to oxidative stress because it increases the activity of oxidation and antioxidation damage repair enzymes through an increase in reactive oxygen species levels [18]. Exercise is well-known as an effective treatment for MS and CVD [18]. Notably, aqua exercise is an ideal form of exercise for overweight and older women, as it is a systemic exercise in which the buoyancy of water decreases the body weight by 90%, thus minimizing the risk of injury [19–21]. In previous studies on older women, aqua exercise was shown to effectively improve blood pressure, insulin resistance, and CVD risk factors [22,23]. Nonetheless, few studies have investigated the effectiveness of aqua exercise in older women with MS.

Recently, as a combined treatment approach involving exercise and nutrition, studies have actively investigated natural products with converged efforts. Burdock is a plant species from the Asteraceae family, which has long been used as food in East Asian regions, including Korea, China, and Japan [20,21,24,25]. Burdock has an 80% water content and is enriched with carbohydrates and dietary fibers. It is considered a healthy food with diverse bioactive compounds and was reported to improve diabetes as well as CVD. Moreover, these compounds can prevent oxidation by suppressing NO overproduction in inflammation and CVD [24,26]. Based on these previous findings, we speculated that combined treatment with aquatic exercise and burdock intake would have a more positive effect than each intervention alone in older women.

Therefore, the aim of this study was to assess the effects of combined aqua exercise and burdock intake on blood pressure, insulin resistance, arterial stiffness, and vascular regulation factors in older women with MS. We hypothesized that a 16-week combined intervention in this population would improve blood pressure and insulin resistance and induce beneficial changes in the level of arterial stiffness through improvement in vascular regulation factors.

2. Materials and Methods

2.1. Participants

This study was conducted according to the guidelines laid down in the Declaration of Helsinki and all procedures involving human participants were approved by the Institutional Review Board of Dongguk University (DUIRB-202009-07). This trial was retrospectively registered in the Clinical Research Information Service (CRIS) (Republic of Korea, KCT0007627). After explaining the study's purpose and contents, written informed consent was obtained from all participants.

The study population included older women aged 70–80 years, who were selected according to the Korea Adult MS Guidelines [27]. The inclusion criteria were as follows:

(1) waist circumference ≥ 85 cm; (2) blood pressure ≥ 130/85 mmHg or taking antihypertensive medication; (3) fasting blood glucose level ≥ 100 mg/dL or taking antidiabetic medication; (4) TG level ≥ 150 mg/dL; and (5) HDL cholesterol level < 50 mg/dL. Individuals satisfying three or more of the above five criteria were selected.

2.2. Study Design

The study was designed as a randomized, double-blind, controlled trial. To determine the effects of a 16-week intervention of burdock intake and aqua exercise, the participants were randomly divided into four groups: placebo control (CON), exercise + placebo (EX), burdock (BD), and exercise + burdock (EXBD). The CON and EX groups took placebo beverages in the same manner in which the BD and EXBD groups took the investigational beverage. The color and odor of the burdock extract and placebo beverage were similar and their containers were identical. Unblinded personnel, who were not involved in any study assessments, labeled the investigational beverage. Investigators, other site personnel, and the participants were blinded to the beverage. The total daily required beverage intake was 300 mL; the participants drank 100 mL of burdock extract or placebo beverage after breakfast, lunch, and dinner. They were instructed not to take any other health supplements or drugs. All measurements were taken twice, before and after the intervention. The study design is presented in Figure 1.

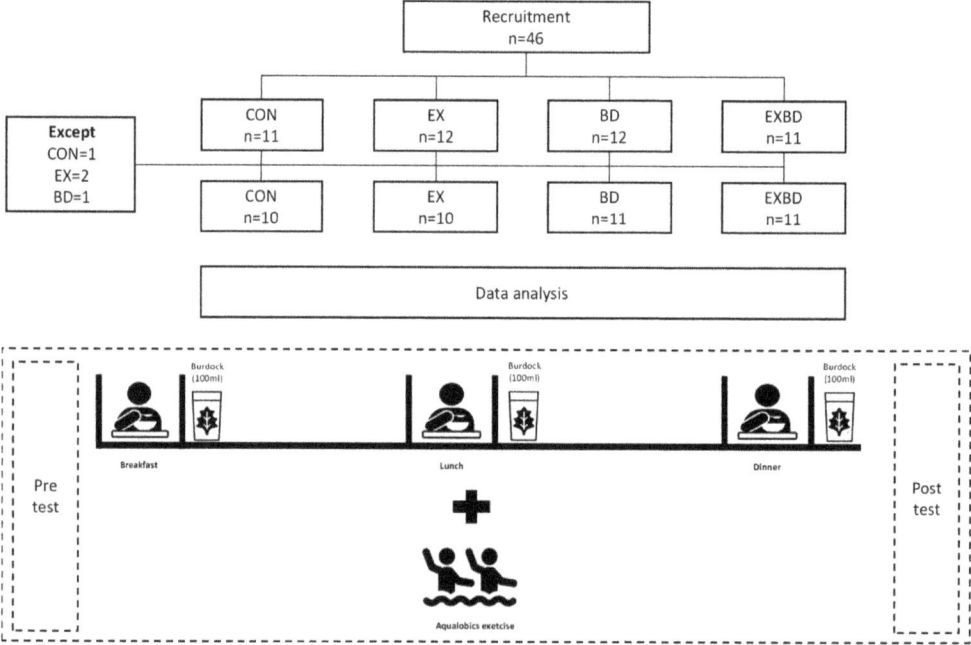

Figure 1. Study design. CON: placebo control, EX: exercise + placebo, BD: burdock, EXBD: exercise + burdock.

2.3. Burdock Extract Preparation and Composition

The burdock extract was prepared according to a method previously described by our research group [20,21,25]. In brief, after harvest in the Sangcheong region (Gyeongnam, Korea), the burdock root was washed and dried, subsequently heated at 100 °C for 3 h, and extracted at 0.7 kg/cm^2 pressure. The main ingredients of the extract were water (98.02% ± 0.02%), crude ash (0.10% ± 0.00%), crude fat (1.12% ± 0.00%), crude protein (0.20% ± 0.00%), crude fiber (0.03%), calcium (0.004% ± 0.00%), and phosphorus

(0.009% ± 0.00%) (Pukyong National University Feed & Foods Nutrition Research Center, Busan, Korea). The burdock extract was placed in small, sealed plastic containers of 100 mL, which were provided to the participants for intake. The composition of the burdock extract is summarized in Table S1.

2.4. Aqua Exercise Program

The aqua exercise program used in this study was developed by revising and complementing the program designed by our research group [20]. The temperature of the swimming pool was maintained at 26–28 °C. The aqua exercise program consisted of 50 min exercise sessions performed three times per week for 16 weeks. Each session included a 5 min warm-up exercise, 40 min of main exercises, and a 5 min cool-down exercise. The exercise intensity was established in the manner conducted in our study group based on the Rating of Perceived Exertion (RPE) scores and the Polar system (RS400sd; model APAC, 90026360; Polar, New York, NY, USA), as follows: W1–5: RPE 9–10 (30–40% heart rate reserve [HRR]), W6–10: RPE 11–12 (40–50% HRR), and W11–16: RPE 13–14 (50–60% HRR) [28]. The details of the aqua exercise program are presented in Table S2.

2.5. Blood Pressure

Blood pressure was measured using a digital blood pressure monitor (Jawon Medical, Daejeon, Korea) after a 10 min rest in the supine position. Measurements were taken twice with a 3 min interval in between. The mean value from the two measurements was used for analysis. When the first and second measurements differed by $\geq$10 mmHg, an additional measurement was taken to obtain the mean value without significant variation.

2.6. Blood Sampling

All participants were instructed to fast for $\geq$8 h before sample collection. At 8–10 a.m., 10 mL of blood was collected from the antebrachial vein by a clinical pathologist. The blood was centrifuged at 3000 rpm for 10 min in Combi-514R (Hanil, Seoul, Korea) for further analysis. All blood analyses were performed according to the procedures described by our research group [29].

2.6.1. Glucose

Glucose levels were measured in serum samples. After marking the sample, reference, and blank, 20 µL of plasma and 20 µL of standard reagent were added to the sample and reference, respectively, with the addition of 3.0 mL of coloring agent. The mixture was then incubated in a 37 °C water bath. Absorbance was measured at 505 nm.

2.6.2. Insulin

Insulin levels were measured in serum samples. After centrifugation, 200 µL of the supernatant was transferred to a test tube coated with anti-insulin antibody. After addition of 1.0 mL of insulin (DPC, Los Angeles, CA, USA), the mixture was incubated at 24 °C for 20 h, followed by aspiration and chemiluminescence immunoassay using an automated immunoanalyzer.

2.6.3. Homeostasis Model Assessment of Insulin Resistance and Quantitative Insulin Sensitivity Check Index

The homeostasis model assessment of insulin resistance (HOMA-IR) and quantitative insulin sensitivity check index (QUICKI) are widely used as simpler and less invasive methods to evaluate insulin resistance based on fasting serum insulin and glucose levels. In this study, the below formulae reported by Matthews et al. and Katz et al. were used to calculate the HOMA-IR [30] and QUICKI [31], respectively.

$$\text{HOMA-IR} = [\text{fasting insulin (mU/L)} \times \text{fasting glucose (mg/dL)}]/22.5$$
$$\text{QUICKI} = 1/[\log(\text{fasting insulin}) + \log(\text{fasting glucose})]$$

2.6.4. PGI$_2$

Whole blood was collected in an anticoagulant tube and added to a plate coated with a PGI$_2$ reagent (Amersham, IL, USA). Next, 50 µL of detection reagent A was added, and the sample was incubated for 1 h at 37 °C. Subsequently, the plate was washed four times with 350 µL of wash buffer, and 100 µL of detection reagent B was added. After incubation at 37 °C for 30 min, the plate was again washed four times with 350 µL of wash buffer and incubated with 90 µL of substrate solution for 15–22 min at ambient temperature in the dark. When the reaction was completed, 50 µL of stop solution was added to each well, and absorbance was measured at 450 nm using Manifold-24 (Amersham, IL, USA).

2.6.5. TXA$_2$

For TXA$_2$ measurement, 0.9 mL of blood was collected and immediately placed in a polystyrene tube. After adding 0.1 mL of 3.8% trisodium citrate, followed by 1 mL of physiological saline and collagen at 2 µL/mL, the mixture was heated for 15 min in a shaking water bath at 37 °C to stimulate the production of TXA$_2$. After a 5 min centrifugation at 2000 rpm, the supernatant was collected for the quantification of thromboxane B$_2$, an unstable product of TXA$_2$ conversion, using a radioimmunoassay kit (Amersham, TRK780, IL, USA).

2.7. Arterial Stiffness

Arterial stiffness was measured using a non-invasive, tonometry-based PW detector (SphygmoCor; AtCor Medical, Sydney, Australia), according to the guidelines described in the Clinical Application of Arterial Stiffness, Task Force III [32]. PWV was measured based on the PW flow from the carotid to the brachial artery. The automated software of the device was used to record the PW on both ends of the artery, and the interdistance was measured using a tape measure. Next, the PWV formula was used to divide the distance (L) by the time variation (Δt) between the PWs recorded on both sides [33].

$$PWV = L/\Delta t$$

For the augmentation index (AIx), we calculated the pressure difference between the highest level of the central blood pressure and the augmentation point that arises at the PW refraction generated by the traveling wave advancing to the periphery to encounter the reflected wave returning to the periphery and divided it by the PWV [34]. In addition, the heart rate-corrected augmentation index at 75 beats per min (AIx@75) was estimated.

2.8. Sample Size Calculation

The sample size was calculated using G-power version 3.1 for Windows (Kiel University, Kiel, Germany). We estimated the sample size for this study as $n = 40$ based on the following conditions: effect size of 0.25 (default), significance of 0.05, and power of 0.70. Considering potential dropouts, a total of 46 participants were recruited.

2.9. Statistical Analysis

All data were statistically analyzed using IBM SPSS Statistics 27.0 (IBM Corp., Armonk, NY, USA) and expressed as means with standard deviations. The level of significance was set at $p < 0.05$. To determine the effects of the 16-week intervention on MS indicators (insulin resistance, vascular regulation factors, and arterial stiffness), two-way repeated measures analysis of variance (ANOVA) was performed with the treatment (CON, EX, BD, and EXBD) and time (pre-test and post-test) as independent variables. The Bonferroni test was used for post-hoc analysis. The post-treatment differences in the response of each variable were analyzed using the pre-test-post-test variation (Δ) by employing one-way ANOVA and Pearson's correlation analysis. The effect size for the pre-test-post-test variation (Cohen's d) was expressed as the mean variation [35].

3. Results

3.1. Participants' Characteristics

Of the 46 enrolled participants, four dropped out of the study owing to personal reasons. Therefore, 42 participants completed the study and were included in the analysis. The characteristics of the participants are presented in Table S3.

3.2. Blood Pressure

The effects of the 16-week intervention of burdock intake and aqua exercise on blood pressure and the relevant variations are shown in Figure 2. A significant time effect was detected for the systolic blood pressure (SBP; $p = 0.039$), but only the BD group showed a significant decrease from 157.13 ± 24.37 mmHg before the intervention to 146.18 ± 17.53 mmHg after the intervention ($p = 0.029$). There was also a significant group effect for the diastolic blood pressure (DBP; $p = 0.05$; Table S4). In addition, one-way ANOVA showed no significant difference in ΔSBP and ΔDBP across all groups (Table S5).

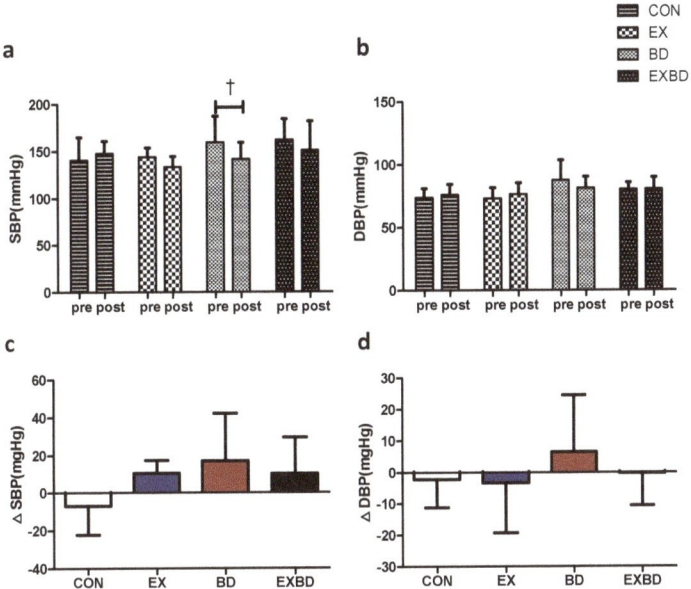

Figure 2. Effect of 16 weeks of aquatic aqua exercise and burdock intake on the blood pressure in older women with metabolic syndrome. (**a**) The systolic blood pressure in the BD group decreased after the 16-week intervention compared with the baseline values. (**b**) No significant changes were detected in the diastolic blood pressure in all groups. Furthermore, no significant differences in systolic (**c**) or diastolic (**d**) blood pressure variation were observed among the groups using one-way analysis of variance. Data are presented as the mean ± standard variation. † $p < 0.05$, significant; before vs. after intervention. SBP, systolic blood pressure; DBP, diastolic blood pressure; CON, placebo control, EX, exercise + placebo, BD, burdock, EXBD, exercise + burdock.

3.3. Insulin Resistance

The effects of the 16-week intervention on insulin resistance and the relevant variation are shown in Figure 3. Insulin levels showed a significant interaction effect ($p = 0.003$). In the within-group analysis, only the EX group showed a significant decrease from 32.77 ± 20.73 mg/dL to 30.17 ± 22.76 mg/dL ($p = 0.002$). Glucose levels showed significant differences both for the time ($p = 0.029$) and interaction effects ($p = 0.004$). In the within-group analysis, the EX and EXBD groups showed significant decreases from 120.24 ± 23.47 mg/dL to 95.48 ± 13.31 mg/dL ($p = 0.001$) and from 103.50 ± 24.19 mg/dL to 88.83 ± 10.76 mg/dL ($p = 0.05$), respectively. The post-hoc test showed significantly smaller ($p = 0.034$) values for the BD group than for the CON group.

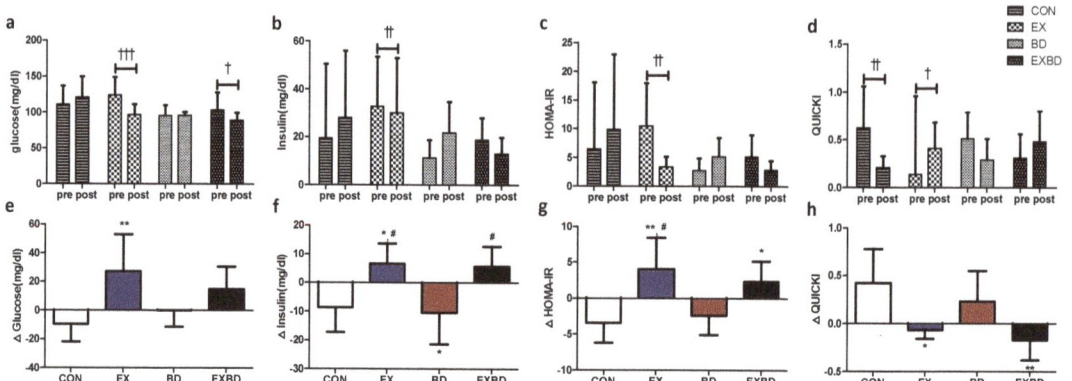

Figure 3. Effect of 16 weeks of aqua exercise and burdock intake on insulin resistance in older women with metabolic syndrome. After the intervention, compared with the baseline values, (**a**) glucose levels were decreased in the EX and EXBD groups, (**b**) insulin levels were decreased in the EX group, (**c**) the HOMA-IR was decreased in the EX group, and (**d**) the QUICKI was decreased in the CON group and increased in the EX group. One-way analysis of variance was used to compare the variation in insulin resistance (**e–h**). Data are presented as the mean ± standard deviation. † $p < 0.01$, †† $p < 0.01$, ††† $p < 0.001$; before vs. after intervention. * $p < 0.05$, ** $p < 0.01$ vs. CON, # $p < 0.05$ vs. BD. HOMA-IR, homeostasis model assessment of insulin resistance; QUICKI, quantitative insulin sensitivity check index; CON, placebo control, EX, exercise + placebo, BD, burdock, EXBD, exercise + burdock.

For the HOMA-IR, the interaction effect was significant ($p = 0.002$) and the within-group analysis showed a significant decrease only in the EX group from 10.45 ± 7.53 to 3.39 ± 1.77 ($p = 0.001$). For the QUICKI, the interaction effect was also significant ($p = 0.002$) and the within-group analysis showed a significant decrease in the CON group from 0.62 ± 0.44 to 0.21 ± 0.12 ($p = 0.005$) and a significant increase in the EX group from 0.14 ± 0.82 to 0.41 ± 0.27 ($p = 0.046$, Table S4). A one-way ANOVA revealed that Δinsulin showed no significant difference per group ($p = 0.002$). The post-hoc test indicated higher values for the EX and EXBD groups than for the CON and BD groups ($p < 0.05$).

Moreover, Δglucose showed a significant between-group difference ($p < 0.007$) and the post-hoc test indicated significantly higher values for the EX group than for the CON group ($p < 0.01$). The ΔHOMA-IR also showed a significant between-group difference ($p = 0.001$), with higher values for the EX and EXBD groups than for the CON group ($p < 0.05$ and $p < 0.01$, respectively) and for the EX group than for the BD group ($p < 0.05$) in the post-hoc test. Similarly, the ΔQUICKI showed a significant difference among groups ($p = 0.003$), with higher values for the EX group than for the CON group ($p < 0.05$) and for the CON group than for the EXBD group ($p < 0.01$) in the post-hoc test (Table S5).

3.4. Vascular Regulation Factors

The effects of the 16-week intervention on vascular regulation factors and the relevant variations are shown in Figure 4. For PGI_2 levels, only the EX group showed a significant increase from 15.98 ± 2.95 pg/mL to 19.32 ± 6.43 pg/mL in the within-group analysis ($p = 0.050$). TXA_2 levels showed a significant interaction effect ($p = 0.002$), and the within-group analysis showed a significant increase in the CON group from 22.43 ± 6.32 pg/mL to 24.73 ± 6.69 pg/mL ($p = 0.003$). Conversely, the EX and EXBD groups showed a significant decrease from 18.39 ± 5.11 pg/mL to 16.88 ± 4.48 pg/mL ($p = 0.049$) and from 22.42 ± 6.66 pg/mL to 20.56 ± 5.88 pg/mL ($p = 0.021$), respectively (Table S6).

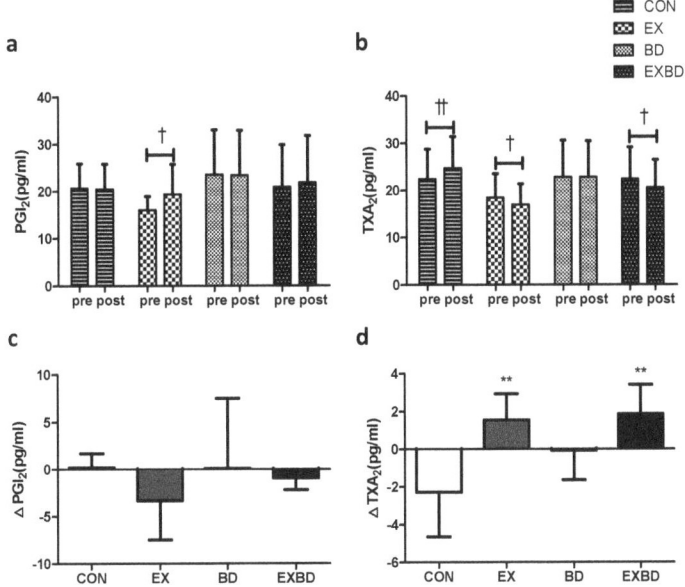

Figure 4. Effect of 16 weeks of aqua exercise and burdock intake on vascular regulation factors in older women with metabolic syndrome. Compared with the baseline values, (**a**) PGI_2 levels were increased in the EX group, and (**b**) TXA_2 levels were decreased in the CON, EX, and EXBD groups after the 16-week intervention. One-way analysis of variance was used to compare the variation in the levels of vascular regulation factors (**c**,**d**). Data are presented as the mean ± standard deviation. $^\dagger p < 0.01$, $^{\dagger\dagger} p < 0.01$; before vs. after intervention. ** $p < 0.01$ vs. CON. PGI_2, prostacyclin, i.e., prostaglandin I2; TXA_2, thromboxane A2; CON, placebo control, EX, exercise + placebo, BD, burdock, EXBD, exercise + burdock.

The one-way ANOVA showed that no significant between-group difference was found for ΔPGI_2, whereas ΔTXA_2 showed a significant difference among groups ($p = 0.002$), with significantly higher values for the CON group than for the EX and EXBD groups ($p < 0.01$; Table S7).

3.5. Arterial Stiffness

The effects of the 16-week intervention of burdock intake and aqua exercise on arterial stiffness and the relevant variations are shown in Figure 5. The AIx showed a significant interaction effect ($p = 0.026$), and the within-group analysis showed a significant increase in the CON group from 33.14 ± 8.09% to 42.00 ± 11.15% ($p = 0.042$) and a significant decrease in the EXBD group from 42.00 ± 11.54% to 31.50 ± 10.09% ($p = 0.027$). For the AIx@75, the within-group analysis showed a significant decrease only in the EXBD group, from 40.00 ± 9.44% to 32.33 ± 7.99% ($p = 0.050$). For the PWV, the interaction effect was significant ($p = 0.023$) and the within-group analysis showed that only the EXBD group had a significant increase from 8.94 ± 1.38 m/s to 9.93 ± 1.12 m/s ($p = 0.015$; Table S8).

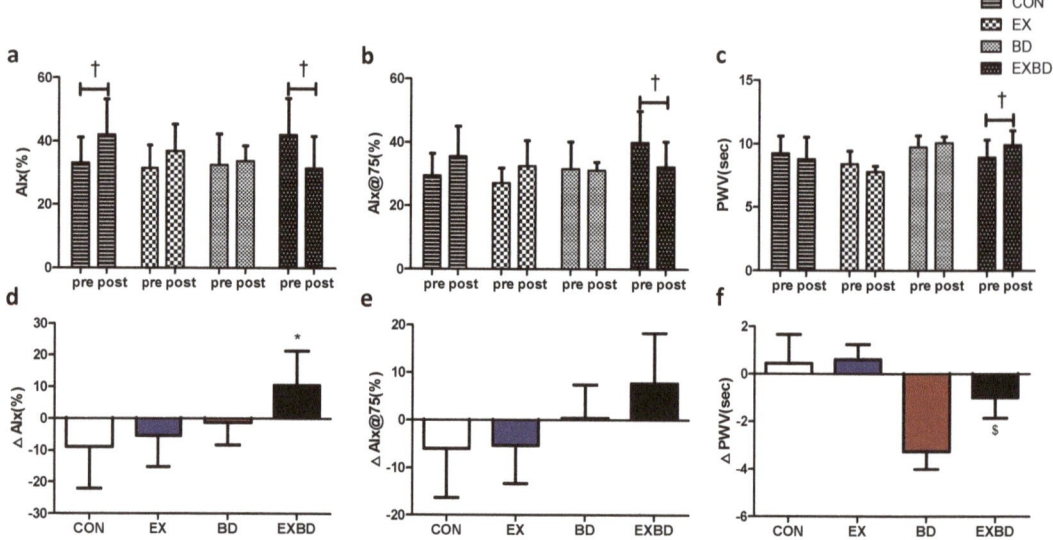

Figure 5. Effect of 16 weeks of aqua exercise and burdock intake on arterial stiffness in older women with metabolic syndrome. Compared with the baseline values, after the 16-week intervention, (**a**) the AIx was decreased in the EXBD group and increased in the CON group, (**b**) the AIx@75 was decreased in the EXBD group, and (**c**) the PWV was increased in the EXBD group. One-way analysis of variance was used to compare the variations in arterial stiffness (**d**–**f**). Data are presented as the mean ± standard deviation. † $p < 0.01$; before vs. after intervention. * $p < 0.05$ vs. CON, $ $p < 0.05$ vs. BD. AIx, augmentation index; AIx@75, heart rate-corrected augmentation index at 75 beats per min; PWV, pulse wave velocity; CON, placebo control, EX, exercise + placebo, BD, burdock, EXBD, exercise + burdock.

The one-way ANOVA indicated that the ΔAIx showed a significant difference among groups ($p = 0.026$), with the post-hoc test indicating significantly higher values for the EXBD group than for the CON group ($p < 0.05$). The ΔAIx@75 showed no significant between-group differences. The ΔPWV showed a significant difference among groups ($p = 0.023$), with the post-hoc test indicating significantly higher values for the EXBD group than for the EX group ($p < 0.05$; Table S9).

3.6. Correlation among Variations

Pearson's correlation analysis for the variations in the measured variables showed a positive correlation between ΔSBP and ΔDBP ($r = 0.657$, $p < 0.001$) and between Δglucose and Δinsulin ($r = 0.674$, $p < 0.001$). A positive correlation was found with the ΔHOMA-IR ($r = 0.860$, $p < 0.001$) and ΔTXA$_2$ ($r = 0.592$, $p < 0.01$); however, there was a negative correlation with the ΔQUICKI ($r = -0.564$, $p < 0.01$). For Δinsulin, there was a positive correlation with the ΔHOMA-IR ($r = 0.892$, $p < 0.001$), ΔAIx ($r = 0.465$, $p < 0.05$), and ΔAIx@75 ($r = 0.461$, $p < 0.05$) and a negative correlation with the ΔQUICKI ($r = -0.760$, $p < 0.001$). For the ΔHOMA-IR, there was a negative correlation with the ΔQUICKI ($r = -0.608$, $p < 0.01$) and a positive correlation with the ΔTXA$_2$ ($r = 0.427$, $p < 0.05$). The ΔQUICKI showed a negative correlation with the ΔAIx ($r = -0.411$, $p < 0.05$), while the ΔPWV negatively correlated with the ΔAIx ($r = -0.622$, $p < 0.001$) and ΔAix@75 ($r = -0.610$, $p < 0.01$). Finally, a positive correlation was found between ΔAIx and ΔAIx@75 ($r = 0.964$, $p < 0.001$). The results of the correlation analysis are summarized in Table S10.

4. Discussion

In this study, we hypothesized that the combined use of aquatic exercise and burdock intake would be more effective than each intervention separately for improving blood pressure, insulin resistance, vascular regulation factors, and arterial stiffness in older women with MS. Our results supported this hypothesis and revealed several novel observations. The 16-week intervention of aqua exercise decreased the levels of insulin, glucose, HOMA-IR, and TXA_2, but increased the levels of QUICKI and PGI_2. Independently, however, the burdock intake intervention did not show significant results for vascular function improvement. Remarkably, the combined use of burdock intake and aqua exercise had an additional effect to improve the AIx, AIx@75, and PWV.

Insulin resistance is the most common risk factor for MS. As it reduces the response of target cells to insulin owing to a decline in their sensitivity to insulin secretion, insulin resistance has a negative effect on the overall metabolism [36,37]. Characteristic outcomes caused by insulin resistance include metabolic disorders, such as type 2 diabetes, obesity, glucose intolerance, and dyslipidemia. Insulin resistance is also recognized as a CVD-related factor in atherosclerosis and hypertension and is characterized by endothelial dysfunction [38].

In older women, the degree of insulin resistance increases with a distinct reduction in physical activity because the hormonal imbalance after menopause results in increased adipose tissue accumulation, as well as increased fasting insulin and glucose levels [39]. Physical exercise is recommended as a solution to these problems and it is associated with minimal side effects. Physical exercise is effective in treating insulin resistance [40], with the levels of insulin resistance and physical exercise being inversely related [41]. In addition, participation in regular exercise not only improves antioxidation in the body but also facilitates glucose absorption in peripheral tissues and enhances insulin sensitivity by increasing the number of insulin receptors [42,43]. In a previous study in patients with type 2 diabetes, an 8-week intervention of aqua exercise significantly reduced insulin resistance [44].

The results of the present study showed a significant decrease in insulin, glucose, and HOMA-IR levels and a significant increase in QUICKI values in the EX group, suggesting that continuous participation in the aqua exercise had a positive effect on insulin resistance. Thus, additional studies should be conducted to further evaluate the preparation and composition of burdock extract for improving insulin resistance in older women with MS.

The risk factors for MS are closely associated with the progression of atherosclerosis, with cytokine secretion from adipocytes exerting a negative effect on insulin sensitivity, thereby resulting in endothelial dysfunction [8,45]. In turn, endothelial dysfunction increases the prevalence of atherosclerosis, while arterial tension is controlled by vasodilators, such as NO and PGI_2, and vasoconstrictors, such as TXA_2 [46].

PGI_2 is known for its powerful role in the induction of vasodilation and in preventing platelet coagulation [47,48]. Gamez-Mendez et al. [49] reported a decline in PGI_2 levels in obese mice, suggesting a role for PGI_2 in endothelial dysfunction. Conversely, TXA_2, which exerts antagonistic effects to those of PGI_2, is a powerful vasoconstrictor with additional roles in inducing platelet coagulation and various physiological responses, such as facilitated thrombosis and endothelial inflammation [50]. Interestingly, a close association was observed between increased platelet activation and coagulation and CVD complications [51].

Regular exercise induces endovascular shear stress and subsequent activation of calcium ion channels and phospholipases, leading to the release of PGI_2 [52]. In a previous study in patients with hypertension, a 16-week exercise intervention was shown to increase the levels of PGI_2 metabolites and decrease those of TXA_2 metabolites [53]. In addition, in a human red blood cell count experiment with burdock extract, an anti-thrombotic effect was reported [54]. Furthermore, in a study in high-fat/cholesterol-diet rats, Lee et al. [55] identified a positive effect of burdock intake on vascular dysfunction.

The results of this study revealed a significant increase in PGI$_2$ levels in the EX group and a significant decrease in TXA$_2$ levels in the EX and EXBD groups, indicating a positive effect of exercise on insulin resistance, by enhancing endothelial function and reducing the risk of CVD in patients with MS. However, no significant effect was shown in the BD group, which highlights the need for further studies to investigate potential markers associated with endothelial dysfunction.

Insulin resistance and hyperglycemia are reported to increase cytokine production and oxidative stress, thereby compromising vascular endothelial function [56,57]. Endothelial dysfunction caused by damage to endothelial cells through structural or functional changes in vascular walls promotes or exacerbates atherosclerosis, an independent predictor of mortality due to coronary artery disease and CVD [58,59]. To detect atherosclerosis, the carotid–femoral PWV is used, whereas the Aix is used for evaluating systemic arterial stiffness [33,60]. Patients with MS are characterized by high PWV values [61].

The increase in shear stress during exercise increases the bioavailability of NO and activates sympathetic nerves to enhance vascular endothelial function [62]. Donley et al. [63] reported that an 8-week intervention of aerobic exercise in patients with MS was associated with a reduction in carotid–femoral PWV levels [64]. Burdock has antioxidant effects due to its caffeoylquinic acid content. This enhanced antioxidation capacity may reduce the content of free radicals and promote endothelial NO synthase expression, thereby increasing NO bioavailability [65]. In addition, Lee et al. [66] performed a principal component analysis of burdock and reported the presence of L-arginine, an NO precursor.

In this study, we found a significant decrease in the AIx and AIx@75 only in the EXBD group after the intervention. In addition, the largest variations in AIx and AIx@75 values (ΔAIx and ΔAIx@75) were observed in the EXBD group. Furthermore, only the BD group exhibited a decline in SBP, although there was no difference in the other variables. These findings indicated that aqua exercise improved insulin resistance and vascular regulation factors in older women with MS, while burdock intake resulted in SBP reduction, with no confirmed effects on other vascular function-related variables. Therefore, it remains unclear whether burdock intake affects vascular function and insulin resistance indicators in older women with MS. However, it was reaffirmed that aquatic exercise can be effective for improving insulin resistance and vascular regulation factors in this population. Moreover, this study revealed that combined burdock intake and aqua exercise can reduce arterial stiffness in individuals with MS.

A potential limitation of this study is that direct markers of antioxidation and NO levels were not measured in response to burdock intake. Thus, additional studies are warranted to investigate the relationship between burdock intake and direct markers of antioxidation and NO. Additionally, there are some limitations pertaining to the generalizability of our findings. First, as the focus of the study was on older women with MS, it is difficult to generalize the results to men or women of other ages. Second, owing to the small sample size, the effect size in our study was limited to 70% of the power. Therefore, future studies should be performed on a larger number of study participants to support our findings.

5. Conclusions

In summary, burdock intake alone cannot be expected to have a significant effect in older women with MS. However, its combined use with aqua exercise, which is effective in decreasing insulin resistance and vascular regulation factors, can additionally improve arterial stiffness.

Supplementary Materials: The following supporting information can be downloaded at: https://www.mdpi.com/article/10.3390/metabo12100970/s1, Table S1: Composition of the burdock root extract; Table S2: Details of the 16-week aqua exercise program for older women with metabolic syndrome; Table S3: Descriptive characteristics of the study participants; Table S4: Effects of the 16-week aqua exercise on blood pressure and insulin resistance in older women with metabolic syndrome; Table S5: Changes in blood pressure and insulin resistance after the 16-week aqua exercise in older women with metabolic syndrome; Table S6: Effects of the 16-week aqua exercise on vascular regulation factors in older women with metabolic syndrome; Table S7: Changes in the vascular regulation factors after the 16-week aqua exercise in older women with metabolic syndrome; Table S8: Effects of the 16-week aqua exercise on arterial stiffness in older women with metabolic syndrome; Table S9: Changes in arterial stiffness after the 16-week aqua exercise in older women with metabolic syndrome; Table S10: Correlation between delta (Δ) values.

Author Contributions: Conceptualization, W.H.S. and M.-S.H.; methodology, W.-M.J. and M.-S.H.; software, J.-H.L.; validation, M.-S.H.; formal analysis, J.-H.L. and H.R.K.; data curation, J.-H.L.; writing—original draft preparation, W.H.S., J.-H.L. and M.-S.H.; writing—review and editing, M.-S.H.; visualization, J.-H.L.; supervision, M.-S.H.; project administration, W.-M.J. and M.-S.H.; funding acquisition, M.-S.H. All authors critically revised the manuscript for important intellectual content and approved the final version for publication. All authors significantly contributed to the research. All authors have read and agreed to the published version of the manuscript.

Funding: This research was supported by the Ministry of Education of the Republic of Korea and the National Research Foundation of Korea (NRF-2019S1A5B5A07106826).

Institutional Review Board Statement: All procedures and protocols performed in this study involving human participants adhered to the ethical standards of the institutional and/or national research committee and the 1964 Helsinki Declaration and were approved by the National Bioethics Committee and Institutional Review Board of Dongguk University (DUIRB-202009-07). This trial was retrospectively registered in the Clinical Research Information Service (CRIS) (Republic of Korea, KCT0007627).

Informed Consent Statement: Written informed consent for participation was obtained from all study participants prior to enrollment. Additionally, written informed consent was obtained from all participants for the publication of this paper.

Data Availability Statement: The authors declare that all data and materials are available to be shared upon formal request to the corresponding author.

Conflicts of Interest: The authors declare no conflict of interest.

References

1. Vega, G.L. Cardiovascular Outcomes for Obesity and Metabolic Syndrome. *Obes. Res.* **2002**, *10*, 27S–32S. [CrossRef] [PubMed]
2. Expert Panel on Detection Evaluation, and Treatment of High Blood Cholesterol in Adults. Executive Summary of the Third Report of the National Cholesterol Education Program (NCEP) Expert Panel on Detection, Evaluation, and Treatment of High Blood Cholesterol in Adults (Adult Treatment Panel III). *JAMA* **2001**, *285*, 2486–2497. [CrossRef] [PubMed]
3. Tillin, T.; Forouhi, N.; Johnston, D.G.; McKeigue, P.M.; Chaturvedi, N.; Godsland, I.F. Metabolic Syndrome and Coronary Heart Disease in South Asians, African-Caribbeans and White Europeans: A UK Population-Based Cross-Sectional Study. *Diabetologia* **2005**, *48*, 649–656. [CrossRef] [PubMed]
4. Mykkänen, L.; Kuusisto, J.; Pyörälä, K.; Laakso, M. Cardiovascular Disease Risk Factors as Predictors of Type 2 (Non-Insulin-Dependent) Diabetes Mellitus in Elderly Subjects. *Diabetologia* **1993**, *36*, 553–559. [CrossRef]
5. Foright, R.M.; Presby, D.M.; Sherk, V.D.; Kahn, D.; Checkley, L.A.; Giles, E.D.; Bergouignan, A.; Higgins, J.A.; Jackman, M.R.; Hill, J.O.; et al. Is Regular Exercise an Effective Strategy for Weight Loss Maintenance? *Physiol. Behav.* **2018**, *188*, 86–93. [CrossRef]
6. Sypniewska, G. Pro-Inflammatory and Prothrombotic Factors and Metabolic Syndrome. *EJIFCC* **2007**, *18*, 39–46. [PubMed]
7. Brook, R.D.; Bard, R.L.; Rubenfire, M.; Ridker, P.M.; Rajagopalan, S. Usefulness of Visceral Obesity (Waist/Hip Ratio) in Predicting Vascular Endothelial Function in Healthy Overweight Adults. *Am. J. Cardiol.* **2001**, *88*, 1264–1269. [CrossRef]
8. McVeigh, G.E.; Brennan, G.M.; Johnston, G.D.; McDermott, B.J.; McGrath, L.T.; Henry, W.R.; Andrews, J.W.; Hayes, J.R. Impaired Endothelium-Dependent and Independent Vasodilation in Patients with Type 2 (Non-Insulin-Dependent) Diabetes Mellitus. *Diabetologia* **1992**, *35*, 771–776. [CrossRef]
9. Furchgott, R.F.; Zawadzki, J.V. The Obligatory Role of Endothelial Cells in the Relaxation of Arterial Smooth Muscle by Acetylcholine. *Nature* **1980**, *288*, 373–376. [CrossRef]
10. Riddell, D.R.; Owen, J.S. Nitric Oxide and Platelet Aggregation. *Vitam. Horm.* **1997**, *57*, 25–48. [CrossRef]

11. Nicosia, S.; Oliva, D.; Bernini, F.; Fumagalli, R. Prostacyclin-sensitive Adenylate Cyclase and Prostacyclin Binding Sites in Platelets and Smooth Muscle Cells. *Adv. Cycl. Nucleotide Protein Phosphorylation Res.* **1984**, *17*, 593–599. [PubMed]
12. Fournier, S.B.; Reger, B.L.; Donley, D.A.; Bonner, D.E.; Warden, B.E.; Gharib, W.; Failinger, C.F.; Olfert, M.D.; Frisbee, J.C.; Olfert, I.M.; et al. Exercise Reveals Impairments in Left Ventricular Systolic Function in Patients with Metabolic Syndrome. *Exp. Physiol.* **2014**, *99*, 149–163. [CrossRef] [PubMed]
13. Scuteri, A.; Najjar, S.S.; Orru', M.; Usala, G.; Piras, M.G.; Ferrucci, L.; Cao, A.; Schlessinger, D.; Uda, M.; Lakatta, E.G. The Central Arterial Burden of the Metabolic Syndrome Is Similar in Men and Women: The SardiNIA Study. *Eur. Heart J.* **2010**, *31*, 602–613. [CrossRef] [PubMed]
14. Safar, M.E.; Thomas, F.; Blacher, J.; Nzietchueng, R.; Bureau, J.M.; Pannier, B.; Benetos, A. Metabolic Syndrome and Age-Related Progression of Aortic Stiffness. *J. Am. Coll. Cardiol.* **2006**, *47*, 72–75. [CrossRef]
15. Malik, S.; Wong, N.D.; Franklin, S.S.; Kamath, T.V.; L'Italien, G.J.; Pio, J.R.; Williams, G.R. Impact of the Metabolic Syndrome on Mortality from Coronary Heart Disease, Cardiovascular Disease, and All Causes in United States Adults. *Circulation* **2004**, *110*, 1245–1250. [CrossRef]
16. Gami, A.S.; Witt, B.J.; Howard, D.E.; Erwin, P.J.; Gami, L.A.; Somers, V.K.; Montori, V.M. Metabolic Syndrome and Risk of Incident Cardiovascular Events and Death. A Systematic Review and Meta-Analysis of Longitudinal Studies. *J. Am. Coll. Cardiol.* **2007**, *49*, 403–414. [CrossRef]
17. Stachowiak, G.; Pertyński, T.; Pertyńska-Marczewska, M. Metabolic Disorders in Menopause. *Prz. Menopauzalny* **2015**, *14*, 59–64. [CrossRef]
18. Golbidi, S.; Mesdaghinia, A.; Laher, I. Exercise in the Metabolic Syndrome. *Oxid. Med. Cell. Longev.* **2012**, *2012*, 349710. [CrossRef]
19. Barbosa, T.M.; Garrido, M.F.; Bragada, J. Physiological Adaptations to Head-out Aquatic Exercises with Different Levels of Body Immersion. *J. Strength Cond. Res.* **2007**, *21*, 1255–1259. [CrossRef]
20. Ha, M.-S.; Kim, J.-H.; Ha, S.-M.; Kim, Y.-S.; Kim, D.-Y. Positive Influence of Aqua Exercise and Burdock Extract Intake on Fitness Factors and Vascular Regulation Substances in Elderly. *J. Clin. Biochem. Nutr.* **2019**, *64*, 73–78. [CrossRef]
21. Ha, M.S.; Yook, J.S.; Lee, M.; Suwabe, K.; Jeong, W.M.; Kwak, J.-J.; Soya, H. Exercise Training and Burdock Root (*Arctium Lappa* L.) Extract Independently Improve Abdominal Obesity and Sex Hormones in Elderly Women with Metabolic Syndrome. *Sci. Rep.* **2021**, *11*, 5175. [CrossRef] [PubMed]
22. Cunha, R.M.; Macedo, C.B.; Araújo, S.F.M.; Santos, J.C.; Borges, V.S.; Soares, A.A.; Ayres, F.; Pfrimer, L.M. Subacute Blood Pressure Response in Elderly Hypertensive Women after a Water Exercise Session: A Controlled Clinical Trial. *High Blood Press. Cardiovasc. Prev.* **2012**, *19*, 223–227. [CrossRef] [PubMed]
23. Kim, J.H.; Ha, M.S.; Ha, S.M.; Kim, D.Y. Aquatic Exercise Positively Affects Physiological Frailty among Postmenopausal Women: A Randomized Controlled Clinical Trial. *Healthcare* **2021**, *9*, 409. [CrossRef] [PubMed]
24. Cao, J.; Li, C.; Zhang, P.; Cao, X.; Huang, T.; Bai, Y.; Chen, K. Antidiabetic Effect of Burdock (*Arctium Lappa* L.) Root Ethanolic Extract on Streptozotocin-induced Diabetic Rats. *African J. Biotechnol.* **2012**, *11*, 9079–9085. [CrossRef]
25. Ha, M.S.; Kim, J.H.; Kim, Y.S.; Kim, D.Y. Effects of Aquarobic Exercise and Burdock Intake on Serum Blood Lipids and Vascular Elasticity in Korean Elderly Women. *Exp. Gerontol.* **2018**, *101*, 63–68. [CrossRef]
26. Wang, B.-S.; Yen, G.C.; Chang, L.W.; Yen, W.J.; Duh, P. Protective Effects of Burdock (*Arctium Lappa* Linne) on Oxidation of Low-Density Lipoprotein and Oxidative Stress in RAW 264.7 Macrophages. *Food Chem.* **2007**, *101*, 729–738. [CrossRef]
27. Kim, B.Y.; Kang, S.M.; Kang, J.H.; Kang, S.Y.; Kim, K.K.; Kim, K.B.; Kim, B.; Kim, S.J.; Kim, Y.H.; Kim, J.H.; et al. 2020 Korean Society for the Study of Obesity Guidelines for the Management of Obesity in Korea. *J. Obes. Metab. Syndr.* **2021**, *30*, 81–92. [CrossRef]
28. Borg, G. Perceived Exertion as an Indicator of Somatic Stress. *Scand. J. Rehabil. Med.* **1970**, *2*, 92–98.
29. Ha, M.-S.; Baek, H. Floor Exercise Improves on Senior Fitness Test, Blood Lipids and Arterial Stiffness in Elderly Women with Metabolic Syndrome. *J. Korean Appl. Sci. Technol.* **2017**, *34*, 899–907. [CrossRef]
30. Matthews, D.R.; Hosker, J.P.; Rudenski, A.S.; Naylor, B.A.; Treacher, D.F.; Turner, R.C. Homeostasis Model Assessment: Insulin Resistance and β-Cell Function from Fasting Plasma Glucose and Insulin Concentrations in Man. *Diabetologia* **1985**, *28*, 412–419. [CrossRef]
31. Katz, A.; Nambi, S.S.; Mather, K.; Baron, A.D.; Follmann, D.A.; Sullivan, G.; Quon, M.J. Quantitative Insulin Sensitivity Check Index: A Simple, Accurate Method for Assessing Insulin Sensitivity in Humans. *J. Clin. Endocrinol. Metab.* **2000**, *85*, 2402–2410. [CrossRef] [PubMed]
32. Van Bortel, L.M.; Duprez, D.; Starmans-Kool, M.J.; Safar, M.E.; Giannattasio, C.; Cockcroft, J.; Kaiser, D.R.; Thuillez, C. Clinical Applications of Arterial Stiffness, Task Force III: Recommendations for User Procedures. *Am. J. Hypertens.* **2002**, *15*, 445–452. [CrossRef]
33. Laurent, S.; Cockcroft, J.; Van Bortel, L.; Boutouyrie, P.; Giannattasio, C.; Hayoz, D.; Pannier, B.; Vlachopoulos, C.; Wilkinson, I.; Struijker-Boudier, H. Expert Consensus Document on Arterial Stiffness: Methodological Issues and Clinical Applications. *Eur. Heart J.* **2006**, *27*, 2588–2605. [CrossRef]
34. Kelly, R.; Hayward, C.; Avolio, A.; O'Rourke, M. Noninvasive Determination of Age-Related Changes in the Human Arterial Pulse. *Circulation* **1989**, *80*, 1652–1659. [CrossRef]
35. Cohen, J. *Statistical Power Analysis for the Behavioral Sciences*; Academic Press: Cambridge, MA, USA, 2013.

36. Morino, K.; Petersen, K.F.; Shulman, G.I. Molecular Mechanisms of Insulin Resistance in Humans and Their Potential Links with Mitochondrial Dysfunction. *Diabetes* **2006**, *55*, S9–S15. [CrossRef]
37. McLaughlin, T.; Abbasi, F.; Cheal, K.; Chu, J.; Lamendola, C.; Reaven, G. Use of Metabolic Markers to Identify Overweight Individuals Who Are Insulin Resistant. *Ann. Intern. Med.* **2003**, *139*, 802–809. [CrossRef] [PubMed]
38. Kim, J.A.; Montagnani, M.; Kwang, K.K.; Quon, M.J. Reciprocal Relationships between Insulin Resistance and Endothelial Dysfunction: Molecular and Pathophysiological Mechanisms. *Circulation* **2006**, *113*, 1888–1904. [CrossRef] [PubMed]
39. Carr, M.C. The Emergence of the Metabolic Syndrome with Menopause. *J. Clin. Endocrinol. Metab.* **2003**, *88*, 2404–2411. [CrossRef]
40. Kitahara, C.M.; Trabert, B.; Katki, H.A.; Chaturvedi, A.K.; Kemp, T.J.; Pinto, L.A.; Moore, S.C.; Purdue, M.P.; Wentzensen, N.; Hildesheim, A.; et al. Body Mass Index, Physical Activity, and Serum Markers of Inflammation, Immunity, and Insulin Resistance. *Cancer Epidemiol. Biomark. Prev.* **2014**, *23*, 2840–2849. [CrossRef]
41. Balkau, B.; Mhamdi, L.; Oppert, J.M.; Nolan, J.; Golay, A.; Porcellati, F.; Laakso, M.; Ferrannini, E. Physical Activity and Insulin Sensitivity: The RISC Study. *Diabetes* **2008**, *57*, 2613–2618. [CrossRef]
42. National High Blood Pressure Education Program Working Group Report on Hypertension in the Elderly. National High Blood Pressure Education Program Working Group. *Hypertension* **1994**, *23*, 275–285. [CrossRef]
43. Sanz, C.; Gautier, J.-F.; Hanaire, H. Physical Exercise for the Prevention and Treatment of Type 2 Diabetes. *Diabetes Metab.* **2010**, *36*, 346–351. [CrossRef] [PubMed]
44. Rezaeimanesh, D.; Farsani, P.A. The Effect of an 8-Week Selected Aquatic Aerobic Training Period on Plasma Leptin and Insulin Resistance in Men with Type 2 Diabetes. *J. Adv. Pharm. Educ. Res.* **2019**, *9*, 121–124.
45. Lupattelli, G.; Lombardini, R.; Schillaci, G.; Ciuffetti, G.; Marchesi, S.; Siepi, D.; Mannarino, E. Flow-mediated Vasoactivity and Circulating Adhesion Molecules in Hypertriglyceridemia: Association with Small, Dense LDL Cholesterol Particles. *Am. Heart J.* **2000**, *140*, 521–526. [CrossRef] [PubMed]
46. Vanhoutte, P.M.; Shimokawa, H.; Tang, E.H.C.; Feletou, M. Endothelial Dysfunction and Vascular Disease. *Acta Physiol.* **2009**, *196*, 193–222. [CrossRef]
47. Bunting, S.; Moncada, S.; Vane, J.R.; Gryglewski, R. Arterial Walls Generate from Prostaglandin Endoperoxides a Substance (Prostaglandin X) Which Relaxes Strips of Mesenteric and Coeliac Arteries and Inhibits Platelet Aggregation. *Prostaglandins* **1976**, *12*, 897–913. [CrossRef]
48. Moncada, S.; Higgs, E.A.; Vane, J.R. Human Arterial and Venous Tissues Generate Prostacyclin (Prostaglandin X), a Potent Inhibitor of Platelet Aggregation. *Lancet* **1977**, *309*, 18–21. [CrossRef]
49. Gamez-Mendez, A.M.; Vargas-Robles, H.; Ríos, A.; Escalante, B. Oxidative Stress-dependent Coronary Endothelial Dysfunction in Obese Mice. *PLoS ONE* **2015**, *10*, e0138609. [CrossRef]
50. Nakahata, N. Thromboxane A2: Physiology/Pathophysiology, Cellular Signal Transduction and Pharmacology. *Pharmacol. Ther.* **2008**, *118*, 18–35. [CrossRef]
51. Erhart, S.; Beer, J.H.; Reinhart, W.H. Influence of Aspirin on Platelet Count and Volume in Humans. *Acta Haematol.* **1999**, *101*, 140–144. [CrossRef]
52. Pahakis, M.Y.; Kosky, J.R.; Dull, R.O.; Tarbell, J.M. The Role of Endothelial Glycocalyx Components in Mechanotransduction of Fluid Shear Stress. *Biochem. Biophys. Res. Commun.* **2007**, *355*, 228–233. [CrossRef] [PubMed]
53. Hansen, A.H.; Nyberg, M.; Bangsbo, J.; Saltin, B.; Hellsten, Y. Exercise Training Alters the Balance between Vasoactive Compounds in Skeletal Muscle of Individuals with Essential Hypertension. *Hypertension* **2011**, *58*, 943–949. [CrossRef] [PubMed]
54. Kim, M.; Lee, Y.; Sohn, H. Anti-Thrombosis and Anti-Oxidative Activity of the Root of *Arctium Lappa* L. *Korean J. Food Preserv.* **2014**, *21*, 727–734. [CrossRef]
55. Lee, Y.J.; Choi, D.H.; Cho, G.H.; Kim, J.S.; Kang, D.G.; Lee, H.S. Arctium Lappa Ameliorates Endothelial Dysfunction in Rats Fed with High Fat/Cholesterol Diets. *BMC Complement. Altern. Med.* **2012**, *12*, 116. [CrossRef]
56. Furukawa, S.; Fujita, T.; Shimabukuro, M.; Iwaki, M.; Yamada, Y.; Nakajima, Y.; Nakayama, O.; Makishima, M.; Matsuda, M.; Shimomura, I. Increased Oxidative Stress in Obesity and Its Impact on Metabolic Syndrome. *J. Clin. Investig.* **2004**, *114*, 1752–1761. [CrossRef]
57. Stocker, R.; Keaney, J.F. Role of Oxidative Modifications in Atherosclerosis. *Physiol. Rev.* **2004**, *84*, 1381–1478. [CrossRef]
58. Malaisseł, W.J.; Conget, I.; Sener, A.; Rorsman, P. Insulinotropic Action of AICA Riboside. II. Secretory, Metabolic and Cationic Aspects. *Diabetes Res.* **1994**, *25*, 25–37. [PubMed]
59. Vlachopoulos, C.; Xaplanteris, P.; Aboyans, V.; Brodmann, M.; Cífková, R.; Cosentino, F.; De Carlo, M.; Gallino, A.; Landmesser, U.; Laurent, S.; et al. The Role of Vascular Biomarkers for Primary and Secondary Prevention. A Position Paper from the European Society of Cardiology Working Group on Peripheral Circulation: Endorsed by the Association for Research into Arterial Structure and Physiology (ARTERY) Society. *Atherosclerosis* **2015**, *241*, 507–532. [CrossRef]
60. Laurent, S.; Boutouyrie, P.; Asmar, R.; Gautier, I.; Laloux, B.; Guize, L.; Ducimetiere, P.; Benetos, A. Aortic Stiffness Is an Independent Predictor of All-cause and Cardiovascular Mortality in Hypertensive Patients. *Hypertension* **2001**, *37*, 1236–1241. [CrossRef]
61. Kim, Y.J.; Kim, Y.J.; Cho, B.M.; Lee, S. Metabolic Syndrome and Arterial Pulse Wave Velocity. *Acta Cardiol.* **2010**, *65*, 315–321. [CrossRef]
62. Padilla, J.; Harris, R.A.; Wallace, J.P. Can the Measurement of Brachial Artery Flow-mediated Dilation Be Applied to the Acute Exercise Model? *Cardiovasc. Ultrasound* **2007**, *5*, 45. [CrossRef] [PubMed]

63. Donley, D.A.; Fournier, S.B.; Reger, B.L.; DeVallance, E.; Bonner, D.E.; Olfert, I.M.; Frisbee, J.C.; Chantler, P.D. Aerobic Exercise Training Reduces Arterial Stiffness in Metabolic Syndrome. *J. Appl. Physiol.* **2014**, *116*, 1396–1404. [CrossRef] [PubMed]
64. Chen, F.A.; Wu, A.B.; Chen, C.Y. The Influence of Different Treatments on the Free Radical Scavenging Activity of Burdock and Variations of Its Active Components. *Food Chem.* **2004**, *86*, 479–484. [CrossRef]
65. Wang, P.; Zweier, J.L. Measurement of Nitric Oxide and Peroxynitrite Generation in the Postischemic Heart: Evidence for Peroxynitrite-mediated Reperfusion Injury. *J. Biol. Chem.* **1996**, *271*, 29223–29230. [CrossRef]
66. Lee, J.; Ha, S.J.; Park, J.; Kim, Y.H.; Lee, N.H.; Kim, Y.E.; Hong, Y.S.; Song, K.M. Arctium Lappa Root Extract Containing L-Arginine Prevents TNF-α-induced Early Atherosclerosis in Vitro and in Vivo. *Nutr. Res.* **2020**, *77*, 85–96. [CrossRef] [PubMed]

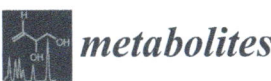

Article

Cheminformatics Identification and Validation of Dipeptidyl Peptidase-IV Modulators from Shikimate Pathway-Derived Phenolic Acids towards Interventive Type-2 Diabetes Therapy

Fatai Oladunni Balogun, Kaylene Naidoo, Jamiu Olaseni Aribisala, Charlene Pillay and Saheed Sabiu *

Department of Biotechnology and Food Science, Faculty of Applied Science, Durban University of Technology, Durban 4001, South Africa
* Correspondence: sabius@dut.ac.za; Tel.: +27-31-373-5330

Abstract: Recently, dipeptidyl peptidase-IV (DPP-IV) has become an effective target in the management of type-2 diabetes mellitus (T2D). The study aimed to determine the efficacy of shikimate pathway-derived phenolic acids as potential DPP-IV modulators in the management of T2D. The study explored in silico (molecular docking and dynamics simulations) and in vitro (DPP-IV inhibitory and kinetics assays) approaches. Molecular docking findings revealed chlorogenic acid (CA) among the examined 22 phenolic acids with the highest negative binding energy (−9.0 kcal/mol) showing a greater affinity for DPP-IV relative to the standard, Diprotin A (−6.6 kcal/mol). The result was corroborated by MD simulation where it had a higher affinity (−27.58 kcal/mol) forming a more stable complex with DPP-IV than Diprotin A (−12.68 kcal/mol). These findings were consistent with in vitro investigation where it uncompetitively inhibited DPP-IV having a lower IC_{50} (0.3 mg/mL) compared to Diprotin A (0.5 mg/mL). While CA showed promising results as a DPP-IV inhibitor, the findings from the study highlighted the significance of medicinal plants particularly shikimate-derived phenolic compounds as potential alternatives to synthetic drugs in the effective management of T2DM. Further studies, such as derivatisation for enhanced activity and in vivo evaluation are suggested to realize its full potential in T2D therapy.

Keywords: chlorogenic acid; diprotin A; dipeptidyl peptidase IV; molecular dynamics simulations; phenolic acids; type-2 diabetes mellitus

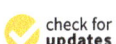

Citation: Balogun, F.O.; Naidoo, K.; Aribisala, J.O.; Pillay, C.; Sabiu, S. Cheminformatics Identification and Validation of Dipeptidyl Peptidase-IV Modulators from Shikimate Pathway-Derived Phenolic Acids towards Interventive Type-2 Diabetes Therapy. *Metabolites* **2022**, *12*, 937. https://doi.org/10.3390/metabo12100937

Academic Editors: Cosmin Mihai Vesa and Dana Zaha

Received: 20 September 2022
Accepted: 29 September 2022
Published: 2 October 2022

Publisher's Note: MDPI stays neutral with regard to jurisdictional claims in published maps and institutional affiliations.

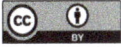

Copyright: © 2022 by the authors. Licensee MDPI, Basel, Switzerland. This article is an open access article distributed under the terms and conditions of the Creative Commons Attribution (CC BY) license (https://creativecommons.org/licenses/by/4.0/).

1. Introduction

Diabetes mellitus is a popular metabolic derangement whose annual impact continues to grow globally; it is anticipated that by 2030, over 764 million people will be suffering from the disease (if no suitable solution is found) [1] as compared to 463 million in 2019 [2]. Type-2 diabetes mellitus (T2D) is characterised by hyperglycaemia resulting from insulin resistance, insensitivity, or both [2,3]. It is noteworthy that prolonged hyperglycaemic conditions in a diabetic state could warrant (excessive) glucose binding covalently to plasma protein (glycation) causing a breakdown of receptor function or alteration of some enzymatic activities. Thus, this leads to the emergence of diabetic complications, such as impairment of vision (retinopathy), kidney dysfunction (nephropathy), and nerve damage (neuropathy), among others. Hence, the ultimate goal for any T2D therapy is to lower the systemic glucose level, and thus prevent the emergence of possible associated diseases, such as hypertension, stroke, etc. [4]. Management options including the use of oral hypoglycaemic agents (OHAs), such as sulphonylureas, biguanides, etc., and insulin have been adopted [3–5]. Sadly, these agents only bring-about normoglycaemia in half of the diabetes sufferers [6]; additionally, they are also characterised by side effects (e.g., obesity, hypoglycaemia, hormonal imbalance, etc.), thus, the clamor for potential alternatives in natural products which are cost-effective and with relatively minimal side effects [7,8].

One of the viable approaches to controlling T2D is via glucagon-like peptide 1 (GLP-1) concerned with the potential of reducing fasting and postprandial glucose in the blood for T2D [3,9,10]. Though, GLP-1 is continuously degraded in the systemic circulation by dipeptidyl peptidase-IV (DPP-IV), a serine aminopeptidase enzyme, inhibitors of DPP-IV would come in handy in preventing this breakdown and thus ensures continuous survival of GLP-1 [3]. Dipeptidyl peptidase-IV (DPP-IV) inhibitors and glucagon-like peptide 1 (GLP-1) are a newer class of antidiabetics [4,6,11]. Dipeptidyl peptidase-IV, widely distributed in tissues and sites (liver, kidney, bone marrow, blood vessels, endo- and/or epithelial cells, etc.) is involved in the inactivation of GLP-1 and glucose-dependent insulinotropic polypeptide (GIP) concerned in the heightened biosynthesis of insulin, the proliferation of β-cells, and the reduction of β-cell apoptosis resulting from postprandial glucose episodes [4]. Hence, inhibiting the action of DPP-IV has been regarded as an important mechanism for systemic glucose control [11,12]. Phenolic acid-derived natural products have been studied and established to elicit various pharmacological effects, such as antioxidative, anticancer, antidiabetic, etc. [3,13–15]. Interestingly, reports of phenolic compounds, such as cyanidin, kaempferol, quercitin, hesperetin, genistein, naringenin, chrysin, methyl p-coumarate as DPP-IV inhibitors from natural products, such as soybeans, grape, *Melicope latifolia*, and citrus have been reported [13–16]. There are numerous submitted in vitro studies that assessed the effects of phytocompounds on glucose reduction via DPP-IV inhibition [13–16], in fact, an in vivo study has also established a reduction in the level of glucose in streptozotocin-induced diabetic rats by the phenolic compound, isoquercitrin isolated from *Apocynum cannabinum* leaves and *Gossypium herbaceum* flower indicating its effectiveness as a DPP-IV inhibitor [17]. However, since there is a dearth of information on the shikimate pathway-derived phenolic acids against DPP-IV, it is envisaged that studying the effect of shikimate pathway-derived phenolic acids as DPP-IV inhibitors could be promising in the development of drug candidates in T2D therapy.

Computational methods have been extensively used to study the interactions between a protein and complementary ligands [18]. The methods can be the prelude step during drug discovery to screen a library of compounds in search of promising bioactive principles with the best therapeutic effect. The methods allow for the elimination of undesirable compounds prior to in vitro and in vivo analyses [18]. Hence, employing computational methods in this study should provide insight into which of the shikimate pathway-derived phenolic acids would afford better interactions with DPP-IV to elicit an effective therapeutic response towards drug discovery prior to in vitro analyses. Based on this background, this study was conceptualised to assess the potential of phenolic acids derived from the shikimate pathway that could be further developed as probable drug candidates against DPP-IV in the management of T2D and to reveal the possible mechanism of inhibition depicted by the best compound through in silico and in vitro methods.

2. Materials and Methods

2.1. Chemicals and Reagents

Chlorogenic acid ($\geq$95%), human DPP-IV, Gly-Pro-4-methoxy-β-naphthylamide ($\geq$98%), and Diprotin A ($\geq$97%) were obtained from Sigma-Aldrich (St. Louis, MO, USA). Unnamed chemicals used for reagent preparation were of analytical grade.

2.2. Methodology
2.2.1. In Silico Study
Molecular Docking

The 22 phenolic acids (chlorogenic acid, ellagic acid, gallic acid, caffeic acid, o-coumaric acid, olivetolic acid, umbellic acid, isoferulic acid, m-coumaric acid, p-coumaric acid, protocatechuic acid, orsellinic acid, ferulic acid, sinapic acid, hypogallic acid, vanillic acid, β-resorcinolic acid, salicyclic acid, syringic acid, veratric acid, gentisic acid, benzoic acid) mined from the shikimate pathway were subjected to molecular docking (MD) adopting the method of Ibrahim et al. [19]. Briefly, the X-ray crystal structure of DPP-IV (ID: 1WCY) was downloaded in PDF format from the Protein Data Bank (https://www.rcsb.org, accessed on 2 August 2021) (Research Collaboratory for Structural Bioinformatics, University of California, San Diego, CA, USA) and optimised using Chimera v1.15 (Resource for Biocomputing, Visualization and Informatics, University of California, San Francisco, CA, USA). The optimisation involves the removal of the co-crystallised ligand and non-standard residues and saving in PDB format for further analyses. PubChem (National Centre for Biotechnology Information, Bethesda, MD, USA) downloaded (https://pubchem.ncbi.nlm.nih.gov, accessed on 2 August 2021) structures of the 22 phenolic acids and Diprotin A three-dimensional (3D), were prepared in Chimera v1.15 software by adding non-polar H atoms and Gasteiger charges. The prepared compounds (optimised) were saved in mol2 format upon being opened in Chimera v1.15 [20]. The PDB version of the DPP-IV and the mol2 version of the phenolic acids and standard were thereafter, subjected to the Autodock Tool (The Scripps Research Institute, San Diego, CA, USA) [21] with all parameters in default settings. The grid sizes were set, and the grid centers were designated at specific dimensions (Centre (Å): 42.4291; 64.2981; 29.9357, Size (Å): 44.834; 34.693; 74.9341, corresponding to x, y, z coordinates, respectively). Based on the docking scores, complexes with the best pose for each phenolic acid were chosen and ranked. The most promising phenolic acid complex was viewed in Discovery Studio v21 to establish the nature of interactions with the amino acid residues of the enzyme at the active site.

However, as molecular docking methods often produce pseudo-positive binding conformations as the most energy-minimised pose, validation of the docking study was conducted by measuring the Root Mean Square Deviation (RMSD) of the docked ligands from the reference position (native inhibitor) in the experimental co-crystal structure of DPP-1V (1WCY) after optimal superimposition [22]. A low RMSD value of 0.8 Å between the docked ligands from the native inhibitor in the crystal structure of DPP-1V suggests the same binding orientation, which lent credence to the docking technique employed (Figure 1).

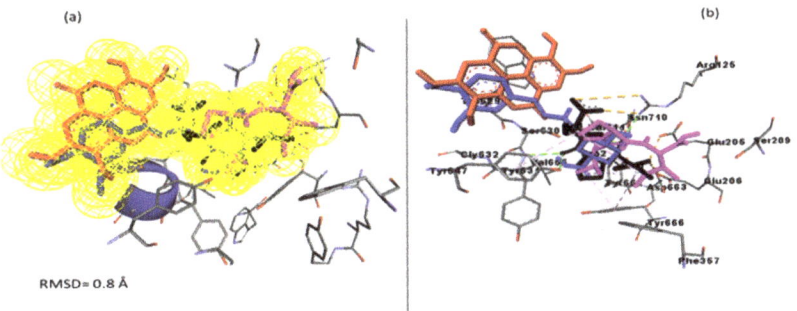

Figure 1. Validation of docking technique and parameters via the superimposition approach against the co-crystal structure of Dipeptidyl peptidase-IV (1WCY). (**a**) The superimposition showed that the docked Diprotin A (purple colour), chlorogenic acid (blue colour), and ellagic acid (red colour) achieved the same orientation with the native inhibitor (black) of 1WCY with a low RMSD value of 0.8 Å. (**b**) showed the investigated compounds and native inhibitors at the binding pocket of DPP-IV displaying active site amino acids.

Molecular Dynamics Simulations

The molecular dynamics simulation (MDS) carried out in 100 ns was performed on the most promising phenolic acid complex as previously reported by Sabiu et al. [23] using the GPU version within the AMBER package. The AMBER LEaP module was neutralised with the inclusion of H atoms and Na^+ and Cl^- counter ions. The system in each case was dipped implicitly within an orthorhombic box of TIP3P water molecules such that all atoms were within 8Å of any box edge. For each simulation, the SHAKE algorithm was used to constrict the hydrogen (H) atoms. The simulations align with the isobaric-isothermal ensemble (NPT), having randomised seeding, 2 ps pressure-coupling constant, 27 Berendsen barostat maintains 1 bar constant pressure, 300 K temperature and Langevin thermostat with a collision frequency of 1.0 ps [24]. Using PTRAJ, the systems were subsequently saved, and each trajectory was analyzed every 1 ps, and the RMSD, Radius of Gyration (RoG), Root Mean Square Fluctuation, Solvent Accessible Surface Area (SASA), and the H-bond flexibility were analysed with AMBER 18 suite of CPPTRAJ module. The Molecular Mechanics/GB Surface Area method (MM/GBSA) was used for the analysis of the negative free binding energy (ΔG) over 100,000 snapshots extracted from the 100 ns trajectory [25].

Pharmacokinetics Assessment

The pharmacokinetic properties comprising the absorption, distribution, metabolism, excretion and toxicity (ADMET) and drug-likeness features of the compound with the most promising complex were predicted with the SWISS ADME (Swiss Institute of Bioinformatics, Lausanne, Switzerland) server (http://swissadme.ch/index.php, accessed on 5 September 2021) while the prediction of probable toxicity was achieved using ProTox (https://tox-new.charite.de/protox_II/, accessed on 6 September 2021) (Structural Bioinformatics Group, CUMIP, Berlin, Germany) [26].

2.2.2. In Vitro Evaluation

DPP-IV Inhibitory Assay

The compound (chlorogenic acid) with the best binding affinity towards DPP-IV was evaluated in vitro and was carried out as reported by Oliveira et al. [27] with modifications. The spectrophotometric assay was based on Gly-Pro-4-methoxy-β-naphthylamide, a chromogenic synthetic DPP-IV substrate, cleavage to β-naphthylamine. In brief, 10 mg chlorogenic acid was suspended in 10 mL of Tris-HCl buffer (50 mM, pH 7.5) in a 15 mL microcentrifuge tube to yield a 1 mg/mL stock solution from where varying concentrations (0.50, 0.40, 0.30, 0.20, 0.10, and 0.05 mg/mL) were prepared. Thereafter, 50 µL of Tris-HCl buffer, 20 µL of DPP-IV (at a final concentration of 17.34 µU/µL in Tris-HCl buffer) and 50 µL of various concentrations of DPP-IV and Diprotin A were released into a 96-well microtiter plate wells and incubated at 37 °C for 10 min. Subsequently, 50 µL of the substrate (0.2 mM in Tris-HCl buffer) was added and further incubated for 30 min at 37 °C. The absorbance readings were taken using a microtiter plate reader (OPTIZEN POP, Apex Scientific, Durban, South Africa) at 405 nm. The experiment was conducted in triplicate and the negative control had no chlorogenic acid. The inhibitory percentage was obtained following the expression [$Abs_0 - bs1/Abs_0 \times 100$ (where Abs_0 is the absorbance of the blank and Abs_1 is the absorbance of either chlorogenic acid or Diprotin A) and thereafter converted to half-maximal inhibitory concentration (IC_{50}) using a linear calibration curve.

Enzyme Kinetics Evaluation

The mode of inhibition of DPP-IV by chlorogenic acid was determined as previously described by Jung et al. [28]. Briefly, 20 µL chlorogenic acid (IC_{50}: 0.3 mg/mL) and DPP-IV were dispensed into five wells of a 96-well plate for a set of experiments. In another set of the experiment (control), a mixture of the buffer (without chlorogenic acid) and DPP-IV with the same volume as the earlier set was prepared. Following this in ascending order, various concentrations (0.1–0.5 mM) of Gly-Pro-4-methoxy-β-naphthylamide were added to the two sets of experiments and subsequently incubated for 20 min at 37 °C. While the experiment was carried out in triplicate, the absorbance of the reacting mixtures was measured at 405 nm using a spectrophotometer (OPTIZEN POP, Apex Scientific, Durban, South Africa) and the calibration curve of Gly-Pro-4-methoxy-β-naphthylamide was used to calculate the amount of produced product (β-naphthylamine) over time and subsequently converted to reaction velocities. A double reciprocal plot of reaction rates (1/V) and substrate concentrations (1/[S]) [29] was carried out for the generation of V_{max}, K_m and K_{cat} parameters of chlorogenic acid.

2.3. Statistical Analysis

Data from the in vitro analysis were analysed using GraphPad Prism 9.2.0 (GraphPad, La Jolla, CA, USA) using a *t*-test (and nonparametric tests), supplemented with a Mann–Whitney test. Results are presented as mean ± standard deviation (SD) of triplicate determinations (n = 3) and mean with *p*-value < 0.05 were considered significant and statistically different. Raw data were analyzed with Origin software V18 (OriginLab Corporation, Northampton, MA, USA) for the in-silico evaluations [30].

3. Results and Discussion

3.1. Computational Analysis

Molecular docking examines the affinity and poses of a compound at an enzyme's active site; compound(s) with the most negative binding score indicate better-posed compounds and a prospective modulator of the enzyme [23]. In this study, the results of the MD of the 22 phenolic compounds against DPP-IV revealed chlorogenic acid as the most promising compound judging by its docking score of −9.0 kcal/mol followed by ellagic acid (−7.8 kcal/mol) relative to the reference standard, Diprotin A, with a score of −6.6 kcal/mol (Table 1). It should be noted that the most negative docking scores of chlorogenic acid and ellagic acid, depicting their better pose in comparison to other compounds and standards, necessitated their further consideration in the study.

Table 1. Binding energy scores of phenolic acids and dipeptidyl peptidase-IV formation.

Compounds	Score (kcal/mol)
Chlorogenic acid	−9.0
Diprotin A	−6.6
Ellagic acid	−7.8
Gallic acid	−6.4
Caffeic acid	−6.3
O-coumaric acid	−6.3
Olivetolic acid	−6.3
Umbellic acid	−6.3
Isoferulic acid	−6.2
M-coumaric acid	−6.2
P-coumaric acid	−6.1
Protocatechuic acid	−6.1
Orsellinic acid	−6.1
Ferulic acid	−6.0
Sinapic acid	−6.0
Hypogallic acid	−6.0
Vanillic acid	−5.9
Beta-resorcinolic acid	−5.7
Salicyclic acid	−5.8
Syringic acid	−5.7
Veratric acid	−5.7
Gentisic acid	−5.6
Benzoic acid	−5.4

Interestingly, the observation with chlorogenic acid regarding its docking score in this study is noteworthy as it interacted more favorably with DPP-IV than other phenolic compounds, such as quercetin and coumarin, previously evaluated against the enzyme [3]. A further probe into the energy component profiles of the chlorogenic acid–DPP-IV and ellagic acid–DPP-IV complexes after the 100 ns MDS further supported the affinity of DPP-IV for chlorogenic acid where its overall binding energy was comparably higher ($p > 0.05$) (−25.74 kcal/mol) compared with ellagic acid (−24.54 kcal/mol) relative to Diprotin A–DPP-IV complex, which was the lowest ($p < 0.05$) (−12.44 kcal/mol) (Table 2).

Table 2. Energy components analyses of the molecular dynamics simulation of the compounds.

Complexes	Energy Components (kcal/mol)				
	ΔE_{vdW}	ΔE_{elec}	ΔG_{gas}	ΔG_{solv}	ΔG_{bind}
DPP-IV + Chlorogenic acid	−28.64 ± 6.84	−49.38 ± 21.85	−78.03 ± 19.96	52.29 ± 15.63	−25.74 ± 6.45 [a]
DPP-IV + ellagic acid	−25.33 ± 4.74	−58.51 ± 18.28	−83.84 ± 16.51	69.30 ± 11.19	−24.54 ± 6.31 [a]
DPP-IV + Diprotin A	−20.32 ± 3.43	−261.44 ± 40.36	−281.76 ± 40.63	269.32 ± 36.75	−12.44 ± 5.48 [b]

DPP-IV: dipeptidyl peptidase-IV; ΔEvdW: van der Waals energy; ΔEelec: electrostatic energy; ΔEgas: gas-phase free energy; ΔGsolv solvation free energy; ΔGbind: total binding free energy. Values with different superscript letters along the same row are significantly ($p < 0.05$) different from each other.

An understanding of the nature of interaction established between the amino acids at the active site of a protein with a ligand is crucial in the development of the ligand as a drug candidate [31]. In this study, chlorogenic acid, ellagic acid and Diprotin A interacted with Ser630 and His740 of the catalytic triad at the active site of DPP-IV (Figure 2) and this observation was in line with the work of Poonam et al. [14] where Ser630 was identified as one of the amino acid residues through which chrysin interacted with DPP-IV. Interaction with the catalytic triad is characteristic of potential DPP-IV inhibitors, preventing endogenous peptides, such as GLP-1 and GIP from interacting with the active site, thus, hindering their subsequent cleavage [32]. The findings from this study regarding the modulatory role of chlorogenic acid on the active site amino acid residues of DPP-IV could provide insights into the possible mechanisms through which chlorogenic acid increased GLP-1 levels, improved the glycaemic index [33], and improved glucose homeostasis and insulin resistance in vivo [34], as previously reported.

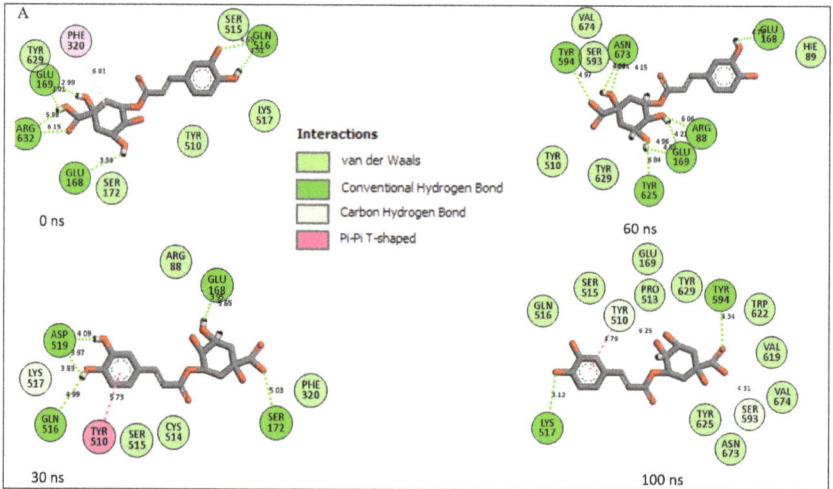

Figure 2. Cont.

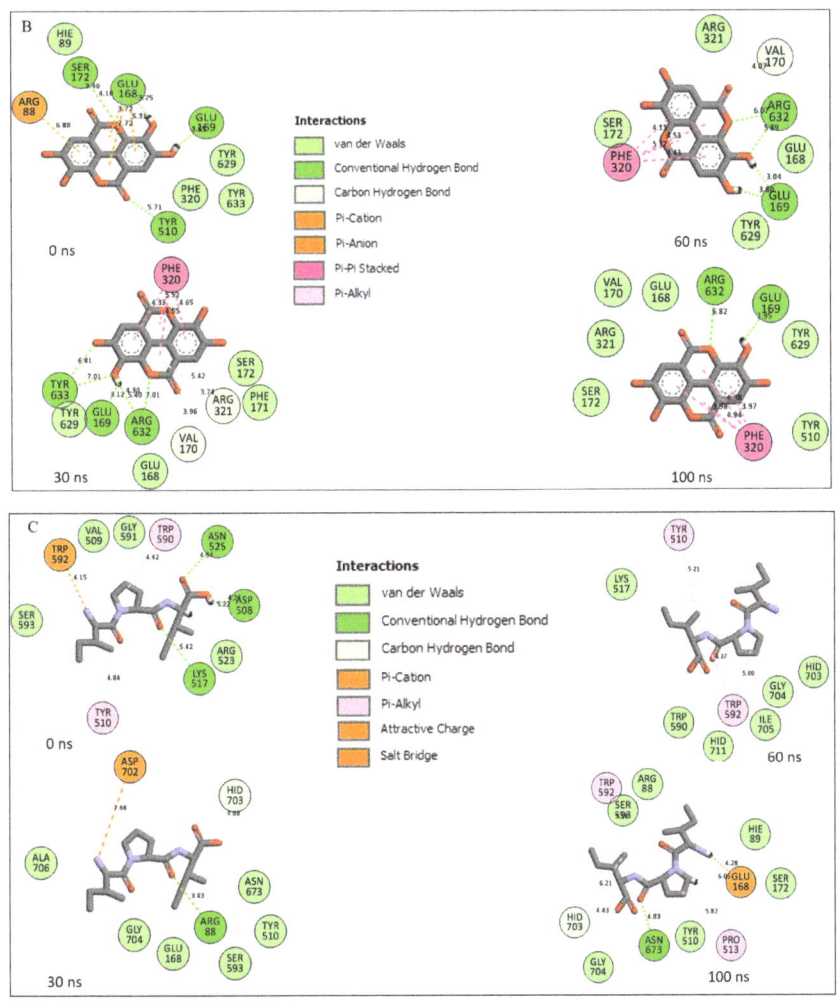

Figure 2. Interaction types and plots of (**A**) Chlorogenic acid–DPP-IV; (**B**) Ellagic acid–DPP-IV and (**C**) Diprotin A–DPP-IV at different time frame during a 100 ns simulation.

Furthermore, the type and number of interactions formed as a result of the binding between the ligand and the amino acid residues of the target protein are crucial in determining the extent of the resulting affinity [35]. In this study, 14 interactions comprising two conventional H-bond (Lys517 and Tyr594), 10 van der Waal forces (Tyr625, Asn673, Val674, Val619, Trp622, Tyr629, Pro513, Glu169, Ser515, Gln516) and two carbon-H bonds (Ser593, Tyr510) were formed with the complexation of chlorogenic acid and DPP-IV (Figure 2A), which is in sharp contrast to the nine interactions [two conventional H-bonds (Arg632 and Glu169), six van der Waal forces (Ser172, Arg321, Val170, Glu168, Tyr629 and Tyr510) and one π-π stacked (Phe320)] from the ellagic–DPP-IV complex (Figure 2B) and eleven interactions [one conventional H-bond (Asn673), six vans der Waal forces (Gly704, Tyr510, Ser172, Hie89, Ser598, Arg88), one carbon-H bond (Hid703), two π-alkyl (Pro513, Trp592) and one salt bridge (Glu168)] observed for the Diprotin A–DPP-IV complex (Figure 2C). The interactions depicted by the three systems are in conformity with the results of the thermodynamics profiles except between ellagic acid and Diprotin A, where the ellagic acid–DPP-IV complex with the most negative binding energy value (which might have been contributed by the two H-bonds) depicted fewer numbers of interactions in comparison with Diprotin A with an H-bond, since it has been reported that H-bonds contribute higher energies to the complex [36]. Additionally, the lowest number of interactions depicted by few numbers of conventional H and van der Waal bonds for the Diprotin A–DPP-IV complex might be suggested as the reason for its lower binding energy score compared to chlorogenic acid–DPP-IV with higher binding energy characterised by a greater number of convention H-bond and van der Waal forces. The higher number of interactions and H-bonds witnessed in this study by chlorogenic acid over Diprotin A was in line with similar work by Tuersuntuoheti et al. [37] where chlorogenic acid isolated from Qingke barley fresh noodles had 19 interactions (nine H-bonds and 10 hydrophobic interactions with amino acids residues of DPP-IV) compared with the used standard (sitagliptin) having 15 interactions (one H-bond and 14 hydrophobic interactions). During the 100 ns simulation period, the conserved residue Tyr510 in the interaction plots of Diprotin A and chlorogenic acid with DPP-IV in each of the time frames studied is relevant to the affinity and stability observed with the two compounds towards the target (Figure 2A,C). This crucial amino acid is missing in the 30 ns and 60 ns time frames in the interaction plot of ellagic acid with DPP-IV (Figure 2C) and may have contributed to the reduced stability observed with ellagic acid compared to the other compound studied with DPP-1V.

Binding energy reflects the totality of all the intermolecular forces or ligand and target interactions and the degree of binding occurring between ligand–protein. It has been reported to be enhanced by H-bonds [38], thus, further corroborating our submission in this study. Additionally, the π-alkyl bond was also among the interactions found in the Diprotin A–DPP-IV complex, possibly contributing to its reduced binding energy. Thus, this finding could be said to be consistent with a previous report [23] where the presence of π-cation interactions of the alpha-glucosidase-acarbose complex was attributed to its lesser binding activity.

Molecular dynamics simulation explores potential changes in the stability, structure, or conformation of a protein–ligand complex following ligand binding [39]. It is, therefore, germane to study parameters, such as RMSD, RMSF, RoG, SASA, and H-bond fluctuations defining whether the overall stability of the complex is maintained. The RMSD measures the changes that the enzyme–ligand structure undergoes over time, and it provides information on the overall stability of the complex [40]. The result of this investigation revealed an average RMSD of DPP-IV after 100 ns to be 1.69 Å while that of chlorogenic acid–DPP-IV, Diprotin A–DPP-IV and ellagic acid–DPP-IV complexes had average RMSD values of 1.75 Å, 1.95 Å and 2.10 Å, respectively (Supplemental Table S1). A lower average RMSD corresponds to a more stable complex over the simulation period [40]. In this study, the mean RMSD values of the three complexes are higher than that of the unbound DPP-IV; however, this might not be taken as an indication of the instability of the complexes during the simulation period. In fact, Rosenberg [41] reported that an RMSD exceeding 3.5 Å may only indicate an unstable complex and an unsuitable inhibitor of the protein. Besides, the average RMSD of the complexes is around 2 Å with the chlorogenic acid–DPP-IV complex revealing superior structural stability (1.75 Å) over the Diprotin A–DPP-IV complex (1.95 Å) and ellagic acid–DPP-IV complex. Interestingly, a study conducted on lac compounds against DPP-IV also showed that the best hit compounds had an average RMSD of 2 Å [42] which is consistent with the observations in the current study. Additionally, it is worth mentioning that the RMSD for the four systems reached an initial convergence at 5 ns and subsequently diverged at 45 ns. It can be noted that the RMSD of the ellagic acid complex saw an increase of around 65–70 ns, while the chlorogenic acid and Diprotin A complexes and the apoenzyme remained stable till the end of the simulation (Figure 3A).

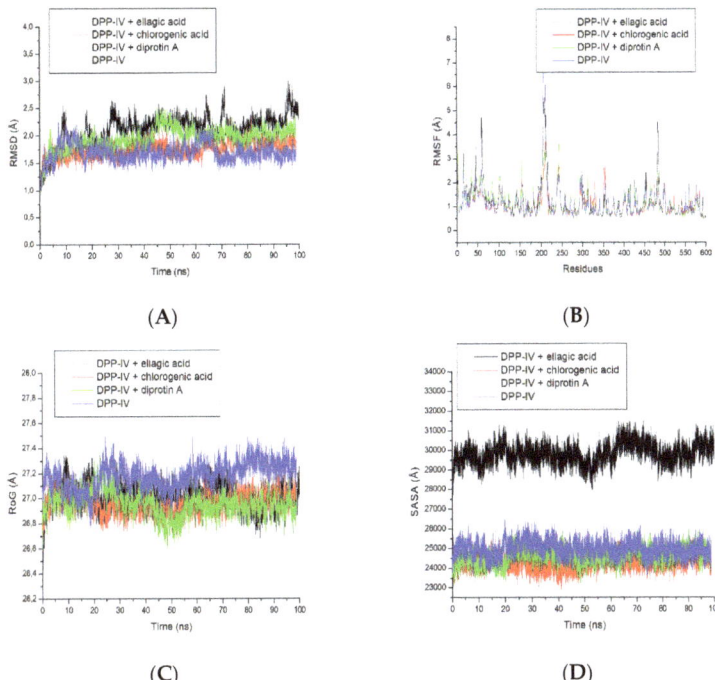

Figure 3. (**A**) Root Mean Square Deviation (RMSD), (**B**) Root Mean Square Fluctuations (RMSF), (**C**) Radius of Gyration (RoG), and (**D**) Solvent Accessible Surface Area (SASA) plots of comparison between Dipeptidyl peptidase-IV (DPP-IV) and chlorogenic acid, ellagic acid and Diprotin A determined over 100 ns molecular dynamics simulations.

Root mean square fluctuation has to do with the flexibility of the ligand and the attitudes of amino acid residues at the binding pocket of the enzyme. The apoenzyme in this study had an average RMSF value of 1.12 Å which is marginally lower than the 1.17 Å for the Diprotin A–DPP-IV complex and significantly higher (1.22 Å) for ellagic acid, suggesting slightly high fluctuations (Supplementary Table S1). However, the lower average RMSF value of the chlorogenic acid–DPP-IV complex (1.08 Å) compared to the unbound DPP-IV is an indication of lesser fluctuation, better flexibility, little or no distortion, and hence indicative of profound stability [43]. The RMSF plot shows similar fluctuations for all four systems (Figure 3B). However, there was a notable increase in the RMSF of the apoenzyme and the chlorogenic acid–DPP-IV complex at residues 225–250 and 475, respectively, (Figure 3B) suggesting the enhanced potential of the ligand to adapt well to the binding pockets of the proteins. This also indicates that binding of the ligand to the receptor allows better stabilisation of the fluctuation of individual amino acid residues, resulting in a more stable complex.

Unlike the RMSF, the RoG signifies the compactness of the complex formed as a result of the interaction between the ligand and enzyme [44]. In this study, both complexes of chlorogenic acid–DPP-IV and Diprotin A–DPP-IV had average RoG values of 26.95 Å and 26.96 Å, respectively, relative to 27.18 Å observed with the apoenzyme (Supplementary Table S1) and ellagic acid–DPP-IV (27.02 Å). Consistent with this observation, the apoenzyme fluctuated the most during the simulation period as evidenced by its highest value compared to the three complexes (Figure 3C and Supplementary Table S1). It was also observed that the three systems reached an initial point of convergence at 10 ns, while the apoenzyme then diverged at 25 ns (Figure 3C). The chlorogenic acid, Diprotin A and ellagic acid complexes on the other hand remained stable with similar fluctuations throughout the simulation (Figure 3C). Since high RoG values are a measure of reduced compactness of the protein–ligand complex and vice versa [45], the exhibited compactness of the three complexes (with chlorogenic acid–DPP-IV being superior) is indicative of their stability. Going by the findings of the current study on the stability, fluctuation, and compactness as expressed with RMSD, RoG, and RMSF values, it is evident that chlorogenic acid competed favorably with Diprotin A, suggesting the potential of chlorogenic acid as a probable DPP-IV inhibitor.

Solvent accessible surface area is a measure of hydrophilic and/or hydrophobicity of the enzyme's amino acid residues on exposure to solvent or water [46], and the degree of variation of exposure could be a result of changes to the protein tertiary structure [47]. Results from the SASA analysis in this study indicated that ellagic acid had the most fluctuations during the simulation; however, consistent fluctuation patterns were noted with all four systems (Figure 3D). Similar fluctuations were observed with the chlorogenic acid–DPP-IV and Diprotin A–DPP-IV complexes, however, at a lower range than the DPP-IV. The reduced average SASA value of the chlorogenic acid–DPP-IV complex (24,324.69 Å) and Diprotin A–DPP-IV (24,625.10 Å) as established in this investigation, (Supplementary Table S1) could be suggestive of the better stability of the compounds, though chlorogenic acid had superior stability over Diprotin A. The complex with a heightened SASA value relative to the unbound protein is a consequence of its reduced solvent access for the non-polar residues preventing its stability [48] which could be attributed to the ill-effect of interruption of the hydrophobic interactions between clustered non-polar amino acid residues and the hydrophobic core during the denaturation or unfolding of the protein [47]. Analysis of the bond interactions between the chlorogenic acid, ellagic acid and Diprotin A complexes indicated that compounds and Diprotin A interacted with non-polar amino acid residues Trp622 (Figure 2A) and Trp592 (Figure 2C), respectively, thus, preventing the amino acid residue from being exposed to the aqueous surrounding as evidenced in the reduced SASA values of both complexes.

The presence of intramolecular H-bonds in a protein structure is germane in its maintenance of stability and conformation (3D) [49]. Hence, H-bond analysis in MD studies is another parameter that provides insight into the stability of the protein structures or resulting complexes formed as a result of protein–ligand binding [49,50]. H-bonds fluctuated mainly around 17–19 H-bonds in the chlorogenic acid complex (Figure 4A) and just below 17–19 H-bonds in the Diprotin A (Figure 4B) and ellagic acid (Figure 4C) complexes. All the complexes showed similar H-bond fluctuation patterns over 100 ns. However, it was noted that after 70 ns, chlorogenic acid tends to form more H-bonds with DPP-IV (in comparison to Diprotin A and ellagic acid) suggesting the reason for the higher binding energy observed with the chlorogenic acid complex, thus, enhancing the affinity of chlorogenic acid for DPP-IV. This observation agrees with the reports of Khan et al. [48] and Al-Humaydhi et al. [51] where there are consistencies in the number of H-bonds that existed between memantine–human serum albumin and galantamine–transferrin complexes post-MDS and docking findings. Above all, the H-bonding patterns of all complexes revealed that chlorogenic acid competes favorably with Diprotin A concerning the hydrogen bonding patterns over the 100 ns simulation and leads to the conclusion that chlorogenic acid could be a potential DPP-IV inhibitor.

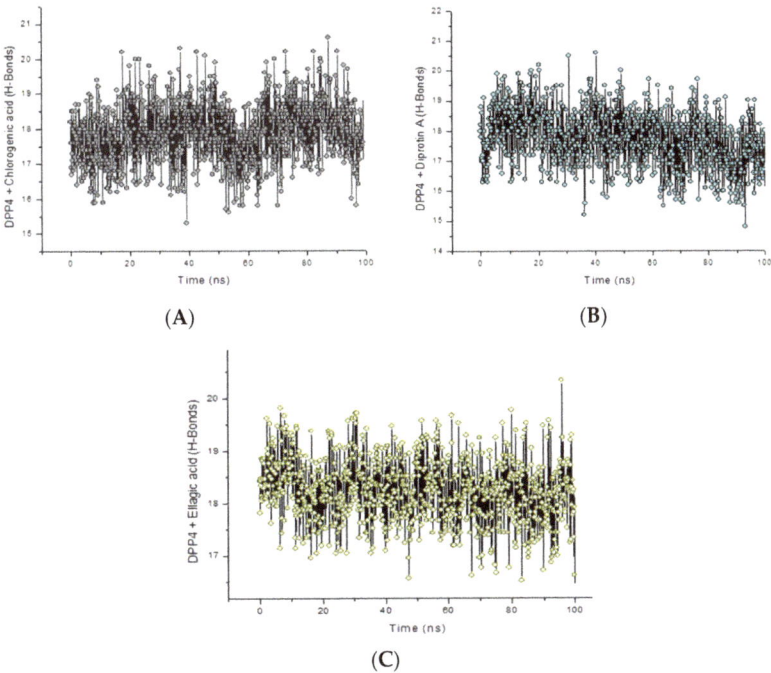

Figure 4. Backbone hydrogen bonds along the 100 ns simulation trajectory for DPP-IV in complex with (**A**) chlorogenic acid, (**B**) Diprotin A and (**C**) ellagic acid.

3.2. Pharmacokinetics Analysis

Based on the computational analyses, it was evident that chlorogenic acid may be a suitable DPP-IV inhibitor that could compete well with a commercial inhibitor, hence was taken for further pharmacokinetics studies. Lipinski's rule of five evaluates the druggability of a drug or molecule and it states that a compound should not possess more than five H-bond donors, 10 H-bond acceptors, a molecular weight not exceeding 500 kilodaltons and the LogP must not be more than 5. Hence, for a compound to be considered an orally available drug, it should not violate two or more of these rules [52].

The findings in the present investigation revealed that chlorogenic acid only violated one rule (having 6 OH) and Diprotin A violated none. Additionally, chlorogenic acid was found to have a low bioavailability score compared to Diprotin A, meaning that the former may be poorly absorbed into the body since the bioavailability score is a measure of the ability of the compound to pass through the systemic circulation in order to elicit its effect at the site of action [53]. The poor absorption of chlorogenic acid witnessed in this study was in contrast to an earlier study by Zhou et al. [54] where they found chlorogenic acid isolated from *Lonicerea japonicae* to be highly absorbed and eliminated following oral administration in Wistar rats. Moreover, poor absorption and excretion of chlorogenic acid have been linked to its co-administration with other components as established in the work of Qi et al. [55] where a comparative study on the bioavailability profile between chlorogenic acid isolated from *Solanum lyratum* and the extract of the same plant was studied. They found the absorption and excretion of the extract to be low following oral administration to Wistar rats, thus, attributing the reduction to the presence of other possible components in the extract. However, it is noteworthy too that a probable drug candidate is only required to have minimally 10% bioavailability [53], which is a condition already fulfilled by chlorogenic acid (11%), (Table 3) although the bioavailability score of Diprotin A was higher (55%) which is expected being a commercially available drug. Additionally, it was observed that chlorogenic acid absorption was low in the GI, which suggests that for it to be a formidable drug candidate that will pass the test of time, it might be necessary for it to be further modified to increase its GI absorption to enhance its possible function as a good DPP-IV inhibitor. Interestingly, the ability of chlorogenic acid (and Diprotin A) not to permeate the blood–brain barrier is a positive indication that it will not cause any complications, such as schizophrenia, anxiety, depression, Alzheimer's, Parkinson's diseases, insomnia, etc., crossing the blood–brain barrier [56].

Table 3. Drug-likeness and absorption, distribution, metabolism, and excretion (ADME) properties of chlorogenic acid and Diprotin A based on gastrointestinal absorption, blood–brain barrier permeation, possible P-gp substrate, and possible cytochromes enzyme inhibition.

Property	Chlorogenic Acid	Diprotin A
Lipinski's rule of five	Yes; 1 violation: NH or OH > 5	Yes; 0 violations
Bioavailability score	0.11	0.55
GI absorption	Low	High
BBB permeant	No	No
P-gp substrate	No	Yes
CYP1A2 inhibitor	No	No
CYP2C19 inhibitor	No	No
CYP2C9 inhibitor	No	No
CYP2D6 inhibitor	No	No
CYP3A4 inhibitor	No	No

CYP: Cytochrome.

Table 4 presents the reports of the various toxicity endpoints that may be potentiated by the test compounds. Except for the immunotoxicity metric, where chlorogenic acid was active, other tested parameters including those of Diprotin A revealed inactivity. Hence, it could be deduced that chlorogenic acid may weaken the immune system when absorbed. Similarly, the lethal dose (LD_{50}) of chlorogenic acid was observed to be in excess of 5000 mg/kg while that of Diprotin A was 3000 mg/kg indicating the possibility of Diprotin A being toxic at a lower dosage, pointing to the fact that the oral administration of the latter at that concentration or above could result in the damage of target organs, such as the liver, kidney, etc.

Table 4. Toxicity classifications and LD_{50} of chlorogenic acid and Diprotin A.

Classification	Chlorogenic Acid	Diprotin A
Hepatotoxicity	Inactive	Inactive
Carcinogenicity	Inactive	Inactive
Immunotoxicity	Active	Inactive
Mutagenicity	Inactive	Inactive
Cytotoxicity	Inactive	Inactive
LD_{50} (mg/kg)	5000	3000

LD: Lethal dose.

3.3. In Vitro Evaluation

Diabetes mellitus is a chronic metabolic disease whose occurrence and dilapidating effects rapidly grow daily arising from chronic hyperglycaemia (elevated glucose level in the blood) as a result of insulin inaction, resistance, or both [6]. Since 764 million people are estimated would be living with the disease by 2030 [1], it then means that the negative impact of the menace would continue to increase if appropriate intervention in terms of management is not provided.

Usually, OHAs and insulin (asides from the other non-convention measures, such as dietary regimen and regular exercise) are the various therapeutic interventions [5] but since they are with side effects, looking for selective, effective management and alternative therapeutic approaches revolving around GLP-1 agonists and DPP-IV inhibitors (among various other targets) is essential [6]. In the present investigation, the activity of DPP-IV was dose-dependently inhibited by chlorogenic acid and Diprotin A, with the most prominent effect observed at the highest investigated concentration in each case (Figure 5A). Judging by their IC_{50} values, chlorogenic acid had the best inhibitory activity against DPP-IV (IC_{50} value: 0.3 mg/mL) relative to 0.5 mg/mL for Diprotin A (Table 5). A further probe into the mode of inhibition of DPP-IV by chlorogenic acid revealed that the enzyme was uncompetitively inhibited (Figure 5B), with the V_{max}, K_m, and K_{cat} values decreasing from 1.09×10^{-3} M/min, 4.42×10^{-4}, and 6.29×10^{-4} M/min, to 3.59×10^{-4} M/min, 1.54×10^{-4} M and 2.07×10^{-4} M/min, respectively, in the presence of chlorogenic acid (Table 5). The implication of this is that chlorogenic acid binds to a site not far from the active site of the enzyme. Incretin (hormone) dually functions by allowing the body to secrete insulin when required while at the same time mopping up excess glucose from the systemic circulation when not required. However, the action of this hormone is terminated by the DPP-IV enzyme, hence, DPP-IV inhibitors, such as Diprotin A block the activity of the DPP-IV enzyme that destroys this vital hormone. The inability of chlorogenic acid to compete with the substrate at binding at the active site of the enzyme as reflected in the uncompetitive inhibition could suggest its possible antidiabetic effect since binding to the enzyme–substrate complex (ESC) might still hinder the activity of the enzyme. Uncompetitive inhibitors bind only to the ESC and not the unbound enzyme [57]. The inhibitor-bound ESC forms when there is a high concentration of substrate present in the environment preventing the release of the product when bound resulting in decreased V_{max}. The inhibitor-bound complex also results in the decrease of ESC concentration which creates a shift towards the formation of the additional ESC to equilibrate the system. The shift results in fewer free enzymes available and more enzymes in the forms of enzyme–substrate and enzyme–substrate–inhibitor complexes [57]. Theoretically, a decrease in the free enzyme corresponds to an enzyme with a greater affinity for the substrate. Thus, uncompetitive inhibition results in both decreased V_{max} and K_m. Since the formation of product is hindered, this also leads to decreased product turnover, and therefore, a decreased K_{cat} value. Some studies established different kinetics of inhibitions (competitive and non-competitive) of DPP-IV by phenolic compounds, such as luteolin, apigenin, resveratrol, flavone, and a phenethylphenylphthalimide analogue, etc., obtained from citrus, berry, etc. [13,58]. However, a peptide (WLQL) among other novel peptides isolated from *Pelodiscus sinensis* was found to have an uncompetitive inhibition against DPP-IV [59] as observed in the study.

Table 5. Inhibitory effect (IC_{50}) and enzyme kinetic parameters of chlorogenic acid against DPP-IV.

Inhibitor	IC_{50} (mg/mL)	V_{max} (M/min)	K_m (M)	K_{cat} (M/min)
Chlorogenic acid	0.3 ± 0.02 [a]	3.59×10^{-4} [a]	1.54×10^{-4} [a]	2.07×10^{-4} [a]
Diprotin A	0.5 ± 0.02 [b]	ND	ND	ND
No inhibitor	ND	1.09×10^{-3} [b]	4.42×10^{-4} [b]	6.29×10^{-4} [b]

ND: Not determined. Values (n = 3) with different superscript letters along the same row are significantly ($p < 0.05$) different from each other.

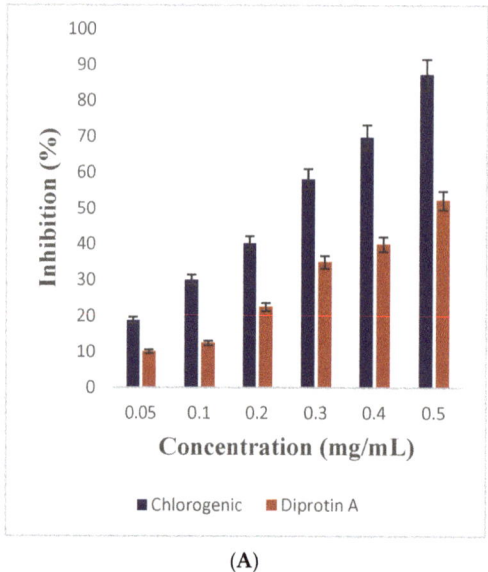
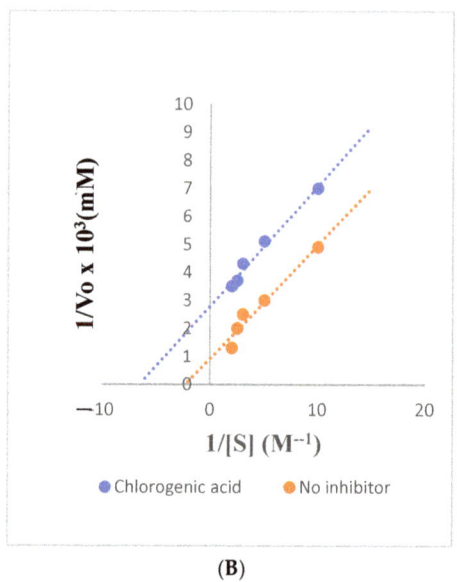

(A) (B)

Figure 5. (**A**) Inhibitory effect of chlorogenic acid and Diprotin A on the activity of DPP-IV, (**B**) Uncompetitive inhibition of DPP-IV by chlorogenic acid.

4. Conclusions

Computational studies are invaluable and significant in screening a library of compounds with potential therapeutic effects in drug discovery and development as evidently shown in this study. Judging by the findings from the computational analyses in this study, chlorogenic acid established superior interaction and affinity with DPP-IV above Diprotin A. Additionally, in vitro investigation revealed the uncompetitive inhibition of DPP-IV by chlorogenic acid indicating both the in-silico result and in vitro assessment being in tandem with one another, demonstrating the potential of chlorogenic acid as a viable candidate in the management of T2D via the inhibition of DPP-IV. Since medicinal plants and/or natural product compounds have continued to find their place as probable alternatives in disease control and management, the laudable activity exhibited by chlorogenic acid in this study attests to the submission about their superiority in the therapeutic effectiveness of natural compounds over some conventional drugs. It is evident that with these findings, diabetes researchers or stakeholders, and sufferers of T2D can be hopeful for the development of chlorogenic acid as a suitable alternative for diabetes management. Further studies are suggested on the optimisation of the compound to enhance its druggability in diabetes therapy as well as in vivo evaluation of its antidiabetic property.

Supplementary Materials: The following supporting information can be downloaded at: https://www.mdpi.com/xxx/s1, Table S1: Average RMSD, RMSF, RoG and SASA values of DPP-IV in complex with chlorogenic acid and Diprotin A.

Author Contributions: S.S. conceptualised and designed the project and revised the draft. F.O.B. interpreted the results and wrote the first draft; K.N. carried out methodology or experimental and analyzed part of the result; J.O.A. co-involved in the experimentation; C.P. supervised the study and revised the draft; All authors have read and agreed to the published version of the manuscript.

Funding: The authors acknowledge the financial assistance of the Directorate of Research and Postgraduate Support, Durban University of Technology, and the National Research Foundation (NRF- research development grant for rated researchers, grant number 120433), South Africa, awarded to S. Sabiu.

Institutional Review Board Statement: Not applicable.

Informed Consent Statement: Not applicable.

Data Availability Statement: The data presented in this study are available in the article.

Acknowledgments: The authors acknowledge the Research and Postgraduate Support of the Durban University of Technology (DUT). The postdoctoral fellowship awarded to Balogun, F.O. by the National Research Foundation (NRF) of South Africa, tenable at the Department of Biotechnology and Food Technology, DUT, is equally acknowledged as well as the Durban University of Technology emerging research grant awarded to Balogun, F.O. Additionally, the NRF is appreciated for funding the Honour's study of K. Naidoo. The Centre for High-Performance Computing (CHPC), South Africa is acknowledged for granting access to the computing systems used in this study.

Conflicts of Interest: The authors declared no conflicting interest regarding the publication of the article. Submitting author is responsible for co-authors declaring their interest.

References

1. Ali, M.Y.; Jannat, S.; Rahman, M.M. Investigation of C-glycosylated apigenin and luteolin derivatives' effects on protein tyrosine phosphatase 1B inhibition with molecular and cellular approaches. *Comput. Toxicol.* **2020**, *17*, 100141. [CrossRef]
2. World Health Organization. Diabetes. Available online: https://www.who.int/news-room/fact-sheets/detail/diabetes (accessed on 13 December 2021).
3. Singh, A.K.; Yadav, D.; Sharma, N.; Jin, J.-O. Dipeptidyl peptidase (DPP)-IV inhibitors with antioxidant potential isolated from natural sources: A novel approach for the management of diabetes. *Pharmaceuticals* **2021**, *14*, 586. [CrossRef] [PubMed]
4. Li, N.; Wang, L.; Jiang, B.; Li, X.; Guo, C.; Guo, S.; Shi, D. Recent progress of the development of dipeptidyl peptidase-4 inhibitors for the treatment of type-2 diabetes mellitus. *Eur. J. Med. Chem.* **2018**, *151*, 145–157. [CrossRef] [PubMed]
5. Chaudhury, A.; Voor, C.; Dendi, R.; Sena, V.; Kraleti, S.; Chada, A.; Ravilla, R.; Marco, A.; Shekhawat, N.S.; Montales, M.T.; et al. Clinical review of antidiabetic drugs: Implications for type-2 diabetes mellitus management. *Front. Endocrinol.* **2017**, *8*, 6. [CrossRef]
6. Singh, A.K.; Patel, P.K.; Choudhary, K.; Joshi, J.; Yadav, D.; Jin, J.-O. Quercetin and coumarin inhibit dipeptidyl peptidase-IV and exhibits antioxidant properties: In silico, in vitro, ex vivo. *Biomolecules* **2020**, *10*, 207. [CrossRef]
7. Abbas, G.; Al-Harrasi, A.; Hussain, H.; Hamaed, A.; Supuran, C.T. The management of diabetes mellitus-imperative role of natural products against dipeptidyl peptidase-4, α-glucosidase and sodium-dependent glucose Co-transporter 2 (SGLT2). *Bioorg. Chem.* **2019**, *86*, 305–315. [CrossRef] [PubMed]
8. Dhameja, M.; Gupta, P. Synthetic heterocyclic candidates as promising α-glucosidase inhibitors: An overview. *Eur. J. Med. Chem.* **2019**, *176*, 343–377. [CrossRef] [PubMed]
9. Müller, T.; Finan, B.; Bloom, S.; D'Alessio, D.; Drucker, D.; Flatt, P.; Fritsche, A.; Gribble, F.; Grill, H.; Habener, J.; et al. Glucagon-like peptide 1 (glp-1). *Mol. Metab.* **2019**, *30*, 72–130. [CrossRef] [PubMed]
10. Gribble, F.M.; Reimann, F. Metabolic messengers: Glucagon-like peptide 1. *Nat. Metab.* **2021**, *3*, 142–148. [CrossRef] [PubMed]
11. Iheagwam, F.N.; Ogunlana, O.O.; Chinedu, S.N. Model optimization and in silico analysis of potential dipeptidyl peptidase IV antagonists from GC-MS identified compounds in *Nauclea latifolia* leaf extracts. *Int. J. Mol. Sci.* **2019**, *20*, 5913. [CrossRef]
12. Gallawitz, B. Clinical use of DPP-4 inhibitors. *Front. Endocrinol.* **2019**, *10*, 389. [CrossRef] [PubMed]
13. Fan, J.F.; Johnson, M.H.; Lila, M.A.; Yousef, G.; Mejia, E.J. Berry and citrus phenolic compounds inhibit dipeptidyl peptidase IV: Implications in diabetes management. *Evid. Based Complement. Altern. Med.* **2013**, *2013*, 479505. [CrossRef]
14. Kalhotra, P.; Chittepu, V.C.S.R.; Osorio-Revilla, G.; Gallardo-Velázquez, T. Structure-activity relationship and molecular docking of natural product library reveal chrysin as a novel dipeptidyl peptidase-4 (DPP-4) inhibitor: An integrated in silico and in vitro study. *Molecules* **2018**, *23*, 1368. [CrossRef]
15. Alexandra, Q.; Nur, K.K.; Pei, C.L.; Dai, C.T.; Muhammad Alif, M.A.; Amin, I.; Khozirah, S.; Khalijah, A. α-Amylase and dipeptidyl peptidase-4 (DPP-4) inhibitory effects of *Melicope latifolia* bark extracts and identification of bioactive constituents using in vitro and in silico approaches. *Pharm. Biol.* **2021**, *59*, 962–971. [CrossRef]
16. Gao, Y.; Zhang, Y.; Zhu, J.; Li, B.; Li, Z.; Zhu, W.; Li, Y. Recent progress in natural products as DPP-4 inhibitors. *Future Med. Chem.* **2015**, *7*, 1079–1089. [CrossRef]
17. Zhang, L. Identification of Isoquercitrin as An Inhibitor Of DPPIV: Implications for Insulin Secretion and Hyperglycemic in Type 2 Diabetes Mice. Ph.D. Thesis, Jilin University, Jilin, China, 2013.
18. Sliwoski, G.; Kothiwale, S.; Meiler, J.; Lowe Jr, E.W. Computational methods in drug discovery. *Pharm. Rev.* **2014**, *66*, 334–395. [CrossRef]
19. Ibrahim, M.A.; Serem, J.C.; Bester, M.J.; Neitz, A.W.; Gaspar, A.R. Multiple antidiabetic effects of three a-glucosidase inhibitory peptides, PFP, YPL and YPG: Dipeptidyl peptidase-IV inhibition, suppression of lipid accumulation in differentiated 3T3-L-1 adipocytes and scavenging activity on methylglyoxal. *Int. J. Biol. Macromol.* **2019**, *122*, 104–114. [CrossRef]
20. Kim, S.; Thiessen, P.A.; Bolton, E.E.; Chen, J.; Fu, G.; Gindulyte, A.; Bryant, S.H. PubChem substance and compound databases. *Nucleic. Acids Res.* **2016**, *44*, 1202–1213. [CrossRef]

21. Forli, S.; Huey, R.; Pique, M.E.; Sanner, M.F.; Goodsell, D.S.; Olson, A.J. Computational protein-ligand docking and virtual drug screening with the AutoDock suite. *Nat. Protoc.* **2016**, *11*, 905–919. [CrossRef]
22. Aribisala, J.O.; Sabiu, S. Cheminformatics Identification of Phenolics as Modulators of Penicillin-Binding Protein 2a of Staphylococcus aureus: A Structure-Activity-Relationship-Based Study. *Pharmaceutics* **2022**, *14*, 1818. [CrossRef]
23. Sabiu, S.; Balogun, F.O.; Amoo, S.O. Phenolics profiling of Carpobrotus edulis (L.) N.E.Br. and insights into molecular dynamics of their significance in type-2 diabetes therapy and its retinopathy complication. *Molecules* **2021**, *26*, 4867. [CrossRef] [PubMed]
24. Gonnet, P. P-SHAKE: A quadratically convergent SHAKE. *J. Comput. Phys.* **2007**, *220*, 740–750. [CrossRef]
25. Sabiu, S.; Idowu, K. An insight on the nature of biochemical interactions between glycyrrhizin, myricetin and CYP3A4 isoform. *J. Food Biochem.* **2022**, *46*, e13831. [CrossRef]
26. Daina, A.; Michielin, O.; Zoete, V. SwissADME: A free web tool to evaluate pharmacokinetics, drug-likeness and medicinal chemistry friendliness of small molecules. *Sci. Rep.* **2017**, *7*, 42717. [CrossRef]
27. Oliveira, V.B.; Araujo, R.L.; Eidenberger, T.; Brandao, M.G. Chemical composition and inhibitory activities on dipeptidyl peptidase IV and pancreatic lipase of two underutilized species from the Brazilian Savannah: *Oxalis cordata* A.St-Hil. and *Xylopia aromatica* (Lam.) Mart. *Food Res. Int.* **2018**, *105*, 989–999. [CrossRef]
28. Jung, H.; Cho, Y.; Oh, S.; Lee, S.; Min, B.; Moon, K.; Choi, J. Kinetics and molecular docking studies of pimarane-type diterpenes as protein tyrosine phosphatase (PTP1B) inhibitors from *Aralia continentalis* roots. *Arch. Pharmacal. Res.* **2013**, *36*, 957–965. [CrossRef] [PubMed]
29. Lineweaver, H.; Burke, D. The determination of enzyme dissociation constants. *J. Am. Chem. Soc.* **1934**, *56*, 658–666. [CrossRef]
30. Seifert, E. Origin Pro 9.1: Scientific Data Analysis and Graphing Software-Software Review. *J. Chem. Inf. Model.* **2014**, *54*, 1552. [CrossRef]
31. Hernández-Santoyo, A.; Yair, A.; Altuzar, V.; Vivanco-Cid, H.; Mendoza-Barrer, C. Protein-protein and protein-ligand docking. In *Protein Engineering—Technology and Application*; Ogawa, T., Ed.; IntechOpen Publishing: London, UK, 2013; Available online: https://www.intechopen.com/chapters/44790 (accessed on 10 January 2022).
32. Lammi, C.; Bartolomei, M.; Bollati, C.; Cecchi, L.; Bellumori, M.; Sabato, E.; Giulio, V.; Mulinacci, A.; Arnoldi, A. Phenolic extracts from extract virgin olive oils inhibit dipeptidyl peptidase IV activity: In vitro, cellular, and in silico molecular modelling investigations. *Antioxidants* **2021**, *10*, 1133. [CrossRef]
33. Jasmine, M.; Tunnicliffe, L.; Eller, K.; Dustin, S.H.; Shearer, J. Chlorogenic acid differentially affects postprandial glucose and glucose-dependent insulinotropic polypeptide response in rats. *Appl Physiol. Nutr. Metab.* **2011**, *36*, 650–659. [CrossRef]
34. Oliveira, L.; Carvalho, M.; Melo, L. Health promoting and sensory properties of phenolic compounds in food. *Rev. Ceres.* **2014**, *61*, 764–779. [CrossRef]
35. Vergara, R.; Romero-Romero, S.; Velázquez-López, I.; Espinoza-Pérez, G.; Rodríguez-Hernández, A.; Pulido, N.O.; Sosa-Peinado, A.; Rodríguez-Romero, A.; Fernández-Velasco, D.A. The interplay of protein-ligand and water-mediated interactions shape affinity and selectivity in the LAO binding protein. *FEBS J.* **2020**, *287*, 763–782. [CrossRef]
36. Adinortey, C.A.; Kwarko, G.B.; Koranteng, R.; Boison, D.; Obuaba, I.; Wilson, M.D.; Kwofie, S.K. Molecular structure-based screening of the constituents of *Calotropis procera* identifies potential inhibitors of diabetes mellitus target alpha glucosidase. *Curr. Issues Mol. Biol.* **2022**, *44*, 963–987. [CrossRef]
37. Tuersuntuoheti, T.; Pan, F.; Zhang, M.; Wang, Z.; Han, J.; Sun, Z.; Song, W. Prediction of DPP-IV inhibitory potentials of polyphenols existed in Qingke barley fresh noodles: In vitro and in silico analyses. *J. Food Process. Preserv.* **2022**, e16808. [CrossRef]
38. Chen, D.; Oezguen, N.; Urvil, P.; Ferguson, C.; Dann, S.M.; Savidge, T.C. Regulation of protein-ligand binding affinity by hydrogen bond pairing. *Sci. Adv.* **2016**, *2*, e1501240. [CrossRef]
39. Childers, M.C.; Daggett, V. Insights from molecular dynamics simulations for computational protein design. *Mol. Syst. Des. Eng.* **2017**, *12*, 9–33. [CrossRef] [PubMed]
40. Martinez, L. Automatic Identification of Mobile and Rigid Substructures in Molecular Dynamics Simulations and Fractional Structural Fluctuation Analysis. *PLoS ONE* **2015**, *10*, e0119264. [CrossRef]
41. Rosenberg, M.S. *Sequence Alignment: Methods, Models, Concepts and Strategies*; University of California Press: Berkeley, CA, USA, 2009. [CrossRef]
42. Nath, V.; Manish, R.; Neeraj, K.; Agrawal, R.; Kumar, V. Computational identification of potential dipeptidyl peptidase (DPP)-IV inhibitors: Structure based virtual screening, molecular dynamics simulation and knowledge-based SAR studies. *J. Mole. Struct.* **2021**, *1224*, 129006. [CrossRef]
43. Cherrak, S.A.; Merzouk, H.; Mokhtari-Soulimane, N. Potential bioactive glycosylated flavonoids as SARS-CoV-2 main protease inhibitors: A molecular docking and simulation studies. *PLoS ONE* **2020**, *15*, e0240653. [CrossRef]
44. Shode, F.O.; Idowu, A.S.K.; Uhomoibhi, O.J.; Sabiu, S. Repurposing drugs and identification of inhibitors of integral proteins (spike protein and main protease) of SARS-CoV-2. *J. Biomol. Struct. Dyn.* **2022**, *40*, 6587–6602. [CrossRef] [PubMed]
45. Chen, J.; Wu, S.; Zhang, Q.; Yin, Z.; Zhang, L. α-Glucosidase inhibitory effect of anthocyanins from *Cinnamomum camphora* fruit: Inhibition kinetics and mechanistic insights through in vitro and in silico studies. *Int. J. Biol. Macromol.* **2020**, *143*, 696–703. [CrossRef]
46. Khan, S.; Bjij, I.; Betz, R.M.; Soliman, M.E. Reversible versus irreversible inhibition modes of ERK2: A comparative analysis for ERK2 protein kinase in cancer therapy. *Future Med. Chem.* **2018**, *10*, 1003–1015. [CrossRef] [PubMed]

47. Zhang, D.; Lazim, R. Application of conventional molecular dynamics simulation in evaluating the stability of apomyoglobin in urea solution. *Sci. Rep.* **2017**, *7*, 1–12. [CrossRef] [PubMed]
48. Khan, S.; Fakhar, Z.; Hussain, A.; Ahmad, A.; Jairajpuri, D.; Alajmi, M.; Hassan, M. Structure-based identification of potential SARS-CoV-2 main protease inhibitors. *J. Biomolec. Struct Dyn.* **2020**, *40*, 3595–3608. [CrossRef] [PubMed]
49. Khan, M.S.; Husain, F.M.; Alhumaydhi, F.A.; Alwashmi, A.S.S.; Rehman, M.T.; Alruwetei, A.M.; Hassan, M.I.; Islam, A.; Shamsi, A. Exploring the molecular interactions of Galantamine with human Transferrin: In-silico and in vitro insight. *J. Molec. Liq.* **2021**, *335*, 1–9.
50. Hubbard, R.E.; Haider, M.K. *Hydrogen Bonds in Proteins: Role and Strength*; eLS John Wiley & Sons, Ltd.: Hoboken, NJ, USA, 2010.
51. Alhumaydhi, F.A.; Aljasir, M.A.; Abdullah, S.M.; Aljohani, S.A.A.; Alwashimi, A.S.S.; Shahwan, M.; Hassan, M.I.; Islam, A.; Shamsi, A. Probing the interaction of memantine, an important Alzheimer's drug, with human serum albumin: In silico and in vitro approach. *J. Molec. Liq.* **2021**, *340*, 116888. [CrossRef]
52. Lipinski, C.A.; Lombardo, F.; Dominy, B.W.; Feeney, P.J. Experimental and computational approaches to estimate solubility and permeability in drug discovery and development settings. *Adv. Drug Deliv. Rev.* **2001**, *46*, 3–26. [CrossRef]
53. Price, G.; Patel, D.A. *Drug Bioavailability*; StatPearls Publishing: Treasure Island, FL, USA, 2020.
54. Zhou, Y.; Zhou, T.; Pei, D.; Liu, S.; Yuan, H. Pharmacokinetics and tissue distribution study of chlorogenic acid from lonicerae japonicae flos following oral administrations in rats. *Evid. Based Complement. Altern. Med.* **2014**, *2014*, 979414. [CrossRef]
55. Qi, W.; Zhao, T.; Yang, W.; Wang, G.; Yu, H.; Zhao, H.; Yang, C.; Sun, L. Comparative pharmacokinetics of chlorogenic acid after oral administration in rats. *J. Pharm. Anal.* **2011**, *1*, 270–274. [CrossRef] [PubMed]
56. Geldenhuys, W.J.; Mohammad, A.S.; Adkins, C.E.; Lockman, P.R. Molecular determinants of blood–brain barrier permeation. *Ther. Deliv.* **2015**, *6*, 961–971. [CrossRef]
57. Ahern, K.; Rajagopal, I. Enzyme Inhibition. Available online: https://chem.libretexts.org/Courses/University_of_Arkansas_Little_Rock/CHEM_4320_5320%3A_Biochemistry_1/05%3A_MichaelisMenten_Enzyme_Kinetics/5.4%3A_Enzyme_Inhibition (accessed on 10 January 2022).
58. Motoshima, K.; Sugita, K.; Hashimoto, Y.; Ishikawa, M. Non-competitive and selective dipeptidyl peptidase IV inhibitors with phenethylphenylphthalimide skeleton derived from thalidomide-related α-glucosidase inhibitors and liver X receptor antagonists. *Bioorg. Med. Chem. Lett.* **2011**, *21*, 3041–3045. [CrossRef]
59. Nong, N.T.P.; Chen, Y.-K.; Shih, W.-L.; Hsu, J.-L. Characterization of novel dipeptidyl peptidase-IV inhibitory peptides from soft-shelled turtle yolk hydrolysate using orthogonal bioassay-guided fractionations coupled with in vitro and in silico study. *Pharmaceuticals* **2020**, *13*, 308. [CrossRef] [PubMed]

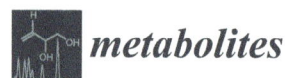

Article

First Report on Comparative Essential Oil Profile of Stem and Leaves of *Blepharispermum hirtum* Oliver and Their Antidiabetic and Anticancer Effects

Muddaser Shah [1,2,†], Saif Khalfan Al-Housni [1,†], Faizullah Khan [1,3], Saeed Ullah [1,4], Jamal Nasser Al-Sabahi [5], Ajmal Khan [1], Balqees Essa Mohammed Al-Yahyaei [1], Houda Al-Ruqaishi [5], Najeeb Ur Rehman [1,*] and Ahmed Al-Harrasi [1,*]

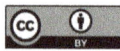

Citation: Shah, M.; Al-Housni, S.K.; Khan, F.; Ullah, S.; Al-Sabahi, J.N.; Khan, A.; Al-Yahyaei, B.E.M.; Al-Ruqaishi, H.; Rehman, N.U.; Al-Harrasi, A. First Report on Comparative Essential Oil Profile of Stem and Leaves of *Blepharispermum hirtum* Oliver and Their Antidiabetic and Anticancer Effects. *Metabolites* **2022**, *12*, 907. https://doi.org/10.3390/metabo12100907

Academic Editors: Cosmin Mihai Vesa and Dana Zaha

Received: 4 September 2022
Accepted: 23 September 2022
Published: 26 September 2022

Publisher's Note: MDPI stays neutral with regard to jurisdictional claims in published maps and institutional affiliations.

Copyright: © 2022 by the authors. Licensee MDPI, Basel, Switzerland. This article is an open access article distributed under the terms and conditions of the Creative Commons Attribution (CC BY) license (https://creativecommons.org/licenses/by/4.0/).

[1] Natural & Medical Sciences Research Center, University of Nizwa, Nizwa 616, Oman
[2] Department of Botany, Abdul Wali Khan University Mardan, Mardan 23200, Pakistan
[3] Department of Pharmacy, Abdul Wali Khan University Mardan, Mardan 23200, Pakistan
[4] Hussian Ebrahim Jamal Research Institute of Chemistry, International Center for Chemical and Biological Sciences, University of Karachi, Karachi 75270, Pakistan
[5] Central Instrument Laboratory, College of Agriculture and Marine Sciences, Sultan Qaboos University, Muscat 123, Oman
* Correspondence: najeeb@unizwa.edu.om (N.U.R.); aharrasi@unizwa.edu.om (A.A.-H.)
† These authors contributed equally to this work.

Abstract: The current research was designed to explore the *Blepharispermum hirtum* Oliver (Asteraceae) stem and leaves essential oil (EO) composition extracted through hydro-distillation using gas chromatography-mass spectrometry (GC-MS) analysis for the first time. The EOs of the stem and leaves of *B. hirtum* were comparatively studied for the in vitro antidiabetic and anticancer potential using in vitro α-glucosidase and an MTT inhibition assay, respectively. In both of the tested samples, the same number of fifty-eight compounds were identified and contributed 93.88% and 89.07% of the total oil composition in the EOs of the stem and leaves of *B. hirtum* correspondingly. However, camphene was observed as a major compound (23.63%) in the stem EO, followed by β-selinene (5.33%) and β-elemene (4.66%) and laevo-β-pinene (4.38%). While in the EO of the leaves, the dominant compound was found to be 24-norursa-3,12-diene (9.08%), followed by β-eudesmol (7.81%), β-selinene (7.26%), thunbergol (5.84%), and caryophyllene oxide (5.62%). Significant antidiabetic potential was observed with an IC_{50} of 2.10 ± 0.57 µg/mL by the stem compared to the EO of the leaves of *B. hirtum*, having an IC_{50} of 4.30 ± 1.56 µg/mL when equated with acarbose (IC_{50} = 377.71 ± 1.34 µg/mL). Furthermore, the EOs offered considerable cytotoxic capabilities for MDA-MB-231. However, the EO of the leaves presented an IC_{50} = 88.4 ± 0.5 µg/mL compared to the EO of the stem of *B. hirtum* against the triple-negative breast cancer (MDA-MB-231) cell lines with an IC_{50} = 123.6 ± 0.8 µg/mL. However, the EOs were also treated with the human breast epithelial (MCF-10A) cell line, and from the results, it has been concluded that these oils did not produce much harm to the normal cell lines. Hence, the present research proved that the EOs of *B. hirtum* might be used to cure diabetes mellitus and human breast cancer. Moreover, further studies are considered to be necessary to isolate the responsible bioactive constituents to devise drugs for the observed activities.

Keywords: *Blepharispermum hirtum*; Asteraceae; GS-MS analysis; essential oils; triple-negative breast cancer; α-glucosidase

1. Introduction

Medicinal plants and their products serve as both traditional and commercial alternative innovative remedies [1]. Due to the efficacy and lower adverse effects, the demand for herbal therapies has increased. Plant based natural products, comprising essential oils (EOs) have gained attention due to their usage in foodstuff, cosmetics, and pharmaceutical productions. Constituting a range of several lipophilic and extremely volatile constituents, obtained from an extensive range of diverse chemical classes, EOs are attributed to multiple health benefits: analgesic, anti-inflammatory, antioxidant, antimicrobial, anticancer, and antidiabetic [2].

Diabetes mellitus is considered as a world health issue, linked to two key features including insufficient insulin secretion or insensitivity to their action. Their high rate of prevalence reflects its severity, and according to the projected statistics of WHO, more than 422 million people have diabetes, 1.5 million deaths are directly attributed to diabetes each year, and the prevalence ratio will increase to 693 million by 2045 [1,3]. The diabetes might lead to several other complications such as polyuria, polydipsia, impaired vision, and skin infections [4]. Therefore, strategies need to be developed to combat these drawbacks. In this context, α-glucosidase (EC 3.2.1.20) has become a promising target for the treatment of diabetes mellitus. The inhibition of these carbohydrates' key metabolic enzymes slows down carbohydrate digestion, resulting in the low absorption of glucose, leading to normalizing the blood glucose levels. Hence, the investigation of new anti-diabetic agents using natural sources is currently of need because of their non-cytotoxic effects [5–7].

Increased interest of users concerning pharmacologically effective plant-based natural products (NPs) as substitute therapies to treat cancer has increased the attention of scientists worldwide [4]. However, an intensifying significance has been observed recently that EOs act as an anticancer medication to overcome the development of multidrug resistance and critical harmful effects linked with available antitumor remedies [5]. Therefore, due to the key role of EOs in cytotoxic therapy, the EOs of unreported plants might be used as a complementary remedy [6].

Blepharispermum hirtum Oliver (family: Asteraceae) is a naturally growing tree, about 2 m in height, and is endemic to Dhofar (Oman). The plant has very broad and soft leaves with a basic inflorescence containing a capitulum of white flowers. The genus *Blepharispermum* comprises 15 species, all of which are shrubs, except for *B hirtum*. *Blepharispermum* species are distributed over different regions of Africa, the Arabian Peninsula, and India [7]. Decoctions as well as the root powder of *B. subsessile* have been used by local practitioners in India for the treatment of various health ailments used in nervous disorders, while the whole plant is used in diarrhea, stomach ache, rheumatic affections, skin diseases, eye troubles, anti-inflammatory diseases, and irregular menstruation [8–10]. Recently, Fatope et al., [9] reported ent-kaurene diterpenoids with larvicidal and antimicrobial activity. It also has promising potential to resist microbes and antifeedant significance [9]. The genus *Blepharispermum* is an affluent basis for many bioactive ingredients including dimethyl isoencecalin and 5-hydroxy-6-acetyl-2-hydroxymethyl-2-methyl chromene [10].

Furthermore, the reported literature of EOs and the traditional uses of the plants growing in Oman have been noticed to have promising potential to cure diabetes and cancer [11,12]. Natural products derived from plants and plant products that have been traditionally used to treat various diseases including cancer and diabetes have advantages in drug discovery [13]. Thus, the current study was designed to profile the constituents of the EOs and determine the in vitro antidiabetic and cytotoxic significance of *B. hirtum*. Hence, the recent study will update the literature on the genus *Blepharispermum* and report on the EOs of *B. hirtum* for the first time.

2. Materials and Methods

2.1. General Instrumentation

The MDA-MB-231 and MCF-7 cell lines were acquired from the American Type Culture Collection (ATCC) and MCF-10A was purchased from the Iranian Biological Resource Center (IBRC) (Tehran, Iran). GC-MS was conducted on a gas chromatography-mass spectrometer (GC-MS-QP2010, Shimadzu Kyoto, Japan). The α-glucosidase enzyme (EC 3.2.1.20, Sigma-Aldrich, Darmstadt, Germany) and spectrophotometer (xMark™ Microplate Spectrophotometer, Bio-Rad, Hercules, CA, USA) were used for the α-glucosidase activity. A

High-Speed Multifunctional Grander (Grand Household, Code. GR-SCG350H) was used for the grinding of the plant. Analytical grade reagents were used in the current study.

2.2. Collection and Identification of Plant Materials

The whole plant material of *B. hirtum* (8.7 kg) was collected from Salalah, the Dhofar region of Oman (April–May 2020). After identification by the plant taxonomist (Syed Abdullah Gilani, Department of Biological Sciences and Chemistry, University of Nizwa, Nizwa, Oman), the leaves (4.0 kg) were separated from the stems (4.2 kg) and placed under shade at room temperature for dryness. The dried samples were ground into fine powder (50–300 mesh) using a stainless-steel blender. A voucher specimen of *B. hirtum* (BHO-03/2020) was deposited in the herbarium of the Natural and Medical Sciences Research Center, University of Nizwa, Oman.

2.3. Essential Oils Extraction

The essential oils extracted through hydro-distillation from the leaves and stem of the *B. hirtum* yielded 1.2 g (0.052%) and 0.95 g (0.045%), respectively, using a Clevenger-type apparatus (three times for at least 6 h) and were observed to be yellow-colored [14,15]. A known quantity of the EOs was collected, dried over anhydrous sodium sulfate (Na_2SO_4), and kept in the refrigerator at 4 °C until further GC-MS analysis and in vitro antidiabetic and cytotoxic assays.

2.4. GC-MS Analysis

The chemical constituents in the stem and leaf samples of the understudy plant were determined through the Perkin Elmer Clarus (PEC) 600 GC System (Perkin Elmer, Waltham, MA, USA) using gas chromatography-mass spectrometry (GC/MS) analysis. The GC/MS instrument was coupled with an Rtx-5MS capillary column (30 m × 0.25 mm, 0.25 µm film thickness) at 260 °C, connected to a PEC 600 mass spectrometer (MS). Electron multiplier (EM) voltage was achieved from autotune with 70 eV ionizing energy (IE). The carrier gas was helium (99.9999%) with a flow rate of 1 mL/min, while temperatures of 260 °C and 280 °C were used for the injection, transfer line, and ion source, respectively, during the whole analysis. The oven temperature was kept at 60 °C, holds for 1 min, at a flow rate of 4 °C/min–260 °C, and stood for 4 min. The essential oil solution (1 µL) was injected with a split ratio of 10:1. The complete chromatographic data were obtained by accumulating the full-scan mass spectra in the range of 45–550 amu. Furthermore, the total processing time of the GC/MS analysis was 55 min.

Identification of the Components

The essential oils extracted from the leaves and stems of *B. hirtum* were identified by their respective chromatogram peaks obtained for each compound through GC-MS analysis. Some of the compounds were identified by comparing their mass spectra with the MS library database (NIST 2011 v.2.3). Compound identification was also made possible by comparing their retention times (Rt) with those of the pure authentic samples and by means of their retention index (RI), relative to the series of n-hydrocarbons [14–16].

2.5. In Vitro α-Glucosidase Inhibitory Assay

Evaluation of the α-glucosidase inhibitory significance of the essential oils of the tested samples proceeded at 37 °C using 0.5 mM phosphate buffer (pH 6.8) [9,10]. High to low doses of the tested samples including (60, 30, 15, 7.8, 3.90, and 1.95 µg/mL), respectively, were incubated with the enzyme (2 U/2 mL) in phosphate buffer for 15 min at 37 °C. After adding the 25 µL substrate, p-nitrophenyl-a-D-glucopyranoside (0.7 mM, final), a spectrophotometer was used to track the changes in absorbance at 400 nm for 30 min. DMSO-d6 (7.5 percent final) was used as a positive control. As a reference standard, acarbose ($IC50$ = 377.7 1.34 µg/mL) was employed. Furthermore, the IC_{50} was calculated by using EZ-fit software, as explained in the statistical analysis section by Equations (2) and (3).

2.6. In Vitro Cytotoxic Potential

In vitro cytotoxicity capacity of EOs was determined by performing an MTT (yellow tetrazolium salt, 3-(4,5-dimethylthizol-2-yl)-2,5-diphenyl tetrazolium bromide) assay by using an aggressive breast cancer cell line (MDA-MB-231) [17]. Human breast normal cell line MCF-10A was kept as a control in the study. Cells were cultured in Dulbecco's modified Eagle medium (DMEM) supplemented with 10% FBS and 1% antibiotics (100 U/mL penicillin). The cells were seeded in a 96-well plate at a density of 1.0×10^4 cells/well and incubated for 24 h at 37 °C in 5% CO_2. The medium was discarded, and both cell lines were treated with different concentrations (3, 10, 30, 100, and 300 µg/mL) of plant EOs [18] after 48 h of incubation (Maher et al. [19]). A total of 20 µL of MTT solution (5 mg/mL) was pipetted into each well and incubated for another 4 h. The medium was later discarded, and the formazan precipitate was dissolved in DMSO. The absorbance of the mixtures was determined using a microplate reader at 570 nm. All experiments were performed in triplicate and the cytotoxicity was expressed as a percentage of cell viability compared to the untreated control cells [18]

$$\% \text{ Viability} = \frac{\text{Absorbance of sample}}{\text{Absorbance of control}} \times 100 \quad (1)$$

2.7. Statistical Analysis

Excel and the SoftMax Pro package were used as the applications to examine the results for biological activity. The following formula was used to determine the % inhibition.

$$\% \text{ Inhibition} = 100 - \left(\frac{O.D_{test\ compound}}{O.D_{control}}\right) \times 100 \quad (2)$$

All of the tested substances' IC_{50} values were calculated using EZ-FIT (Perrella Scientific, Inc., Amherst, MA, USA). All experiments were carried out in triplicate to reduce the likelihood of mistakes, and differences in the results are reported as the standard error of mean values (SEM).

$$SE = \frac{\sigma}{\sqrt{n}} \quad (3)$$

The cytotoxic activity was estimated via IBM SPSS Statistics 26 software and utilized to analyze the dose response and computation of IC_{50}.

3. Results and Discussion

3.1. Composition of Essential Oil

The role of essential oils in the therapy of human health complications from ancient times to date cannot be denied. The promising potential attributed to EOs is due to the presence of valuable ingredients. In the current study, through the GC-MS analysis, fifty-eight compounds were identified in the EOs of the stems and leaves of *B. hirtum* (Table 1). The compounds identified in the stem through GC-MS screening contributed 93.88% of the total oil composition among which camphene was noticed as the dominant compound having 23.63%, followed by β-selinene with 5.33%, β-elemene (4.66%), and laevo-β-pinene (4.38%) (Table 1 and Figure 1). While the same number of compounds were identified in the EOs of the leaves of the *B. hirtum* sample, which contributed 89.07% of the total composition, with major compounds of 24-norursa-3,12-diene at 9.08%, followed by β-eudesmol (7.81%), β-selinene (7.26%), thunbergol (5.84%), and caryophyllene oxide (5.62%) (Figures 1 and 2). The compound camphene was earlier reported in the EOs of *Piper cernuum*, as presented by Girola et al. [20], while β-selinene was previously noticed in *Litsea cubeba* and *Lanthana camara*, as stated by Si et al. [21] and Sarma et al. [22], respectively. Furthermore, our data consented to the outcomes elaborated by Quassinti et al. [23] in *Hypericum hircinum* and *Ferulago macrocarpa*, as described by Sajjadi et al. [24]. In addition, our data are also supported by the outcomes earlier reported by Akpulat et al. [25] and Hulley et al. [26] in the EOs of some plants belonging to the family Asteraceae, which might be due to the presence of the common chemical ingredients. However, our findings do not match the

EOs reported by Mejia et al. [27] in *Brassica nigra* and also with the literature documented by Oroojalian et al. [28] in some Apiaceae species. Many factors are responsible for the variation among the contents present within a plant species including the difference in plant family and environmental gradients [29].

Table 1. The GC-MS analysis of the EOs of *Blepharispermum hirtum* Oliver.

S. No.	Compounds	RT$_{min}$	RI$_{cal}$	RI$_{rep}$	% Stem	% Leaves
1	5,5-Dimethyl-1-vinylbicyclo [2.1.1] hexane	7.44	927	920	0.12	0.03
2	3-Thujene	7.65	935	928	3.11	0.06
3	Camphene	7.88	944	935	23.63	2.19
4	2,4(10)-Thujadiene	8.39	963	957	0.53	0.03
5	Sabinene	8.91	982	964	2.21	0.14
6	Laevo-β-Pinene	9.01	986	978	4.38	0.12
7	β-Myrcene	9.37	999	981	0.91	0.25
8	α-Phellandrene	9.75	1013	997	0.39	0.05
9	3-Carene	9.92	1019	1005	0.11	0.04
10	p-Cymene	10.30	1033	1011	1.46	0.14
11	D-Limonene	10.42	1037	1018	2.79	0.46
12	γ-Terpinene	11.25	1067	1047	1.51	0.11
13	Linalool	12.34	1106	1082	0.49	0.32
14	Perillen	12.40	1108	1086	0.04	0.08
15	α-Campholenal	13.10	1134	1102	0.42	0.31
16	2,9-Dimethyl-5-decyne	13.10	1136	1103	0.31	0.03
17	L-Pinocarveol	13.46	1147	1108	0.85	0.84
18	cis-Verbenol	13.52	1149	1110	0.25	0.36
19	trans-Verbenol	13.61	1153	1128	0.71	2.51
20	p-Mentha-1,5-dien-8-ol	14.18	1174	1148	0.56	0.69
21	Terpinen-4-ol	14.47	1185	1175	0.67	0.46
22	Myrtenol	15.00	1205	1174	0.45	0.49
23	Levoverbenone	15.34	1218	1191	0.26	0.86
24	cis-Carveol	15.54	1226	1208	0.08	0.37
25	Bornyl acetate	17.26	1292	1269	1.23	0.83
26	α-Terpinyl acetate	18.78	1354	1322	0.91	0.97
27	Copaene	19.48	1383	1376	0.47	0.44
28	β-Bourbonene	19.71	1392	1386	0.84	1.57
29	β-Elemene	19.84	1398	1398	4.66	4.52
30	Caryophyllene	20.54	1428	1421	3.73	4.35
31	Humulene	21.32	1462	1454	1.31	1.55
32	Alloaromadendrene	21.49	1469	1459	0.39	0.59
33	γ-Muurolene	21.80	1483	1471	1.05	1.01
34	Germacrene D	21.94	1489	1480	3.26	1.31
35	β-Selinene	22.08	1495	1509	5.33	7.26
36	α-Selinene	22.26	1503	1500	2.92	4.63

Table 1. Cont.

S. No.	Compounds	RT$_{min}$	RI$_{cal}$	RI$_{rep}$	% Stem	% Leaves
37	Cubebol	22.64	1521	1512	0.33	0.99
38	δ-Cadinene	22.82	1529	1514	1.59	2.93
39	Elemol	23.38	1554	1535	0.63	1.42
40	Germacrene D-4-ol	23.99	1582	1570	0.09	0.31
41	Caryophyllene oxide	24.19	1991	1575	2.89	5.62
42	Humulene 1,2-epoxide	24.743	1617	1596	0.61	1.16
43	γ-Eudesmol	24.786	1619	1627	0.58	1.18
44	Cubenol	25.09	1634	1631	0.13	0.38
45	tau-Cadinol	25.341	1946	1637	0.77	1.78
46	β-Eudesmol	25.57	1657	1644	2.73	7.81
47	Benzyl Benzoate	27.77	1767	1765	0.12	0.54
48	α-Phellandrene, dimer	28.32	1794	1801	0.43	0.76
49	m-Camphorene	31.11	1945	1960	0.09	0.31
50	Cembrene A	31.41	1961	1970	0.32	0.58
51	p-Camphorene	31.68	1978	1977	0.08	0.41
52	Geranyl-α-terpinene	32.21	2007	1990	0.05	0.13
53	Verticillol	32.70	2036	2036	0.29	0.38
54	Cembrenol	34.55	2046	2161	0.25	0.29
55	Thunbergol	34.71	2156	2173	3.32	5.84
56	24-Norursa-3,9(11),12-triene	46.48	2156	3042	1.23	3.17
57	24-Noroleana-3,12-diene	46.645	3013	3057	1.55	4.03
58	24-Norursa-3,12-diene	47.198	3060	3105	3.46	9.08
	Total % of the identified compounds				93.88	89.07

RI$_{calc}$ = Retention index calculated. RI$_{rep}$ = Retention index obtained from database (NIST, 2011). RT = Retention time (min).

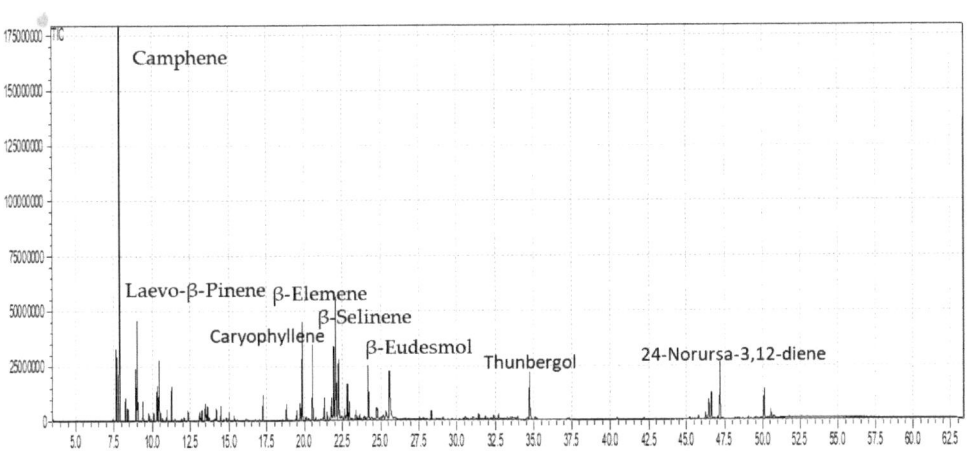

Figure 1. The GC chromatogram of the essential oils of the stem of *B. hirtum*.

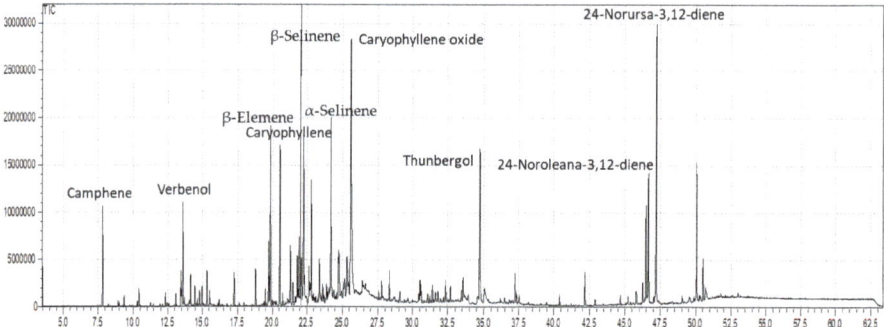

Figure 2. The GC chromatogram of the essential oils of the leaves of B. hirtum.

3.2. In Vitro Antidiabetic Significance

It is very clear that in recent times, natural products have been considered as untapped diamonds because of their invaluable medicinal use and lower side effects. The recent studies were designed to keep these key features of new drug candidates. The reported pharmacotherapeutic importance of EOs in the treatment of diabetes encouraged us to identify anti-diabetic agents via evaluating natural resources [30]. Therefore, in the current studies, two samples of EOs extracted from B. hirtum were subjected to, due to their crucial role in the inhibition of the key anti-diabetic targeted enzyme, α-glucosidase. Interestingly, both samples displayed overwhelming anti-diabetic potential with very high potency IC_{50} = 2.10 ± 0.57 µg/mL (stem) and 4.30 ± 1.56 µg/mL (leaves) when compared with the marketed drug acarbose IC_{50} = 377.71 ± 1.34 µg/mL (Figure 3). This invaluable high potency of these natural products further showed and strengthened their role as anti-diabetic agents. The stem EOs contained camphene in a higher quantity (23.63%) compared to the leaves (2.19%), which has a significant role in curing diabetes, as reflected in the literature stated by Mishra et al. [31] and Hachlafi et al. [32], and this might be the reason for which the EOs of the stem depicted a significant capacity to act as an antidiabetic agent. In addition, our findings were in agreement with the data reported by Majouli et al. [33] for Hertia cheirifolia and Ceylan et al. [34], which documented the significance of Thymus spathulifolius due to the presence of common constituents and the same technique used in the mentioned plant species and understudy plant samples. However, our results did not match the previously described outcome of Ahmad [35] for M. spicata and Basak et al. [36], which revealed the significance of the EOs of Laurus nobilis. Variation in the capacity of the plants mainly depends upon the chemical ingredients that might be altered due to the edaphic, climatic, quality, and availability of water, as stated by Shah et al. [37], and is also affected by the elemental and other ingredients present in the water available for plants.

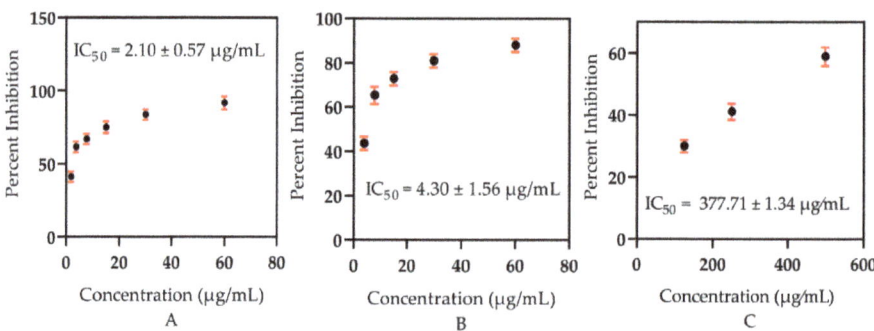

Figure 3. The in vitro antidiabetic significance of B. hirtum essential oils: (**A**) Stem, (**B**) leaves, and (**C**) standard acarbose.

3.3. In Vitro Cytotoxicity Capacity

The cytotoxic potential of the tested samples of *B. hirtum* EOs was evaluated from low to high doses using human breast cancer cell line MDA-MB-231 compared to human normal breast epithelial cell lines; Michigan cancer foundation (MCF) MCF-10A was used as a control in the experiment. The MTT [3-(4,5-dimethylthiazol-2-yl)-2,5-diphenyltetrazolium bromide] assay was used to determine the decrease in the cancer cell viability induced by cytotoxic agents. For MDA-MB-231, the IC_{50} values, % inhibition, and viability of the tested EOs are presented in Table 2. Our findings show that the EOs of the leaves and stem have promising capabilities against MDA-MB-231 cells with IC_{50} values of 88.4 ± 0.5 and 123.6 ± 0.8 µg/mL, respectively. To determine whether the cytotoxic effects of the oils were selective for malignant cells in comparison to the non-malignant cells, the non-tumorigenic MCF-10A cells were screened through the tested EOs from low to high doses (3, 10, 30, 100, and 300 µg/mL) in a similar manner as the cancer cells. After the MTT assay, the results of the % inhibition and viability for the MCF-10A cell lines by essential oils are presented in Table 3. The results showed that these cells were less susceptible to the actions of the essential oil, particularly at a higher dose of 300 µg/mL. The data in this study revealed that the triple negative MDA-MB-231 cells, which bear an aggressive phenotype, responded more favorably to EOs, and showed greater cytotoxicity. The significant potential for cytotoxicity was observed when non-tumorigenic MCF-10A cells were exposed to this plant's EOs, which suggested that EOs have the potential in offering promising treatment for patients with breast cancer. Some valuable constituents were noticed in the understudy plant samples due to which they offered promising potential cancer therapy. Our findings agreed with the report described by Ortiz et al. [38] of the plant species belonging to the genus *Santalum* and Furtoda et al. [39] in the *Blepharocalyx salicifolius*. Our findings also favor the study of Loizzo et al. [40], who described the significance of the EOs of some plants of the family Lamiaceae and Lauraceae.

Table 2. The % viability and inhibition of *B. hirtum* essential oil on the breast cancer cell line MDA-MB-231.

Tested Samples	Conc. (µg/mL)	% Viability	% Inhibition	IC50 (µg/mL)
Leaves	3	94.33	5.66	88.4 ± 0.5
	10	82.41	17.58	
	30	71.09	28.90	
	100	47.85	52.14	
	300	26.26	73.73	
Stem	3	96.49	3.50	123.6 ± 0.8
	10	85.43	14.56	
	30	72.65	27.34	
	100	53.04	46.95	
	300	37.05	62.94	

Table 3. The % Viability and inhibition of *B. hirtum* essential oil on the normal breast cell line MCF-10A.

Tested Samples	Conc (µg/mL)	% Viability	% Inhibition	IC50 (µg/mL)
Leaves	3	96.29	3.70	>300
	10	93.04	6.99	
	30	89.34	10.65	
	100	86.96	13.03	
	300	78.07	23.99	

Table 3. *Cont.*

Tested Samples	Conc (μg/mL)	% Viability	% Inhibition	IC$_{50}$ (μg/mL)
Stem	3	97.50	2.49	>300
	10	95.28	4.71	
	30	89.93	10.06	
	100	85.10	14.89	
	300	79.22	20.77	

4. Conclusions

The comparative analysis of the *B. hirtum* stem and leaves EOs revealed that the understudy plant is an affluent source of responsible bioactive chemical constituents that are intended to produce as useful properties as the plant. Fifty-eight constituents were observed in the EOs of the stem and leaves of *B. hirtum* and contributed 93.88% and 89.07% of the total amount, respectively. Camphene was observed as a major compound (23.63%), followed by β-selinene (5.33%), β-elemene (4.66%), and laevo-β-pinene (4.38%) in the stem EO. While the 24-norursa-3,12-diene (9.08%), β-eudesmol (7.81%), β-selinene (7.26%), thunbergol (5.84%), and caryophyllene oxide (5.62%) were noted as the dominant constituents. Considerable potential to cure diabetes was offered by the tested samples compared to the standard. Moreover, the EOs of *B. hirtum* produced significant cytotoxicity effects against the breast cancer cell line MDA-MB-231 and were non-toxic to the normal cell line MCF-10A. The occurrence of the chemical constituents and promising α-glucosidase and cytotoxic activities of the EOs validate their pharmaceutical and nutraceutical importance. Hence, the analysis revealed that *B. hirtum* EOs can be used as an alternative promising natural remedy to cure diabetes mellitus and cancer.

Author Contributions: M.S., S.K.A.-H. and B.E.M.A.-Y. conducted the collection, extraction, and wrote the original manuscript. J.N.A.-S. and H.A.-R. extracted the EOs and performed the GC-MS analysis and interpreted the data. F.K. performed the anticancer activity, while S.U. and A.K. screened the samples against α-glucosidase activity. N.U.R. and A.A.-H. designed and supervised the project and, in addition, assisted in reviewing and editing the manuscript. All authors have read and agreed to the published version of the manuscript.

Funding: This research was funded by The Research Council through the funded project (BFP/RGP/CBS/21/002). The APC was funded by the same project.

Institutional Review Board Statement: Not applicable.

Informed Consent Statement: Not applicable.

Data Availability Statement: The data presented in this study are available in the article.

Acknowledgments: The authors would also like to give their sincere appreciation to The Research Council through the funded projects (BFP/GRG/EBR/20/014) and (BFP/RGP/CBS/21/002).

Conflicts of Interest: The authors declare no conflict of interest.

References

1. World Health Organization. Global Report on Diabetes. Available online: http://www.who.int/diabetes/en/ (accessed on 28 November 2018).
2. Shah, M.; Bibi, S.; Kamal, Z.; Al-Sabahi, J.N.; Alam, T.; Ullah, O.; Murad, W.; Rehman, N.U.; Al-Harrasi, A. Bridging the Chemical Profile and Biomedical Effects of *Scutellaria edelbergii* Essential Oils. *Antioxidants* **2022**, *11*, 1723. [CrossRef]
3. Hundal, R.S.; Krssak, M.; Dufour, S.; Laurent, D.; Lebon, V.; Chandramouli, V.; Inzucchi, S.E.; Schumann, W.C.; Petersen, K.F.; Landau, B.R.; et al. Mechanism by which metformin reduces glucose production in type 2 diabetes. *Diabetes* **2000**, *49*, 2063–2069. [CrossRef] [PubMed]
4. Yin, Z.; Zhang, W.; Feng, F.; Zhang, Y.; Kang, W. α-Glucosidase inhibitors isolated from medicinal plants. *Food Sci. Hum. Wellness* **2014**, *3*, 136–174. [CrossRef]

5. Fitsiou, E.; Pappa, A. Anticancer activity of essential oils and other extracts from aromatic plants grown in Greece. *Antioxidants* **2019**, *8*, 290. [CrossRef] [PubMed]
6. Sharma, M.; Grewal, K.; Jandrotia, R.; Batish, D.R.; Singh, H.P.; Kohli, R.K. Essential oils as anticancer agents: Potential role in malignancies, drug delivery mechanisms, and immune system enhancement. *Biomed. Pharmacother.* **2022**, *146*, 112514. [CrossRef]
7. Eriksson, T. The genus *Blepharispermum* (Asteraceae, Heliantheae). *Plant Syst. Evol.* **1992**, *182*, 149–227. [CrossRef]
8. Jadhav, A.; Acharya, R.; Harisha, C.R.; Shukla, V.J.; Chandola, H. Pharmacognostical and preliminary physico-chemical profiles of *Blepharispermum subsessile* DC. root. *Ayu* **2015**, *36*, 73.
9. Fatope, M.O.; Varma, G.B.; Alzri, N.M.; Marwah, R.G.; Nair, R.S. ent-Kaurene Diterpenoids from *Blepharispermum hirtum*. *Chem. Biodivers.* **2010**, *7*, 1862–1870. [CrossRef] [PubMed]
10. Agarwal, S.; Verma, S.; Singh, S.S.; Tripathi, A.; Khan, Z.; Kumar, S. Antifeedant and antifungal activity of chromene compounds isolated from *Blepharispermum subsessile*. *J. Ethnopharmacol.* **2000**, *71*, 231–234. [CrossRef]
11. Ahamad, J.; Uthirapathy, S.; Mohammed Ameen, M.S.; Anwer, E.T. Essential oil composition and antidiabetic, anticancer activity of *Rosmarinus officinalis* L. leaves from Erbil (Iraq). *J. Essent. Oil Bear. Plants* **2019**, *22*, 1544–1553. [CrossRef]
12. Rashan, L.; Hakkim, F.L.; Idrees, M.; Essa, M.; Velusamy, T.; Al-Baloshi, M.; Al-Bulushi, B.; Al Jabri, A.; Alrizeiki, M.; Guillemin, G. Boswellia gum resin and essential oils: Potential health benefits—An evidence based review. *Int. J. Nutr. Pharmacol. Neurol. Dis.* **2019**, *9*, 53–71. [CrossRef]
13. Ahamad, J.; Naquvi, K.J.; Mir, S.R.; Ali, M.; Shuaib, M. Review on role of natural alpha-glucosidase inhibitors for management of diabetes mellitus. *Int. J. Biomed. Res.* **2011**, *2*, 374–380.
14. Rehman, N.U.; Alsabahi, J.N.; Alam, T.; Khan, A.; Rafiq, K.; Khan, M.; Al-Harrasi, A. Chemical Constituents and Carbonic Anhydrase II Activity of Essential Oil of *Acridocarpus orientalis* A. Juss. in Comparison with Stem and Leaves. *J. Essent. Oil Bear. Plants* **2021**, *24*, 68–74. [CrossRef]
15. Rehman, N.U.; Alsabahi, J.N.; Alam, T.; Rafiq, K.; Khan, A.; Hidayatullah; Khan, N.A.; Khan, A.L.; Al Ruqaishi, H.; Al-Harrasi, A. Chemical Composition and Biological Activities of Essential Oil from Aerial Parts of *Frankenia pulverulenta* L. and *Boerhavia elegans* Choisy from Northern Oman. *J. Essent. Oil Bear. Plants* **2021**, *24*, 1180–1191. [CrossRef]
16. Sarma, N.; Gogoi, R.; Loying, R.; Begum, T.; Munda, S.; Pandey, S.; Lal, M. Phytochemical composition and biological activities of essential oils extracted from leaves and flower parts of *Corymbia citriodora* (Hook.). *J. Environ. Biol.* **2021**, *42*, 552–562.
17. Welsh, J. Animal models for studying prevention and treatment of breast cancer. *Anim. Mod. Hum. Dis.* **2013**, *3*, 997–1018.
18. Sakhi, M.; Khan, A.; Iqbal, Z.; Khan, I.; Raza, A.; Ullah, A.; Nasir, F.; Khan, S.A. Design and Characterization of Paclitaxel-Loaded Polymeric Nanoparticles Decorated with Trastuzumab for the Effective Treatment of Breast Cancer. *Front. Pharmacol.* **2022**, *13*, 85529. [CrossRef] [PubMed]
19. Maher, M.; Kassab, A.E.; Zaher, A.F.; Mahmoud, Z. Novel pyrazolo [3,4-d] pyrimidines: Design, synthesis, anticancer activity, dual EGFR/ErbB2 receptor tyrosine kinases inhibitory activity, effects on cell cycle profile and caspase-3-mediated apoptosis. *J. Enzy. Inhib. Med. Chem.* **2019**, *34*, 532–546. [CrossRef] [PubMed]
20. Girola, N.; Figueiredo, C.R.; Farias, C.F.; Azevedo, R.A.; Ferreira, A.K.; Teixeira, S.F.; Capello, T.M.; Martins, E.G.; Matsuo, A.L.; Travassos, L.R. Camphene isolated from essential oil of *Piper cernuum* (Piperaceae) induces intrinsic apoptosis in melanoma cells and displays antitumor activity in vivo. *Biochem. Biophy. Res. Commun.* **2015**, *467*, 928–934. [CrossRef] [PubMed]
21. Si, L.; Chen, Y.; Han, X.; Zhan, Z.; Tian, S.; Cui, Q.; Wang, Y. Chemical composition of essential oils of Litsea cubeba harvested from its distribution areas in China. *Molecules* **2012**, *17*, 7057–7066. [CrossRef] [PubMed]
22. Sarma, N.; Begum, T.; Pandey, S.K.; Gogoi, R.; Munda, S.; Lal, M. Chemical profiling of leaf essential oil of *Lantana camara* Linn. from North-East India. *J. Essent. Oil Bear. Plants* **2020**, *23*, 1035–1041. [CrossRef]
23. Quassinti, L.; Lupidi, G.; Maggi, F.; Sagratini, G.; Papa, F.; Vittori, S.; Bianco, A.; Bramucci, M. Antioxidant and antiproliferative activity of *Hypericum hircinum* L. subsp. majus (Aiton) N. Robson essential oil. *Nat. Prod. Res.* **2013**, *27*, 862–868. [CrossRef]
24. Sajjadi, S.; Shokoohinia, Y.; Jamali, M. Chemical composition of essential oil of *Ferulago macrocarpa* (Fenzl) Boiss. fruits. *Res. Pharm. Sci.* **2012**, *7*, 197.
25. Akpulat, H.A.; Tepe, B.; Sokmen, A.; Daferera, D.; Polissiou, M. Composition of the essential oils of *Tanacetum argyrophyllum* (C. Koch) Tvzel. var. argyrophyllum and *Tanacetum parthenium* (L.) Schultz Bip.(Asteraceae) from Turkey. *Biochem. Syst. Ecol.* **2005**, *33*, 511–516. [CrossRef]
26. Hulley, I.; Özek, G.; Sadgrove, N.; Tilney, P.; Özek, T.; Başer, K.; Van Wyk, B.-E. Essential oil composition of a medicinally important Cape species: *Pentzia punctata* (Asteraceae). *S. Afr. J. Bot.* **2019**, *127*, 208–212. [CrossRef]
27. Mejia-Garibay, B.; Palou, E.; López-Malo, A. Composition, diffusion, and antifungal activity of black mustard (*Brassica nigra*) essential oil when applied by direct addition or vapor phase contact. *J. Food Prot.* **2015**, *78*, 843–848. [CrossRef]
28. Oroojalian, F.; Kasra-Kermanshahi, R.; Azizi, M.; Bassami, M.R. Phytochemical composition of the essential oils from three Apiaceae species and their antibacterial effects on food-borne pathogens. *Food Chem.* **2010**, *120*, 765–770. [CrossRef]
29. Mubin, N.; Rehman, N.U.; Murad, W.; Shah, M.; Al-Harrasi, A.; Afza, R. *Scutellaria petiolata* Hemsl. ex Lace & Prain (Lamiaceae).: A New Insight in Biomedical Therapies. *Antioxidants* **2022**, *11*, 1446.
30. Heghes, S.C.; Filip, L.; Vostinaru, O.; Mogosan, C.; Miere, D.; Iuga, C.A.; Moldovan, M. Essential oil-bearing plants from Balkan Peninsula: Promising sources for new drug candidates for the prevention and treatment of diabetes mellitus and dyslipidemia. *Front. Pharmacol.* **2020**, *11*, 989–996. [CrossRef]

31. Mishra, C.; Code, Q. Comparative anti-diabetic study of three phytochemicals on high-fat diet and streptozotocin-induced diabetic dyslipidemic rats. *Int. J. Biomed. Adv. Res.* **2018**, *9*, 8–21.
32. Hachlafi, N.E.; Aanniz, T.; Menyiy, N.E.; Baaboua, A.E.; Omari, N.E.; Balahbib, A.; Shariati, M.A.; Zengin, G.; Fikri-Benbrahim, K.; Bouyahya, A. In vitro and in vivo biological investigations of camphene and its mechanism insights: A review. *Food Rev. Int.* **2021**, 1–28. [CrossRef]
33. Majouli, K.; Hlila, M.B.; Hamdi, A.; Flamini, G.; Jannet, H.B.; Kenani, A. Antioxidant activity and α-glucosidase inhibition by essential oils from *Hertia cheirifolia* (L.). *Ind. Crops Prod.* **2016**, *82*, 23–28. [CrossRef]
34. Ceylan, R.; Zengin, G.; Uysal, S.; Ilhan, V.; Aktumsek, A.; Kandemir, A.; Anwar, F. GC-MS analysis and in vitro antioxidant and enzyme inhibitory activities of essential oil from aerial parts of endemic *Thymus spathulifolius* Hausskn. et Velen. *J. Enzym. Inhib. Med. Chem.* **2016**, *31*, 983–990. [CrossRef]
35. Ahamad, J. Aroma profile and α-glucosidase inhibitory activity of essential oil of *Mentha spicata* leaves. *J. Essent. Oil Bear. Plants* **2021**, *24*, 1042–1048. [CrossRef]
36. Basak, S.S.; Candan, F. Effect of Laurus nobilis L. essential oil and its main components on α-glucosidase and reactive oxygen species scavenging activity. *Iran. J. Pharm. Res.* **2013**, *12*, 367–382.
37. Shah, M.; Murad, W.; Ur Rehman, N.; Halim, S.A.; Ahmed, M.; Rehman, H.; Zahoor, M.; Mubin, S.; Khan, A.; Nassan, M.A. Biomedical applications of *Scutellaria edelbergii* Rech. f.: In vitro and in vivo approach. *Molecules* **2021**, *26*, 3740. [CrossRef] [PubMed]
38. Ortiz, C.; Morales, L.; Sastre, M.; Haskins, W.E.; Matta, J. Cytotoxicity and genotoxicity assessment of sandalwood essential oil in human breast cell lines MCF-7 and MCF-10A. *Evid. Based Comp. Altern. Med.* **2016**, *2*, 1–13. [CrossRef] [PubMed]
39. Furtado, F.B.; Borges, B.C.; Teixeira, T.L.; Garces, H.G.; Almeida Junior, L.D.d.; Alves, F.C.B.; Silva, C.V.d.; Fernandes Junior, A. Chemical composition and bioactivity of essential oil from *Blepharocalyx salicifolius*. *Int. J. Mol. Sci.* **2018**, *19*, 33. [CrossRef] [PubMed]
40. Loizzo, M.R.; Tundis, R.; Menichini, F.; Saab, A.M.; Statti, G.A.; Menichini, F. Cytotoxic activity of essential oils from Labiatae and Lauraceae families against in vitro human tumor models. *Anticancer Res.* **2007**, *27*, 3293–3299. [PubMed]

MDPI
St. Alban-Anlage 66
4052 Basel
Switzerland
www.mdpi.com

Metabolites Editorial Office
E-mail: metabolites@mdpi.com
www.mdpi.com/journal/metabolites

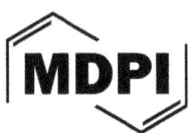

Disclaimer/Publisher's Note: The statements, opinions and data contained in all publications are solely those of the individual author(s) and contributor(s) and not of MDPI and/or the editor(s). MDPI and/or the editor(s) disclaim responsibility for any injury to people or property resulting from any ideas, methods, instructions or products referred to in the content.

www.ingramcontent.com/pod-product-compliance
Lightning Source LLC
LaVergne TN
LVHW070152120526
838202LV00013BA/917